Promoting Continence

A Clinical and Research Resource

Edited by

Kathryn Getliffe BSc(Hons) MSc PhD RGN DN PGCEA

Professor of Nursing, School of Nursing & Midwifery, University of Southampton, Southampton, UK

Mary Dolman BSc(Nurs) RGN ET ENB978 ResCert CounsCert

Independent Nurse Specialist, Continence and Stoma Care, Bath, UK

Foreword by

Katherine N. Moore PhD RN CCCN

Professor Faculty of Nursing, Adjunct Professor Faculty of Medicine/Division of Urology, University of Alberta, Edmonton, Canada

THIRD EDITION

Baillière Tindall

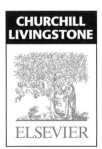

CHURCHILL LIVINGSTONE

ELSEVIER

EDINBURGH LONDON NEW YORK OXFORD PHILADELPHIA ST LOUIS SYDNEY TORONTO 2007

BAILLIÈRE
TINDALL
ELSEVIER

An imprint of Elsevier Limited

© Baillière Tindall 1997 except chapter 7 © 1977, Reckitt & Benckiser
© Elsevier Science Limited 2003 except chapter 8 © 2003, Reckitt & Benckiser
© 2007, Elsevier Limited. All rights reserved.

First edition 1997
Second edition 2003
Third edition 2007

ISBN: 9780443103476

British Library Cataloguing in Publication Data
A catalogue record for this book is available from the British Library

Library of Congress Cataloging in Publication Data
A catalog record for this book is available from the Library of Congress

Note

Knowledge and best practice in this field are constantly changing. As new research and experience broaden our knowledge, changes in practice, treatment and drug therapy may become necessary or appropriate. Readers are advised to check the most current information provided (i) on procedures featured or (ii) by the manufacturer of each product to be administered, to verify the recommended dose or formula, the method and duration of administration, and contraindications. It is the responsibility of the practitioner, relying on their own experience and knowledge of the patient, to make diagnoses, to determine dosages and the best treatment for each individual patient, and to take all appropriate safety precautions. To the fullest extent of the law, neither the Publisher nor the editors assume any liability for any injury and/or damage to persons or property arising out or related to any use of the material contained in this book.

The Publisher

Promoting Continence

For Baillière Tindall

Commissioning Editor: Mairi McCubbin
Development Editor: Gill Cloke/Katrina Mather
Project Manager: Kerrie-Anne Jarvis
Design Direction: George Ajayi
Illustrators: H.L. Studios, David Banks
Illustration Manager: Merlyn Harvey

Contents

Contributors

Angela C. Billington DipHV RGN SCM
Director of Continence Services, Bournemouth Teaching Primary Care Trust, Bournemouth, UK

Mary Dolman BSc(Nurs) RGN ET ENB978 ResCert CounsCert
Independent Nurse Specialist, Continence and Stoma Care, Bath, UK

Sharon Eustice BPhil MSc DNCert RN Nurse Practitioner
Diploma Independent and Supplementary Prescriber
Nurse Consultant, Cornwall and Isles of Scilly Primary Care Trust, Cornwall, UK

Mandy Fader BSc(Hons) PhD RN
Continence Technology and Skin Health Group, School of Nursing and Midwifery, University of Southampton, Southampton, UK

Kathryn Getliffe BSc(Hons) MSc PhD RGN DN PGCEA
Professor of Nursing, School of Nursing & Midwifery, University of Southampton, Southampton, UK

Collette Haslam BSc(Hons) RGN
Clinical Nurse Specialist in Uroneurology, Department of Uroneurology, National Hospital for Neurology and Neurosurgery, London, UK

Gaye Kyle BA(Hons) RGN MA
Senior Lecturer, Faculty of Health and Human Science, Thames Valley University, Slough, UK

Mary R. Kennedy RMN RGN
Nurse Consultant, North Essex Mental Health Partnership NHS Trust, Colchester, Essex, UK

Karen Logan MSc Dip Leadership and Management RGN
Nurse Consultant, Director of Continence Services, Llanfrecfa Grange, Cwmbran, Torfaen, UK

Phil Prynn BA(Hons) CertEd RGN ONC
Continence Services Manager, Continence Advisory Service, Wokingham Hospital, Wokingham, Berkshire, UK

Deborah Rigby MSc OND RGN FEATC ENB978
Continence Service Manager, Bristol Primary Care Trust, Knowle Clinic, Bristol, UK

June Rogers MBE BA(Hons) MSc RN RSCN ENB216 ENB978
Paediatric Continence Adviser, Director PromoCon, Disabled Living, Manchester, UK

Linda J. Smith MA MSc PhD
Consultant Clinical Psychologist, Northumberland Tyne & Wear NHS Trust, Newcastle upon Tyne, UK

Paul S. Smith MA MSc PhD
Consultant Clinical Psychologist, Tees Esk and Wear Valleys NHS Trust, Earls House Hospital, Durham, and University of Newcastle upon Tyne, Newcastle upon Tyne, UK

Sue Thomas BA(Hons) RGN RM DN CPT
Royal College of Nursing Practice and Policy Adviser for Chronic Disease and Disability, Royal College of Nursing, London, UK

Foreword

The *Oxford English Dictionary* defines a textbook as: *a book used as a standard work for the study of a particular subject; . . . a manual of instruction in any science or branch of study, esp. a work recognized as an authority.* The emphasis for *Promoting Continence* should be on the final phrase: '*a work recognized as an authority*'. This book transmits scholarly knowledge on the topic of continence care whilst comprehensively summarising the current state of the science, identifying many areas of knowledge gaps and encouraging critical thinking through case studies and examples. Herein, *Promoting Continence* transmits the established body of knowledge through instruction and with authority. This strong combination renders the material meaningful to undergraduate students (and would be a welcome addition to a curriculum on chronic health issues) and to professional practitioners alike.

Promoting Continence will challenge readers to explore the topics further – particularly those where research evidence is lacking – and it will encourage nursing leadership in the field of continence care within a scholarly framework of theory and research. Credible and responsible, the authors have been conscious of their professional and scholarly roles to present the evidence on which claims of effectiveness are based and to note that there is a paucity of well-designed research on many topics related to continence. Even in the areas in which there is evidence, theory does not necessarily translate into practice for a host of reasons. This book will help bridge that disparity. When continence care is not proactive and patients suffer as a result, the ethical precept 'First do no harm' is violated. Pressure ulcers, skin irritation, odour, extra laundry, personal shame and loss of self-esteem are all associated with incontinence. Indeed, staff attitudes can also be affected and be imposed on the patient. If *Promoting Continence* could be integrated into the curriculum of certificate programmes, the level of competency, and ability to initiate research-based treatment programmes may be significantly enhanced.

Any book of the calibre of *Promoting Continence* is a work of dedication, commitment and challenge. The highly relevant chapters will keep the reader focused and provide much information. Not only does the book address the clinical assessment of people suffering from incontinence but also considers issues related to leadership, management, nurse prescribing, and evidence-based care. It should be required reading for nurses at various levels of healthcare provision and could easily be used as a reference source for others outside the discipline of nursing. The authors have gone to considerable effort to produce an authoritative textbook which is applicable to UK and international healthcare professionals alike. It behoves administrators everywhere to ensure best care based on the evidence – *Promoting Continence* provides them with that starting point.

Katherine Moore
Professor Faculty of Nursing
Adjunct Professor Faculty of Medicine/
Division of Urology
University of Alberta
Edmonton
Canada

Preface

The third edition of *Promoting Continence* has been extensively revised and updated by an experienced and knowledgeable team, including both new contributors and colleagues from earlier editions. The aim of the book, as always, is to give providers and purchasers of health and social care a deeper understanding of the promotion of continence and to enable them to be comfortable and confident with a subject that is not easy to talk about. Incontinence is a global issue and the book's content is designed to have relevance for all readers wherever they may be. Although the policy context inevitably centres on the UK, the evidence base that underpins care strategies remains internationally applicable.

We have reorganised the book's structure in several areas in an attempt to maintain a clear focus for practitioners and their patient groups, whilst at the same time endeavouring to minimise overlap between chapters. For the first time we have included a section on mental illness and incontinence, and this is linked with consideration of other vulnerable groups in a chapter that also addresses incontinence in the frail elderly and those with neurological dysfunction (Chapter 6). Management of incontinence through the use of catheters and other containment products has also been combined in a single chapter (Chapter 10) and we are indebted to colleagues in the international team which provided detailed and up-to-date analysis of this subject for the 3rd International Consultation on Incontinence in 2004 and the subsequent publication (Cottenden et al 2005).

Although the term 'incontinence' has been used throughout the book to refer to urinary incontinence unless otherwise stated, Chapter 8 has been devoted to bowel care and faecal incontinence, although some consideration of this problem also occurs in other chapters. Case studies are included in most chapters to help demonstrate the application of research or other sources of evidence-based knowledge in clinical practice. Early recognition of continence problems and underlying causes, together with planning and provision of appropriate treatment, is fundamental to promoting continence. Equally important is the need for professional knowledge to be linked with understanding of the impact of incontinence on the individual's life and for decisions on care to be made together wherever possible.

Translating research evidence into clinical practice and the dissemination and implementation of the scientific knowledge that underpins care is a challenge for health services and a number of important factors which impact on success have been identified. These include the following key points:

1. Management of change at organisational and individual levels
2. Nature of the intervention
3. Methods and styles of communication

4. Change agents and leaders
5. Outreach experts
6. Organisational and social context system contexts
7. Users of the innovation
8. Characteristics of nurses
9. Education and clinical experience of nurses
10. Use of audit and feedback

(Bero et al 1998, Estabrooks et al 2003)

Many of these factors are addressed in various ways within this book but readers are encouraged to keep this overview in mind when thinking about their own services and individual practice. Research evidence is of little value if it is not translated into best practice.

The following sections summarise the key features of each chapter:

Chapter 1 – Incontinence in perspective – begins with a comprehensive overview of incontinence from a range of perspectives, including epidemiological, historical, individual and policy viewpoints. In this new edition, there is increased emphasis on quality of life measures and international perspectives, as well as recognition of governmental policy drivers.

Chapter 2 – Assessing bladder function – examines the anatomical and physiological processes that control normal bladder filling and emptying and compares these with the pathophysiology of bladder dysfunction. The most common causes of continence problems are considered and the chapter goes on to discuss the principles of assessment of patients' bladder function. We acknowledge that there are contrasting views on whether to refer to people with continence problems as patients, clients or some alternative term, when many are basically well apart from their continence-related symptoms. However, we have chosen to use the term 'patient' in most places for consistency.

Chapters 3 and 4 – as in earlier editions, the subject of promotion of continence and management of incontinence in adults has been divided into two chapters, entitled Mainly women and Mainly men. Whilst it is recognised that many causes of incontinence and approaches to treatment are common to both men and women, some conditions are far more common in one sex than the other. For example, genuine stress incontinence is considerably more common in women than in men, but urinary retention is more frequently experienced by men. This strategy allows in-depth discussion of theory and research underpinning practice, particularly where anatomical differences are important or where other sexual differences such as childbirth or enlargement of the prostate gland exert an influence. Issues or problems that could overlap into both chapters, such as problems of overactive bladder and urge incontinence, are discussed principally in *Chapter 3* since the overall prevalence of incontinence is relatively higher in women than in men.

Chapter 5 – Mainly children – highlights many of the practical issues associated with toilet training difficulties and problems of daytime and nighttime wetting and faecal soiling, which occur most commonly in childhood.

A new inclusion in this third edition is *Chapter 6 – Vulnerable groups* – which brings together discussion of some of the particular groups at risk of continence problems: frail elderly people, those with mental illness and incontinence, and those with neurological dysfunction. Prevalence of incontinence is known to increase with advancing age but assessment and care options are largely similar for adults of any age. The frail elderly do represent a different challenge and one where the goal of continence care is not always to achieve full continence but may be to manage incontinence more effectively. However, the most important message is that incontinence is not an inevitable part of growing older and that age alone should not prevent people receiving appropriate assessment and treatment.

People with mental illness and incontinence are vulnerable to the double stigma associated with mental illness and also with incontinence. Physical care sometimes comes second to mental health care for these people and this section of the chapter raises awareness of the issues involved. The third group of vulnerable people included in this chapter are those with neurological disabilities for whom bladder and bowel problems are very common. This section examines the relationship between the site of neurological damage and the symptoms experienced, together with key aspects of assessment and treatment.

Chapter 7 – Continence training in intellectual disability – provides a comprehensive account of the state of knowledge in this field. It addresses the principles of behavioural modification in depth, together with numerous examples of its practical application.

Chapter 8 – Bowel care – provides a focus on management of constipation and faecal incontinence in adults. This topic is also discussed in other chapters where the emphasis is on particular patient groups, notably Chapter 5 for children, Chapter 6 for people with neurological dysfunction and Chapter 7 for people with intellectual disability.

Chapter 9 – Medication for continence – is written by a new contributor and nurse prescriber, and brings direct experience of the impact of medications on continence. The chapter includes not only medications that may be used as part of planned care to treat either urinary or faecal incontinence, but also medications that can contribute to these problems. The developing role of nurse prescribing in continence care provides a key element and is supported by a series of case studies derived from practice.

In *Chapter 10 – Catheters and containment products* – the use of catheters and management of catheter-associated problems is addressed in detail, including clean intermittent self-catheterisation and long-term, indwelling, urethral or suprapubic catheterisation. This chapter includes information on the careful selection of equipment and on patient monitoring, together with practical advice in the form of a 'troubleshooting' guide. However, non-invasive approaches to dealing with incontinence are preferable to catheterisation or surgery in most cases, and for some patients alternative containment products are more suitable. There is no single product which is suitable for all individuals and the continually changing range of products can make selection difficult. The second part of this chapter examines the available product groups together with clear guidance on the principles underpinning selection of the most appropriate product for each individual patient.

In the final chapter, *Chapter 11 – Service organisation and delivery* – the emphasis is on practical aspects of continence service development. Critical issues for service leaders are highlighted and discussed and include the importance of being politically aware and understanding the varied agendas of others in managerial or leadership roles. The chapter also offers some insight into ways of mapping current services to enable them to be documented and then improved upon.

In this edition we have no longer included a chapter on Resource Information as in previous editions, although some of this information occurs within specific chapters. This is because of the wealth of information now available directly from websites, internet searches, electronic databases and libraries. In addition, some websites change their addresses or cease to be available for various reasons and therefore it is difficult to ensure their currency for readers.

In conclusion, this book is written for all health professionals and other carers with an interest in continence. It is hoped that it will be of value to clinical specialists, community and hospital-based nurses and those working in nursing homes. It may also be a resource for students at all levels undertaking general or specialist courses. In addition, it may be useful to other members of the multidisciplinary team, including general practitioners, physiotherapists and occupational therapists, health promotion departments and social services.

Whatever your role or interest in incontinence, we hope this third edition contributes to your knowledge, enhances your practice and stimulates you to discover more.

Kathy Getliffe
Mary Dolman
Southampton and Bath, 2007

References

Bero L A, Grilli R, Grimshaw J M et al 1998 Closing the gap between research and practice: an overview of systematic reviews of interventions to promote the implementation of research findings. British Medical Journal 317:465–468

Cottenden A, Bliss D, Fader M et al 2005 Management with continence products. In: Abrams P, Cardozo L, Khoury S, Wein A (eds) Incontinence. Health Publication, Plymouth, p 149–253

Estabrooks C A, Floyd J A, Scott-Findlay S et al 2003 Individual determinants of research utilization; a systematic review. Journal of Advanced Nursing 43:506–520

Chapter 1

Incontinence in perspective

Kathryn Getliffe and Sue Thomas

A little rebellion now and then is a good thing . . .

Thomas Jefferson (1787)

INTRODUCTION

Living with incontinence can shatter lives, but people are often unwilling to seek help and too many remain unaware that continence problems can often be cured and almost always improved.

Incontinence is a common problem worldwide, affecting people of all ages and from all social and cultural backgrounds. Although the physical effects may not be clinically life threatening, the symptoms can have a devastating impact on the quality of life of individuals, their families and friends. Incontinence is a symptom with many causes, but any failure to adequately assess, treat and support those with a continence problem robs people of their dignity and imposes limitations on lifestyles, employment opportunities and social functioning. Embarrassment and ignorance about the subject prevent many people seeking help but with correct diagnosis and appropriate treatment, incontinence is a condition that can often be cured and mostly improved, often by relatively simple, non-invasive methods delivered outside of hospital settings.

This chapter provides an overview of con–tinence issues and continence care from his–torical, epidemiological, individual and policy

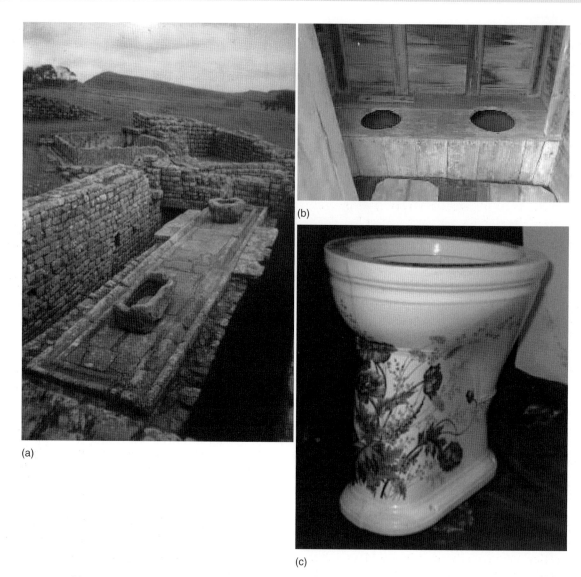

Figure 1.1   (a) Roman latrines excavated near Hadrian's Wall, Northumberland, UK. (b) Earth closet (usually located in an out-house). (c) Decorated Victorian toilet: 'The Progress – a restrained and elegant design'.

perspectives. It explores the impact of living with incontinence on quality of life (QoL) and provides a synopsis of approaches to enhancing the evidence base to underpin treatments and care strategies. The chapter concludes with a brief discussion of the promotion of continence care in the international arena. Although much of the policy discussion centres on the UK context, there are core themes and lessons to be learnt which have much wider relevance. The chapter focuses primarily on urinary incontinence except where faecal incontinence is specifically stated. Chapter 8 looks at bowel care and faecal incontinence in detail.

SOME HISTORICAL PERSPECTIVES

The importance attached to bladder and bowel control is as old as the human race. Latrine-like receptacles thought to date back 10 000 years have been excavated in the Orkney Isles and Figure 1.1a shows Roman remains near Hadrian's Wall,

Northumberland. Earth closets (Fig. 1.1b) have been used for centuries and although the forerunner of the modern flush toilet was invented by Sir James Harrington in 1596 it was almost another 200 years before a flushing water closet was first patented by Alexander Cummings in 1775. In 1848 a Public Health Act ruled that every new house should have a water closet, privy or ash pit and it was during the Victorian era that the decorated toilet became a 'work of art' (Fig. 1.1c).

Although often an 'unmentionable' subject, urine has been utilised for a variety of practical purposes through the ages and Robert Record, in his *Urinal of the Physik* (1651), recommends human urine as a cure for spots on the face, canine urine as a cure for corns and warts, and male ass's urine to reduce baldness and stimulate new hair growth. The urea in urine has been used for centuries as a fixing agent in dyeing cloth and until recently urine was stored for the treatment of wool in the tweed industry. Even today, in some countries, human excreta are preciously collected and used to manure the crops.

The oldest known medical record of a remedy for urinary incontinence comes from ancient Egyptian medicine. The Papyrus Ebers (1550 BC) recommends a mixture of juniper berries, cypress and beer 'to remove constant running of urine'. Since then, a wide range of methods for treating people to control this basic bodily function have been recommended, including hydrotherapies, vaginal douches and various external devices such as body-worn urinals, penile clamps and vaginal pessaries. One remedy used in the Middle Ages included tying a frog around the waist, but the success of this treatment is not recorded! By the nineteenth century pilgrimage and prayer were increasingly employed to achieve a cure. St Catherine of Alexandria was considered to be the patron saint of urinary incontinence and St Vitus from western Germany the patron saint for constipation. Also during this time the avoidance of certain foods was strongly advocated including salt, sharp and sour foods, malt liquor, tea and coffee. Some of these remedies, such as limiting tea and coffee, remain in common use today.

Incontinence continues to be a significant problem worldwide, affecting the lives of millions of individuals and families, with associated impact on quality of life and burden on health and social care services. The prevalence and characteristics of continence problems in different populations are examined in the following sections.

EPIDEMIOLOGICAL PERSPECTIVES

Defining incontinence

Continence can be described as having the ability to store urine in the bladder or faeces in the bowel and to excrete voluntarily where and when it is socially appropriate. In children, continence is about being able to alternate voluntarily and comfortably between the storing and emptying phases of the bladder and bowel. The age of achieving continence varies according to the individual's physical and social development, the natural maturation of the central nervous system and the cultural background (see Chs 5 and 8).

Urinary incontinence can be defined, in its simplest terms, as 'the complaint of any involuntary leakage of urine' (Abrams et al 2005; Box 1.1). Faecal incontinence is the involuntary loss of liquid or solid stool that is a social or hygienic problem (Box 1.1). Studies on the prevalence of incontinence are important for many reasons which include awareness of the size of the problem

> **Box 1.1 International Continence Society definitions (Abrams et al 2005)**
>
> - *Urinary incontinence** is the complaint of any involuntary leakage of urine
> - *Stress urinary incontinence* is the complaint of involuntary leakage on effort or exertion, or on sneezing or coughing
> - *Urge urinary incontinence* is the complaint of involuntary leakage accompanied by or immediately preceded by urgency
> - *Mixed urinary incontinence* is the complaint of involuntary leakage associated with urgency and also with exertion, effort, sneezing or coughing
> - *Faecal incontinence* is the involuntary loss of liquid or solid stool that is a social or hygienic problem
>
> * In infants and small children this definition is not applicable.

to inform service development and provide a baseline against which to measure progress. However, prevalence studies frequently use differing definitions of incontinence (or sometimes do not state their definition at all). This presents difficulties in making comparisons between study outcomes and/or populations and it is important to have a clear understanding of the definition used when assessing the results of any epidemiological study. The International Continence Society (ICS) promotes the use of common definitions and common data collection criteria where possible to facilitate such comparisons (Box 1.1).

These recently revised and simplified definitions are helpful but do not give any indication of the severity of the continence problem or its impact on the individual, and many studies incorporate some time frame for incontinence such as daily episodes of incontinence, any incontinence in the preceding month, etc. Severity can be considered in terms of objective measures (e.g. frequency, volume, pad weighing) and/or in subjective terms as the degree of 'bother' experienced by the individual.

Prevalence studies

It is difficult to measure and compare the prevalence of incontinence accurately because not only are there real differences between population groups, but the way that data are collected can also have a notable effect (Thom 1998). People may underreport the problem because of associated embarrassment, particularly in an interview situation. By contrast, positive responses to a postal questionnaire which asks 'Have you ever wet your underclothing' are likely to overinflate the prevalence figures by inclusion of individuals who admit to infrequent loss of very small quantities of urine. If questions are directed to professionals or carers rather than the individual with incontinence the perceptions may be different again. Depending on the ultimate way in which the prevalence figures are to be used, it may also be useful to distinguish between different types of incontinence or those with an incontinence problem which is managed effectively with aids such as a catheter and those without satisfactory management.

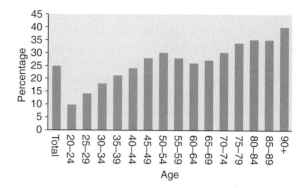

Figure 1.2 Prevalence of UI (any leakage) in women 20 years+. Data from the EPINCONT study (Hannestad et al 2000). Reproduced with permission from Abrams et al 2005.

Urinary incontinence is a frequently occurring symptom affecting people of all ages, but with increasing prevalence in older age groups, and most commonly in women (Hunskaar et al 2004, McGrowther et al 2004). In Hunskaar et al's large cross-sectional study of women in four European countries, 35% of those responding reported urinary loss in the preceding 30 days. Stress incontinence seems to be the predominant type in younger and middle ages, with the prevalence of urge/mixed incontinence increasing in older women (Hunskaar et al 2005). Overall, the prevalence of incontinence in women appears to increase up to middle age with a further increase as age advances beyond 70 years (Hannestad et al 2000, Hunskaar et al 2004) (Fig. 1.2). The epidemiology of incontinence in men has not been investigated to the same extent as in women and it is important to recognise that it is rarely an isolated problem in men, but more often a component of a multifactorial problem which commonly includes other lower urinary tract symptoms (e.g. weak stream, hesitancy, dribbling, erectile dysfunction) (see Ch. 4). Most epidemiological studies of urinary incontinence have been on Caucasian populations and much less is known about other ethnic groups.

Prevalence figures for the UK are summarised in Boxes 1.2–1.4. The results of a survey of over 10 000 adults aged over 40, which included a high response rate of over 70%, showed that more than one in three had clinically significant symptoms of bladder problems (Perry et al 2000). More than

Box 1.2   UK prevalence of urinary incontinence (DH 2000a)

FOR PEOPLE LIVING AT HOME
- Between 1 in 20 and 1 in 14 women aged 15–44
- Between 1 in 13 and 1 in 7 women aged 45–64
- Between 1 in 10 and 1 in 5 women aged 65 and over
- Over 1 in 33 men aged 15–64
- Between 1 in 14 and 1 in 10 men aged 65 and over

FOR PEOPLE (BOTH SEXES) LIVING IN INSTITUTIONS
- 1 in 3 in residential homes
- Nearly 2 in every 3 in nursing homes
- Between 1 in 2 and 2 in 3 in wards for the elderly and elderly mentally infirm

Table 1.1   Perceptions of continence symptoms

Symptom severity	Women (%)	Men (%)	Total (%)
Bothersome	8.0	6.2	7.2
Want help	3.8	3.8	3.8
Socially disabling	3.2	2.2	2.8

Percentages of 10 226 adults over 40 whose symptoms of urinary incontinence were a problem to them (Perry et al 2000).

Box 1.4   UK prevalence of faecal incontinence (DH 2000a)

Information about faecal incontinence is less extensive than for urinary incontinence, but current best estimates suggest:

ADULTS
- 1 in 100 in adults at home
- 17 in 100 in the very elderly
- 1 in 4 in people in institutional care

CHILDREN
- 1 in 30 children aged 4–5 years
- 1 in 50 children aged 5–6 years
- 1 in 75 children aged 7–9 years
- 1 in 100 children aged 11–12 years

Box 1.3   UK prevalence of nocturnal enuresis (DH 2000a)

It is estimated that about 500 000 children in the UK suffer from nocturnal enuresis (persistent bedwetting). The prevalence decreases with age as follows:
- 1 in 6 children aged 5 years
- 1 in 7 children aged 7 years
- 1 in 11 children aged 8 years
- 1 in 50 teenagers.

The persistence of nocturnal enuresis into adulthood is frequently unacknowledged, but it is estimated that 1 in 100 adults continues to have lifelong bedwetting problems (ERIC 1995).

20% of women and nearly 15% of men had incontinence several times a month and approximately 20% of both men and women had nocturia requiring them to get up twice a night or more. Most people with clinically significant symptoms did not find them bothersome or want help but those who did are shown, as percentages of the total sample, in Table 1.1.

Nocturnal enuresis is widespread in children (Johnson 1998) and is more common in boys (Chiozza et al 1998). It is characterised by complete emptying of the bladder during sleep without any symptoms indicating bladder dysfunction (see Ch. 5). Urinary symptoms tend to decrease with age but are still experienced by a significant number of healthy teenagers (Swithinbank et al 1998) and can persist into adulthood.

Faecal incontinence is far less common than urinary incontinence but the social consequences can be more severe. Faecal incontinence affects people of all ages, but its prevalence is particularly difficult to estimate because it is seen by professionals and the public to be more embarrassing, resulting in reluctance by the former to ask questions and the latter to seek help (Johanson & Lafferty 1996). However, it is more common in the general population than is often realised. Although prevalence increases with advancing age and/or disability, there are also large numbers of younger people who experience symptoms. A postal survey in the UK which included 10 000 respondents (Perry et al 2002) found that 5.7% of women and

> **Box 1.5 Comparing incontinence with prevalence of other conditions (from data compiled by the Continence Foundation 2000a)**
>
> - Urinary incontinence affects up to 4 million people in the UK compared to:
>   - asthma, up to 3.4 million
>   - diabetes, up to 2.4 million.
> - Faecal incontinence affects up to 600 000 people in the UK compared to:
>   - dementia, 700 000
>   - epilepsy, 420 000
>   - Parkinson's disease, 120 000
>   - multiple sclerosis, 85 000.

6.2% of men over 40 years of age living in their own homes report some degree of faecal incontinence. Overall, 1.4% of adults reported major faecal incontinence (at least several times a month) and 0.7% had disabling incontinence (with a major impact on their life). The commonest cause of faecal incontinence in healthy women is childbirth trauma (Kamm 1994).

Comparing incontinence with prevalence of other conditions

Prevalence data are important in planning service provision and resources but for those not involved in such activities the meaning or usefulness of prevalence figures can often be quite difficult to grasp. The Continence Foundation (2000a) make a notable comparison between the prevalence of incontinence and that of other 'common' conditions which helps to put the numbers into context (Box 1.5).

Risk factors for incontinence

Some individuals have greater potential for developing incontinence or prolapse of pelvic organs than others. There is evidence that age, pregnancy, parity and body mass index are all recognisable risk factors (Sampselle et al 2002, Rortveit et al 2003, Hunskaar et al 2005), with more variable evidence for smoking, hysterectomy and menopause. Obesity is an acknowledged risk factor for incontinence in women, with a 4.2 times risk asso-

ciated with stress incontinence and a 2.2 times risk associated with urge incontinence (Hunskaar et al 2005) (see Chs 2 and 3). Given that obesity is an increasing problem and now affects 20% of the population in the UK, this factor needs greater attention.

Women employed in certain occupations that constrain free access to toilet facilities, including nurses, teachers and women in the military, have also been shown to be at increased risk of developing urinary incontinence (Fitzgerald et al 2002). The experiences of these women raise important questions about the long-term effects of prolonged periods between voiding and self-management strategies, such as fluid restriction and absorbent pad use.

INDIVIDUAL (PATIENT) PERSPECTIVES

Incontinence and quality of life (QoL)

> Incontinence is soul shattering. It can completely ruin the lives of those of us who are affected by it.

> I've not gone out for years for fear of wetting someone's chair or car seat.

These words illustrate the depth of feeling and distress that can accompany incontinence. Although it is no longer the 'prohibited' subject it once was, lack of understanding of the condition and embarrassment continue to be major factors stopping people seeking help. It is not easy for an adult to say 'I wet myself'. Symptoms such as persistent headaches or fever will prompt people to seek medical help, whilst leaking urine or faeces is still often hidden.

The physical signs of incontinence are objectively demonstrable, but the effects on the quality of life of the individual, their understanding of the condition and their ability to cope vary subjectively. Incontinence impacts strongly on how people feel about themselves, their choice of clothing (e.g. dark colours and loose clothing to hide wet patches or bulky absorbent pads) and the way in which they interact with others at home, at work or in the wider social setting (Box 1.6).

The day-to-day activities that the majority of people take for granted can become a major plan-

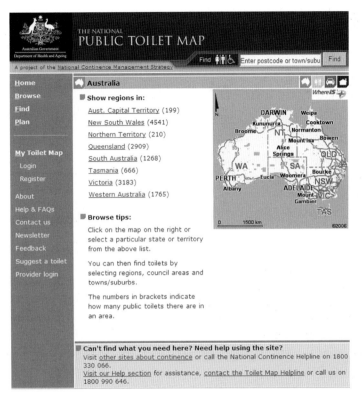

Figure 1.3   The Australian Public Toilet Map website. Reproduced with permission. (http://www.toiletmap.gov.au)

Box 1.6   Living with incontinence: some comments made by women in a recent study on use of absorbent pads for incontinence (Getliffe et al 2007)

I don't wear tight clothes in case the outline of the pad can be seen. It would be embarrassing. I have different clothes for different occasions but all tend to be baggy and they are chosen for the incontinence problem.

I'm terrified the pad will smell. If I was out with friends I would have to leave. I couldn't be next to them in case they could smell me and I would be utterly mortified.

Sometimes it affects being with friends because you just don't trust yourself and don't want to leave a wet patch on their seat, so you tend to leave early so it spoils the time with them and they often don't understand why you are leaving earlier than you should.

You prepare yourself before going out anywhere, wash before going and carry wipes in a bag. You tend to go over the top with padding . . . but then you worry about discreetness . . .

---

ning exercise, or just impossible for people with incontinence. Journeys on public transport are frequently avoided, making going to work, visiting places of public entertainment or socialising impossible. Being 'caught short' in a public place is a major concern. Finding accessible public toilets is a cause of anxiety for many people and coping strategies may include detailed mapping of public toilets and planning ahead for regular toilet stops. In Australia these needs have been acknowledged and facilitated by a national public toilet map website (Fig. 1.3). Public toilet access can be a particular problem for women and Goldsmith (1992) drew attention to shortcomings in a study which showed that there was a higher ratio of public toilets for men, toilets were not wide enough to accommodate the child's buggy and mother, travellers at main-line stations had to struggle down flights of stairs with their luggage and local authorities often closed public toilets on financial grounds.

Incontinence and enuresis can contribute to marital and family breakdown. People avoid making social contacts and lose their confidence in personal relationships. Disgust or fear of wetting or soiling partners can cause frigidity and impotence, and catheters and appliances can have a devastating effect on body image. Men and women have been known to refuse surgery because they were worried that the consequences could have a detrimental effect on their sex life. Professionals rarely initiate advice on sexual activity and have been known to be uncertain as to whether sexual intercourse is possible for people with an indwelling catheter. (Advice on sexual activity in relation to incontinence is offered in several later chapters, including with a catheter in situ; see Ch. 10).

The experience of being incontinent is unique to each individual and healthcare professionals need to understand this and work with each person to determine 'patient-centred goals' and the most appropriate strategy to try to attain them (Dougherty et al 2002, Williams et al 2002). It is also important to recognise that QoL is an indicator of the individual's perception of their physical, psychological and social well-being and that this is also influenced by personal and cultural values and beliefs.

Quality of life measures

QoL measures are becoming increasingly important in evaluations of treatment interventions, particularly in clinical trials where differences in measurable clinical outcomes may be small, but where patient morbidity is reduced or patient/carer satisfaction is increased (Kelleher 2000). As many studies are now multicentre and sometimes multinational it is essential to identify the most widely acceptable tool to facilitate comparisons

between studies. QoL measures can also be an important outcome in economic evaluations of continence care and provide the most obvious effectiveness measure from the patient's point of view.

An acknowledgement of the multidimensional nature of QoL helps to emphasise the importance of considering individuals' needs and experiences in relation to their own circumstances and the concept of QoL can be considered to encompass:

> ... those attributes valued by patients, including their resultant comfort or sense of well-being; the extent to which they are able to maintain reasonable physical, emotional and intellectual function; the degree to which they retain their ability to participate in valued activities within the family, in the workplace and in the community.
> Quoted in Naughton & Shumaker (1996).

Measures of health-related QoL include both generic (e.g. the SF-36) and continence-specific tools. Donovan et al (2005) reviewed a range of continence-specific tools and Box 1.7 indicates those recommended on the basis of research evi-

---

Box 1.7   Recommended QoL instruments (adapted from Donovan et al 2005)

QoL IMPACT OF UI
- Men and women
  - I-QoL
  - SEAPI-QMM
- Women
  - King's Health Questionnaire
  - Incontinence Impact Questionnaire
  - Urinary Incontinence Severity Score (UISS)
  - CONTILIFE
- Men
  - none

COMBINED SYMPTOMS AND QoL IMPACT OF UI
- Men and women
  - ICIQ
- Women
  - Bristol female LUTS-SF
  - SUIQQ
- Men
  - ICS male SF

dence. A QoL measure for faecal incontinence has been developed by Rockwood et al (2000).

When selecting any QoL measure to use as part of a study or evaluation of incontinence it is important to check what patient group (e.g. male, female or both), what age group and which particular continence problem (e.g. urge incontinence) it was originally designed for and whether it has been tested and validated for the group you wish to use it with. As with prevalence studies (addressed above), it can be difficult to make comparisons between studies where different measures of QoL have been used. One of the most recent developments in continence-specific QoL measures is the International Consultation on Incontinence Modular Questionnaire (http://www.iciq.net). The I-QoL is a validated 0–100 scale, with lower scores indicating higher impact on QoL. It consists of 22 items divided into three domains of related effects:

- avoidance and limiting behaviours (8 items)
- psychosocial effects (9 items)
- social embarrassment (5 items).

Each item is scored according to how applicable it is to the respondent's current situation using a Likert scale from 1 (not at all) to 5 (extremely) (Boxes 1.8 and 1.9).

Other useful websites associated with developments in quality of life and patient reported outcome measures (PROMS) include the International Society for Quality of Life Research (http://www.isoqol.org) and the National Centre for Health Outcomes Development (http://nchod.uhce.ox.ac.uk/incontinence.pdf).

Fears about urine leakage and exposure of continence problems to others are common to most people with incontinence symptoms (Margalith et al 2004, Papanicalaou et al 2005, Irwin et al 2006). People with incontinence have been found to be more depressed, have higher levels of anxiety, feel more stigmatised and have poorer life satisfaction compared to people who are continent (Shaw 2001). Although this can apply to all types of incontinence (see Ch. 2), people with symptoms of overactive bladder (OAB) with urge incontinence or mixed incontinence appear to experience greater psychological distress than those with symptoms of stress incontinence (Sandvik et al 1993). Other

---

> **Box 1.8 Research study 1: Assessment of bothersomeness and impact on quality of life of incontinence in women in France, Germany, Spain and the UK**
>
> The I-QoL was used in a large postal questionnaire-based study, designed by Papanicolaou et al (2005) to assess the bothersomeness and impact on the quality of life of incontinence in women in four European countries. The women in the sample (1573 respondents) were known (from earlier work) to have experienced incontinence during the previous 30 days.
>
> Over 80% of the 1573 women who responded reported that their urinary incontinence was bothersome and nearly half (45%) were 'moderately' to 'extremely' bothered. The greatest negative effect appeared to be on physical activities, confidence, self-perception and social activities, with a direct, statistically significant correlation between increase in bothersomeness and severity of symptoms. Younger women appeared to be more bothered by their symptoms, perhaps because they were more likely to be balancing the demands of a career and personal life than those over 60 years of age.

studies have concurred with this and Irwin et al (2006) reported an investigation of the impact of OAB symptoms on employment, social interactions and social well-being in six European countries (Box 1.9). It is interesting to note that despite debilitating effects, 43% of respondents did not consider it worth discussing their symptoms with a doctor, suggesting that OAB remains an under-reported and undertreated condition.

Help-seeking behaviour

There are a number of key themes which are recurrent in studies of the psychological impact of incontinence (Button et al 1998). These include:

- distress
- embarrassment
- inconvenience
- threat to self-esteem
- loss of personal control
- desire for normalisation.

Box 1.9   Research study 2: Impact of overactive bladder symptoms on employment, social interactions and emotional well-being in six European countries

This study by Irwin et al (2006) was a two-stage, telephone-based survey of 11 521 individuals aged 40–64 years in six European countries (France, Germany, Italy, Spain, Sweden, UK). In stage one, individuals were screened for reported symptoms suggestive of an overactive bladder (OAB) and in stage two those with OAB (1272) were asked questions about the impact of their symptoms on their emotional well-being, social interactions and productivity at home and at work. Overall, three-quarters of those with OAB (1272) stated that this condition interfered with or made it more difficult to perform daily activities, with a third reporting that their symptoms made them feel depressed and more than a quarter had stress or concern due to symptoms. (Prevalence of depression in the general population is thought to be around 8.5%.)

Men were significantly more likely to report these symptoms as something they have to learn to live with (79% men, 74% women) and a natural part of the ageing process (76% men, 67% women). Men were also significantly more likely to report OAB with urge incontinence as having an impact on their daily work life (38% men, 22% women), including worry about interrupting meetings, impact on decisions made about work location and hours, and voluntary termination or early retirement.

The study concluded that OAB is a highly prevalent condition in the general population, few patients are treated and OAB symptoms have a significant detrimental effect on QoL. Those with OAB should be encouraged to seek help from healthcare professionals.

Despite the burden of their symptoms, most people with urinary incontinence do not seek help and often develop coping strategies, such as avoiding social contact and physical activities, limiting fluid intake, making frequent toilet visits and wearing protective pads (Hannestad et al 2000, Kinchen et al 2003, O'Donnell et al 2005). In the large European prevalence survey of incontinence in women (Hunskaar et al 2004) only a quarter of respondents in the UK and Spain had consulted a doctor about their symptoms, with slightly higher percentages in France (33%) and Germany (40%). Many women delay seeking help for reasons that include lack of time, shame and fear of surgery (Margalith et al 2004). This reluctance to seek help highlights the need to actively promote better knowledge and understanding of treatment options and cure prospects within the general public.

The severity of symptoms is an important factor in promoting help-seeking behaviour but is strongly related to the individual's own perception of severity rather than direct measures of severity. A number of studies have examined reasons for people not seeking treatment. One of the main reasons seems to be that incontinence is not viewed as a legitimate medical condition but rather as a normal part of the ageing process (Shaw 2001). It can also be viewed as something which is somehow the individual's own fault, perhaps through being a woman and giving birth (Ashworth & Hagan 1993). In the absence of an 'illness identity' it is often not considered or recognised as appropriate for discussion with a health professional.

Coping mechanisms

Coping mechanisms vary from person to person but are almost always directed towards concealing the problem from others (see Box 1.6). A complex set of behavioural strategies can sometimes take up much of the individual's time and energy but failure to conceal results in social isolation and loss of self-esteem. There is evidence that self-management programmes for a number of chronic conditions can result in tangible benefits in terms of reduced severity of symptoms, improved life control and activity, and improved resourcefulness and life satisfaction. The self-help book *Don't Make Me Laugh* (Astbury & White 2001) is a good example of effective partnership working (including active listening to people living with incontinence!). This book resulted from discussions during a series of focus groups with people experiencing continence problems. The group participants identified important and common concerns, which were then addressed in the resulting user-focused book. Group members were invited to review the early drafts and contribute to the book's final content and format. This approach fits well with the concept of the Expert Patient Pro-grammes (DH 2001c) which is about developing the confidence and motivation of patients to work in partnership with health professionals and to use their own skills and knowledge to take effective control over their condition.

Professionals also have their own coping styles and strategies. It is generally assumed that nurses are comfortable with all aspects of care, but it can be as embarrassing assisting people to perform intimate tasks as it is for those receiving the help. Although it is important that all health and social care workers recognise their own feelings and reactions, it is equally important that effective ways of managing them are developed. A report on incontinence in residential care by the Royal College of Physicians (1995) recommended that carers should be given the opportunity to share their own feelings with staff and to be aware of the effects of social and cultural differences in their own lives.

POLICY AND SERVICE PERSPECTIVES

The costs of incontinence

The widespread prevalence of incontinence cannot be ignored but true measures of the costs of incontinence are difficult to assess (Hu et al 2005). However, health economists are increasingly being called to:

- estimate the cost of treating an illness or problem such as incontinence
- evaluate the economic consequences of not treating that illness
- compare the costs and benefits (cost-effectiveness) of alternative treatments.

In the UK alone there are more than 5 million people with incontinence and a 'health economy' with a population of 250 000 people is likely to have around 14 000 individuals with urinary incontinence (UI) and around 2250 with faecal incontinence (FI). The associated costs to that health economy are in the order of £1.8 million per year (Continence Foundation 2000a). This is indicative of a total expenditure for the UK of more than £420 million (approximately 1/120th of the total cost of the NHS) (Continence Foundation 2000b).

As pressures on scarce resources increase, good economic evaluations become even more important. For example, payment by results (PbR) is a new NHS financial structure that represents a reformed financial flow system for the UK National Health Service; instead of funding treatment through block contracts, from 2006 onwards NHS service providers will receive payment through each case treated on a single tariff cost with no variation for provider. Precise costs of treatment or effects of not treating a patient will be required to make a strong case for high-quality, cost-effective care.

There can be no question that the overall cost of continence care is set to rise substantially as demographic changes increasingly impact on service provision. Aside from the economic burden to services, however, there are personal costs to individuals and carers. Lack of effective continence treatment or containment strategies can lead to breakdown in overall health, economic problems for the families affected and increasing difficulties in coping with incontinence from physical, psychological and social perspectives. The contribution provided by informal carers should not be underestimated and such 'hidden costs' may be transferred to public costs if adequate support is unavailable and/or when informal carers become unable to cope. Incontinence has often been cited as the final straw that influences whether a patient can be managed at home or is admitted to institutional care (Thom 1997). People with congenital and acquired disabilities are now surviving into old age and, together with the very large numbers of elderly people in the population, these represent the largest client groups and have perhaps the greatest need for these resources.

Developing continence services

Gaining momentum and promoting public awareness

The opening phrase of the chapter suggests that 'A little rebellion now and then is a good thing . . .'. It is certainly true that some degree of rebellion is always needed to generate large-scale change in services and Box 1.10 provides a summary of progress in gaining momentum and promoting

Box 1.10   Gaining momentum – early development of continence services in the UK

A concerted approach to promoting continence in the UK began to gain strength during the 1970s as attitudes towards incontinence gradually changed, together with greater awareness of treatments and potential cure. Health professionals, scientists and bioengineers were working together, pioneering assessment tools and interventions, and at the same time nurses were being appointed to specialist posts, mainly in urodynamics units. The momentum continued during the 1980s with the setting up of continence services and the appointment of continence advisors. The Incontinence Action Group, comprising representatives from the health and social care professions and from industry, was charged with reviewing the provision of continence services and the training of professionals. Their report, *Action on Incontinence* (King's Fund 1983), highlighted the absence of continence as a topic in the pre- and postregistration training of doctors and nurses and the need to educate professionals and the public. It also recommended that an incontinence clinic with some form of urodynamics assessment and a continence nurse advisor should be available in each district. This was followed by a report from the Royal College of Physicians (1986), entitled *Physical Disability in 1986 and Beyond*, which set out the general principles for the operation of a urinary continence service and advocated a written district policy.

Within a decade there were over 300 nurses and two physiotherapists in these specialist posts (Mandelstam 1990). The development of the posts and the services provided varied around the country, depending on the way in which the posts were initially created and funded (Roe 1990). In many instances the services were based on economic grounds rather than the needs of the local population, and the role of the advisor depended on the source of funding for the post. As continence services developed, professionals and the public saw a greater need for information, education and support. In 1981 over 100 healthcare professionals from across the UK met in response to a questionnaire asking health authorities to identify professionals concerned with continence. From this meeting the Association of Continence Advisors (now the Association for Continence Advice) was founded. A few years later the Royal College of Nursing set up a special interest group for continence (now the Continence Care Forum). In 1988 the Enuresis Resource and Information Centre (ERIC) emerged as a support group for children with nocturnal enuresis and their parents and carers. This service has extended to include daytime wetting, encopresis, and physical and learning needs (see Ch. 5). In the following year a group of patients established a self-help group called the

National Action on Incontinence (now known as *In*contact – Action on Incontinence). This consumer-led group continues to play a major role in developing government policy and public awareness. The Continence Foundation was formed in 1994 as an umbrella group and focuses on advice, awareness and advocacy, campaigning for improvements in policy and services. Two years later PromoCon was established as a joint initiative of the Continence Foundation and the Disabled Living Centres Council, Manchester, providing a national resource of continence products, coordinating resources within Disabled Living Centres and piloting public awareness campaigns. This network of continence organisations meets twice a year as the UK Continence Alliance – 'a forum to aid clarification, communication, collaborations and support between continence organisations'.

PUBLIC AWARENESS CAMPAIGNS
The first major, government supported, publicity campaign took place in 1994, led by the Continence Foundation and their affiliated organisations. The slogan was *Don't Suffer in Silence* and the aim was to increase public knowledge about incontinence and to encourage people to seek help. More than 1.5 million leaflets, posters and toilet stickers were distributed to healthcare professionals, relevant voluntary organisations, libraries, national rail and coach companies, fast-food chains and a host of other organisations. In addition, press packs which included case histories of people willing to be interviewed were sent to journalists in the professional and public media, and a booth at London's Waterloo station offered information to commuters. The national Incontinence Information Helpline was given government funding to extend its opening times and remained open for 12 h a day throughout the week-long campaign. The annual Continence Awareness Week has continued each year, with a range of themes.

CONTINENCE PUBLIC AWARENESS CAMPAIGNS
- 1994 Don't suffer in silence
- 1995 Dry day – dry night
- 1996 Your baby, your bladder, your bowels
- 1997 The pelvic floor
- 1998 Dispelling myths about bladder problems
- 1999 The well-behaved bladder
- 2000 Women and childbirth
- 2001 Helping you to help yourself
- 2002 Functional incontinence
- 2003 Male incontinence
- 2004 It's no laughing matter
- 2005 Overactive bladder
- 2006 Do you know what can be done today?

the development of continence services in the UK.

Opportunities for raising public awareness are increasing as the taboos on mentioning bladder and bowel disorders gradually decrease in most cultures. Previous stringent restrictions on content and timing of advertisements on sensitive issues, such as incontinence, have been revised and incontinence pads are now advertised on television at peak times. Other advertisements – once tucked away on the back pages of weekly papers, offering plastic pants and male appliances and guaranteeing discreet mailing – are now replaced by high-profile glossy pictures in women's magazines, national papers and the Internet. Although there is relatively little research-based evidence to evaluate the effectiveness of public awareness campaigns, and indeed it is difficult to identify appropriate measurable outcomes other than increased numbers of people seeking help or further information, there are several key components of any programme designed to promote public awareness. Some of these are summarised in Box 1.11. Many continence-related commercial companies continue to invest substantially in raising public awareness through products and non-product initiatives such as self-help leaflets, videos and helplines. Partnership working is often beneficial to ensure accurate, informative material. All information, however, needs to be medically accurate and easy to read. Reliable sources include the Continence Foundation, *Incontact*, community pharmacies, NHS Direct, the Department of Health, the National Library for Health and professionally endorsed websites.

Towards a comprehensive, integrated, continence service

Increasing demand has placed incontinence higher on the political and public agenda. In recognition of the extent of need and rising costs to the NHS, and as a result of an extensive lobbying campaign, the Department of Health (England) published its guidance on *Good Practice in Continence Services* in 2000 (DH 2000a) (subsequently referred to as the Guidance). This document set out a model of good practice to help achieve more responsive, equitable and effective continence services. The empha-

---

Box 1.11 Some key components for developing public awareness campaigns

PURPOSE/FOCUS
- Clear key message(s)

TARGET POPULATION
- Generic approach to whole population or directed towards a specific group; local, regional or national campaign

TIME FRAME
- Preparation
- Duration of campaign
- Evaluation period/follow-up

COMMUNICATION CHANNELS
- Media (e.g. TV, radio, newspapers, magazines), phone-in lines, billboards
- Via health and social care professionals, consumer groups, commercial companies (product manufacturers), professional marketing agencies

PROMOTIONAL MATERIAL
- Posters, fliers, bookmarks
- Information for clients: clear purpose; focus (too little, too much?); ethically acceptable; accurate, up-to-date information; relevant to consumers; easy to understand, large print, English and other languages; contact numbers/addresses etc.

PLANNED RESPONSE
- Plans to cope with increased demand for help. It is important to be realistic about what services are able to provide

EVALUATION
- Pilot plans and promotional materials in advance
- Identify appropriate outcomes to be measured (is there a base-line measure for comparison?)
- Which communication channels worked best for particular groups?

This table is by no means exhaustive and experienced professional help in campaign design and delivery is recommended where possible.

---

sis is on primary care to be the first contact point for people with incontinence and a number of targets are suggested, together with effective interventions which can be implemented at minimum cost but maximum gain for primary care. The Guidance also calls for proactive identification of people with continence problems and stresses the need to help carers understand incontinence and possible treatments. Promoting inde-pendence is a fundamental theme throughout this policy (and throughout this book), and the goal is that people with a continence problem can access high-quality, effective, timely assessment, diagno-sis, advice and treatment to enable them to fulfil their health potential and remain independent.

Although incontinence has gained greater rec-ognition within the UK healthcare agenda in recent years, increasing competition for scarce resources, together with reorganisation of services and commissioning processes, means that persist-ent efforts are required to maintain/increase the level of awareness and support. Incontinence will continue to present a major challenge to individu-als and to commissioners and providers of health and social care, both now and for the foreseeable future.

The review of continence services which led to the publication of the Guidance on *Good Prac-tice in Continence Services* (DH 2000a) identified a number of problems across the country including:

- lack of involvement of users at all levels of service planning and delivery
- geographical variations in the range and quanti-ties of treatment provided and the time spent waiting
- geographical variations in the number of staff trained and the quality of the education and the training given
- gross differences in the NHS Trust policies for the provision of continence supplies. For example, the most common maximum pad allowance per 24 h was five, with the lowest two and the highest seven (Anthony 1998).

The Guidance called for integrated continence services 'based upon and evolved from existing local continence services' (see Ch. 11). These serv-ices are expected to be 'cohesive and comprehen-sive', covering urinary and faecal incontinence in all age groups – children to older people – in hospi-tal, at home or in care. Services should be provided at different levels and through different bodies, not necessarily the NHS, and based on agreed evi-dence-based policies, procedures and guidelines with group audit and review (Fig. 1.4). Within this integrated service, primary practice is viewed as

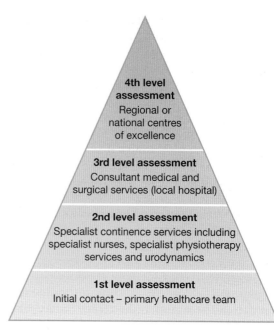

Figure 1.4   Continence service pathways. Local integrated services, led by a Director of Continence Services, will include levels 1–3. Local services should have specific referral arrangements with level 4 provision.

responsible for: (1) identifying the local population with incontinence; (2) ensuring appropriate resources; (3) providing first-line assessment and treatment, using agreed care pathways; (4) audit-ing the service, and (5) making the results available for research. In order to fulfil this role, primary care and community professionals need to be trained appropriately to implement the prevention, assess-ment and treatment of incontinence.

The Guidance set out clear targets, interven-tions and indicators for the following:

- primary health care and community teams
- health authorities and primary care trusts
- joint targets for health and local authorities with respect to children, and to residential care and nursing homes
- inpatient care.

It recognises the need for continence products and recommends that supplies should be governed by clinical need and not cost alone (see Ch. 10). However, it is also noted that a better knowledge and understanding by health professionals is needed about products such as hand-held urinals (especially female urinals) and lifestyle aids and adaptations which can often prevent the need for continence products such as pads.

Leading and delivering continence services

The Guidance recommends that a Director or Head of Continence Services, usually a specialist nurse or physiotherapist, leads the service, coordinating continence specialist nurses, physiotherapists and hospital-based specialists and services. The Director/Head is expected to take a lead in developing shared policies, protocols and pathways that will make for a cohesive and comprehensive service and to coordinate all staff across the whole health economy in primary, secondary and tertiary care with outside agencies including social services, education authorities, care home providers, users and carers. Informed and effective commissioning is crucial in developing continence services but the absence of time-related performance targets has resulted in variable priorities and progress in service development within different health economies (Thomas et al 2004). The Continence Foundation (2000b) published a resource book *Making the Case for Investment in an Integrated Continence Service* which offered comprehensive advice on getting incontinence on the agenda, including compilation and analysis of population profiles, and estimating costs to the service (see Ch. 11).

Traditional roles such as the continence nurse specialist and specialist physiotherapist remain central to service delivery but in order to manage the magnitude of the problem of incontinence within the population other professionals are increasingly being encouraged to develop their skills in continence assessment and management. Nurse consultants were introduced in 1999 (*Making a Difference*, DH 1999) as part of the modernisation of career frameworks. The nurse consultant, whilst retaining clinical expertise, has a central role in initiating and leading significant development in practice, education and research. Although there are still relatively few nurse consultants in continence, these posts have the potential to offer great opportunities (and also present

great challenges). Physiotherapists have well-recognised expertise in continence care and occupational therapists are increasingly working across continence services to address functional continence issues. The role of pharmacists in raising awareness of continence problems and sources of help and/or medication advice is also increasingly acknowledged.

More specific expanding role opportunities, which can be linked to continence care, are those of 'practitioners with special interests' (PwSI), including allied health professionals (AHPwSI) as well as GPs and nurses. PwSI services may encompass delivering clinical services and/or undertaking procedures, and aim to bridge the interface between hospitals and primary care, thus increasing the range of care provided in the community. These roles do not conform to any particular grade or specialty, but relate to the need to redesign services to address population needs (http://www.dh.gov.uk/PolicyAndGuidance/OrganisationPolicy/PrimaryCare/fs/en).

Aside from this aspect of workforce modernisation, the NHS is undergoing a revolution in terms of information management through the NHS 'Connecting for Health' national programme (http://www.connectingforhealth.nhs.uk). It is envisaged that eventually all patients' records will be held on computer and made accessible to health professionals and carers as well as patients themselves. The same technology will be used to provide all professionals with up-to-date information on the treatment of problems such as incontinence, so that a range of professionals are competent to treat patients. A key issue for the future relates to competence to assess, treat and manage incontinence and Skills for Health (http://www.skillsforhealth.org) are currently developing a range of continence competencies for the workforce.

Patient care pathways

Patient care pathways, or integrated care pathways, are a main feature of current healthcare policies. Their emphasis is on prevention and self-care, with the patient as an active agent rather than a passive recipient, and on services coordinated seamlessly from public health information to the initial points of contact in primary care and referral on to more specialist services. Care pathways also provide an effective strategy to support evidence-based assessment, treatment and management (Bayliss et al 2000). Although published tools can provide a strong (and often well-tested) framework for audit and monitoring, different strategies may be appropriate in different settings and in order to achieve local ownership and commitment some local adaptation of published tools can be helpful.

Continence care and other healthcare priorities

Continence care contributes directly and indirectly to a broad range of healthcare priority areas even when continence is not explicitly identified. Much of the care can be delivered by nurses, to build capacity into each health economy (e.g. through advanced nursing practice which includes nurse prescribing; see Ch. 9), nurse-led clinics, nurse management of caseloads, receiving referrals and ordering diagnostic investigations, all of which may be delivered through integrated care pathways (see Ch. 11). Good continence care contributes directly to priorities such as the National Service Frameworks (NSFs) for Older People (DH 2001a); Children, Young People and Maternity services (DH 2004a); and for Long Term Conditions (LTC) (DH 2005), which focuses on neurological conditions. For example, there is evidence that 42% of stroke survivors are incontinent and 18% are still incontinent on leaving hospital (Rudd et al 1999); however, good continence care can reduce the effects of the stroke and enhance self-esteem and rehabilitation. Accidents and injuries not only have a major impact on the health of individuals but also lead to large numbers of attendees at Accident and Emergency departments and admissions to hospital, often to trauma and orthopaedic facilities. Incontinence can lead to falls as people hurry to get to a toilet and urge incontinence in particular has been associated with a 30% increased risk of falls and a 3% increased risk of fractures (Brown et al 2000).

The NSF for LTC has outlined a series of quality requirements for service delivery that include what people with LTC say that they need. Many of these are also relevant to continence (Box 1.12).

> **Box 1.12   Quality requirements relevant to continence: NSF for long-term conditions (DH 2005)**
>
> 1. A person-centred service where people are offered an integrated assessment and planning of their health and social care needs
> 2. Early recognition and prompt diagnosis
> 3. Emergency and acute management
> 4. Early and specialist rehabilitation
> 5. Community rehabilitation and support
> 6. Provision of equipment and accommodation
> 7. Personal care and support
> 8. Palliative care
> 9. Supported family and carers
> 10. Care when in hospital or other health or social care setting.

There are also clear connections with national benchmarking programmes, initiated in the *Essence of Care* (DH 2001b). The latter programme focuses on the 'fundamental and essential aspects of care' and continence, including bladder and bowel care, was one of eight areas of health concerns identified by patients, carers and healthcare professionals. The programme aims to improve the quality of care by a process of benchmarking, which identifies good practice and continuous development through comparison and sharing and documents. For example, the NSF for LTC has stimulated benchmarking to take place for conditions which may not previously have elicited a specific interest in continence issues such as Parkinson's disease (Bowron 2006). There is increasing guidance published by the National Institute for Health and Clinical Excellence (NICE) on incontinence. In October 2006 NICE and the National Collaborating Centre for Women's and Children's Health published a clinical guideline on the management of urinary incontinence in women. The Healthcare Commission assesses the implementation of NICE guidance as a component of National Standards.

Healthcare policy drivers

The current governmental reform agenda is driven by a series of interlinked policies to ensure the NHS offers efficiently delivered, high-quality, patient-centred care. *National Standards, Local Action: Health and Social Care Standards and Planning Framework 2005/6–2007/8* follows on from *The NHS Plan* (DH 2000b) and *The NHS Improvement Plan* (DH 2004b). This framework aims to put people at the heart of public services and sets out the level of quality and development standards for all organisations in England providing NHS care, together with priorities and targets. It defines four priorities for the NHS:

1. Health and well-being of the population (covering health promotion and ill-health prevention)
2. Patient user experience (promoting maximum information and choice as well as positive experience so that the service is more consumer focused)
3. Access to services (to ensure people have prompt access to care)
4. Long-term conditions (to support health by promoting self-care and treatment in the community setting, avoiding hospital wherever possible).

This policy increases the focus on care outside of hospital settings with strong emphasis on self-care and personal choice and should, in the future, contribute to more people coming forward for help with their continence problems. This underpinning theme also provides the foundation for the White Paper on community services *Our Health, Our Care, Our Say: A New Direction for Community Services* (DH 2006) which proposes stronger working links between health and social care professionals to provide a more personal service.

The emphasis of incontinence management is moving from containment (Audit Commission 1999) to the promotion of continence through conservative or more complex treatments to reduce the prevalence of treatable incontinence and improve the quality of life in those with intractable incontinence. Collaboration and commitment by policy-makers and professionals is essential and the Guidance on *Good Practice in Continence Services* (DH 2000a) argues for investment in integrated continence services to bring together a multidisciplinary, multiagency team across health and social care services. The extent to which development of integrated services for incontinence has taken place, together with an examination of some

of the practical issues involved, is the subject of further discussion in Chapter 11.

Ethnic minority communities and other minority groups

There is a particular need to ensure fair access to services for groups who may experience difficulties in making contact with them, including:

- ethnic minority communities
- children in foster care and at boarding schools
- travelling people
- people with long-term physical difficulties, neurological conditions and learning disabilities
- prisoners, asylum seekers and refugees
- homeless people and those living in hostels
- older people in residential care and nursing homes.

Promoting health care in a multicultural society is challenging on a number of accounts, particularly around cultural issues and language barriers (DH 1998, O'Neale 2000), and it is now widely acknowledged that more equitable continence services need to be provided to minority ethnic communities as there is low uptake of services from these groups. The taboos and inhibitions connected with continence demand understanding, respect and provision for religious and cultural needs. For example, douching facilities are required for Muslims who cleanse with water after toileting, and women from certain cultures require a female doctor. Language is frequently a barrier and multilingual co-workers are required to improve communication and assessment. Describing incontinence symptoms and treatments in any language is problematic: clinical terminology may not be easy to translate, advice easy to understand or treatments culturally acceptable, and a range of information in differing languages and media is necessary. The Continence Foundation has translated some of its material into other European, Asian and African languages.

The needs of prisoners who have incontinence of either urine or faeces has in the past been a neglected area of care. Historically, prison healthcare services were provided by the prison service and not the NHS, which led to suboptimal care in some prisons as a result of inadequate training for prison healthcare staff. In 1999 a formal partnership was established between the prison service and the NHS in an effort to secure better health care in prisons and in 2003 the commissioning responsibility for prison health care moved to the NHS. Community continence services are now taking a lead in the provision of continence clinics in prisons and offering access to training in continence assessment and management to staff.

Chapters 6 and 7 address some of the particular issues for other vulnerable groups.

Ethical issues

The ability to have bladder and bowel control is a basic right for each one of us. However, an ethical conflict can sometimes arise when there are differences between consumer and professional choices. People are encouraged to make choices, but the resources are not always available to cope with demand or the services offered are not acceptable to the potential users.

Differing perceptions of treatments from professionals' and carers' perspectives can also be a source of concern. Some procedures are simply intended to relieve symptoms and although the outcome may be satisfactory to the professional, it can be a bitter disappointment to the person who had expected to be cured. For example, some surgical procedures may resolve incontinence but can result in voiding difficulty. Having to self-catheterise several times a day for the remainder of one's life may not be an acceptable price to pay. Other procedures such as botulinum toxin injections into the bladder wall to reduce involuntary contractions will need to be repeated at regular intervals. Intermittent catheterisation is recommended as a highly effective way of controlling some forms of incontinence but although it is generally seen as a simple procedure by nursing staff, it may be quite frightening to the client or carer. Carers may sometimes be expected to perform this procedure on a partner or relative when one or both find this unacceptable.

Diagnostic tools used for urinary and faecal investigations are not always understood by or acceptable to clients. Urodynamics (see Ch. 2) is frequently cited as an example. This investigation is used for the accurate diagnosis of dysfunction and has an important role to play in research; however, it is a highly invasive procedure, which many people find embarrassing and undignified.

Although the broad concerns highlighted by these issues are not exclusive to continence care, this does not make them any the less important.

The evidence base for effective continence care

Although there are still many questions unanswered, the evidence base for effective care is growing, with increases in the number of well-designed, multicentred studies to validate assessment and treatment standards and procedures. The 3rd International Consultation on Incontinence, held in 2004, brought together experts from around the world to analyse and disseminate the best available evidence on incontinence (Abrams et al 2005). Other groups or agencies, including the National Institute for Health and Clinical Excellence (NICE), the Cochrane Library and the Scottish Intercollegiate Guidelines Network (SIGN), provide critical reviews of published literature and clinical guidance. Box 1.13 provides descriptors of levels of evidence and grades of recommendation.

Box 1.13 Levels of evidence and grades of recommendation (ICI assessments 2004: Oxford guidelines, modified; Abrams et al 2005)

LEVELS OF EVIDENCE
Level 1: systematic reviews, meta-analyses, good quality randomised controlled trials (RCTs)
Level 2: RCTs, good prospective cohort studies
Level 3: case control studies, case series
Level 4: expert opinion

GRADES OF RECOMMENDATION
Grade A: based on level 1 studies. Highly recommended
Grade B: consistent level 2 or 3 evidence. Recommended
Grade C: level 4 studies or majority evidence. Optional
Grade D: evidence inconsistent/inconclusive. No recommendation possible

CONTINENCE EDUCATION

Lack of education and knowledge relating to continence within the health and social care professions is a limiting factor in service development and delivery. This deficit often results in avoidance of the subject of continence promotion, the use of inappropriate management methods (e.g. indiscriminate use of pads) or inappropriate referrals to more expensive services that are already overloaded (RCP 1995). Most nurses receive some formal educational input on managing incontinence in their preregistration programmes but often little on continence promotion. A report by the Audit Commission (1999) found that assessment skills were inadequate and that 20% of district nurses had not received training in continence assessment. In a study of continence care in the community (Bignell & Getliffe 2001), continence training in general nursing training was only reported by 25% of 171 respondents. Similarly, continence training as part of training for district nursing or health visiting qualifications was only reported by 25% of respondents. Only 7% had taken a formal postregistration course on Promotion of Continence (ENB 978). The RCP (1995) reported that a high percentage of staff nurses working in elderly care settings had received no formal education or training in continence since qualifying yet only 12% of nurses surveyed identified lack of knowledge as a problem. It is questionable how much change in attitudes and approaches to continence care can be expected when education input continues to remain low. The RCP report (1995) recommended the inclusion of continence training as a core subject in medical schools and a later RCP report (1998) emphasised the necessity for continence promotion and management to be included in training programmes for medical, nursing, social work and paramedical professions.

Healthcare support workers (HCSWs) are now encouraged to complete National Vocational Qualifications (NVQ) in Care and some employers insist on HCSWs holding at least the NVQ in Care Level II before employment. The Level II and III programmes contain comprehensive units on continence promotion for both urinary and bowel problems, but the potential benefit of these programmes is reduced by the fact that they are not compulsory for attainment of the award. However, as management of incontinence is often delegated to HCSWs, it is important to encourage completion of this unit.

CONTINENCE ORGANISATIONS WORLDWIDE

Internationally, continence care provision in urinary incontinence has developed at different rates, within differing care models, resulting in scattered and inconsistent services (Milne & Moore 2003). Peer group support and self-help are generally strong in the continence arena and in many countries user groups provide the driving force for improved services. The UK is well represented by interdisciplinary and consumer non-profit-making organisations, most having charitable status. In the UK, professionals took the lead in setting up such organisations, whereas in North America similar groups were consumer led. The first gathering of continence organisations from around the world was held in Rome in 1993, during the International Continence Society (ICS) meeting. Fourteen organisations from 10 countries focused their discussion on public awareness, fund raising and avenues for international collaboration. This grouping evolved to become the Continence Promotion Committee (CPC) of the ICS. The CPC produces an annual newsletter, *Continence Worldwide*, and hosts a website at http://www.continenceworldwide.org.

There are now continence organisations in many more countries worldwide (Box 1.14) and details are available on the website above. In 1998 the Asia Pacific Continence Advisory Board (APCAB) was established to support the development of continence promotion programmes within countries of the Asia Pacific Rim. The sharing of information, ideas and materials was very effective in helping more countries begin to establish new organisations.

An English-language questionnaire survey of continence organisations conducted by the CPC in 2003 (Newman et al 2005) provided one of the most comprehensive sources of information about the activities of various continence organisations. Twenty-four responses were received from 19

Box 1.14   Continence organisations worldwide (adapted from Newman et al 2005)

Australia	India	Philippines
Austria	Indonesia	Poland
Belgium	Israel	Singapore
Brazil	Italy	Spain
Canada	Japan	Sweden
China (Hong Kong)	Korea	Taiwan
Czech Republic	Malaysia	Thailand
Denmark	Netherlands	UK
Germany	New Zealand	USA
Hungary	Norway	

countries (67% response rate). The survey identified that, in most organisations (16/24 respondents), membership included both professionals and consumers. Eleven countries have a 'continence advisor' in their healthcare services; however, more than 80% of the respondents (from 19 different countries) felt their government had relatively little interest in continence services and that the understanding of incontinence by the general public was very limited.

It seems clear that the primary mission for all continence services remains focused on raising awareness of continence issues with the general public, the government and healthcare services.

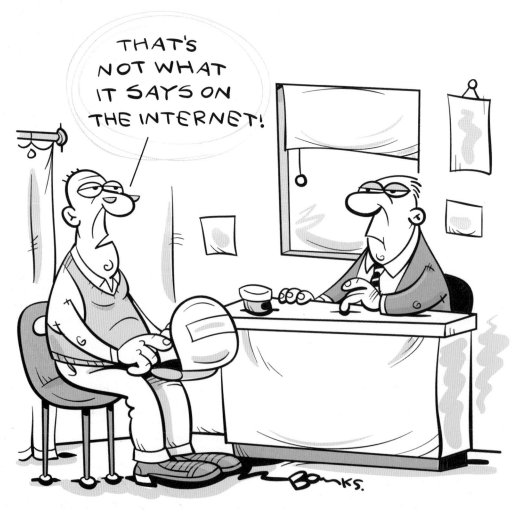

Figure 1.5   Who knows best?

Information technology

Information technology and the Internet have opened unlimited opportunities to share continence information worldwide and electronic information has become an essential tool for the public, professionals and industry. There are more than 15 000 websites across the world dealing with continence issues and in many ways this readily available source of information is changing the relationship between the public and professionals (Fig. 1.5). It is vital that patients and the general public are guided towards information that is accurate, reliable and up to date. The Center for Applied Special Technology (CAST) – an educational, non-profit-making organisation – uses information technology to expand opportunities for ALL people to access information through information technology. Websites such as http://easyinfo.org.uk and www.inspiredservices.co.uk. advise on the most beneficial way to present information to people with special needs and offer guidance on accessing information for people with visual impairment.

CONCLUSIONS

Although incontinence is a common condition, it is one that can be cured in around 70% of cases (RCP 1995) and significantly improved in the majority of others. Nationally and internationally, continence services are gaining a higher profile and there is active collaboration and commitment by policy-makers and professionals to reducing the prevalence of treatable incontinence. The media are now more receptive to issues surrounding incontinence, helping to break down the myths and taboos which surround the subject, and the expansion in information technology provides new sources of information for the general public and health professionals. However, continence problems continue to be underreported and undertreated in many cases and the challenges remain to increase awareness and promotion of continence and to advance understanding of continence problems and effective interventions.

ACKNOWLEDGEMENTS

With acknowledgements to Helen White for her contribution to earlier editions

References

Abrams P, Cardozo L, Khoury S, Wein A 2005 Incontinence, vol 1. Health Publication, Paris, p 11, 266, 1632

Anthony B 1998 Provision of continence supplies by NHS trusts. Middlesex University, London

Ashworth P, Hagan M 1993 The meaning of incontinence: a qualitative study of non-geriatric urinary incontinence sufferers. Journal of Advanced Nursing 18:1415–1423

Astbury N, White H 2001 Don't make me laugh. Northumbria Healthcare NHS Trust, North Shields

Audit Commission 1999 First assessment: a review of district nursing services in England and Wales. Audit Commission, London

Bayliss V, Cherry M, Locke R, Salter L 2000 Pathways for continence care. British Journal of Nursing 10(2):87–90

Bignell V, Getliffe K A 2001 Clinical guidelines for promotion of continence in primary care: community nurses' knowledge, practice and perceptions of role. Primary Health Care Research and Development 2:163–176

Bowron A 2006 Professional care guide. Northumbria Healthcare Parkinson's Disease Service, Tyne and Wear

Brown J, Vittinghoff E, Wyman J et al 2000 Urinary incontinence: does it increase risk for fall and fractures? Journal of the American Geriatric Society 48:721–725

Button D, Roe B, Webb C et al 1998 Continence: promotion and management by the primary care health team. Consensus guidelines. Whurr, London

Chiozza M, Bernardinelli P, Caione R et al 1998 An Italian epidemiological multicentre study of nocturnal enuresis. British Journal of Urology 81(supplement 3):86–89

Continence Foundation 2000a Incontinence: a challenge and an opportunity for primary care. Continence Foundation, London

Continence Foundation 2000b Making the case for investment in an integrated continence service. Continence Foundation, London

Department of Health 1998 They look after their own, don't they? DH, London

Department of Health 1999 Making a difference. DH, London

Department of Health 2000a Good practice in continence services. DH, London

Department of Health 2000b The NHS Plan. DH, London

Department of Health 2001a National Service Framework for older people. DH, London

Department of Health 2001b The essence of care. DH, London

Department of Health 2001c Expert patient programme. DH, London

Department of Health 2004a National Service Framework for children, young people and maternity services. DH, London

Department of Health 2004b The NHS improvement plan. DH, London

Department of Health 2005 National Service Framework for long term conditions. DH, London

Department of Health 2006 Our health, our care, our say: a new direction for community services. DH, London

Donovan J, Bosch R, Gotoh M et al 2005 Symptom and quality of life assessment. In: Abrams P, Cardozo L, Khoury S, Wein A (eds) Incontinence. Health Publication, Paris

Dougherty M C, Dwyer J W, Pendergast J E et al 2002 A randomised trial of behavioural management in continence with older rural women. Research in Nursing and Health 25:3–13

ERIC 1995 Incontinence promotional leaflet. Enuresis Resource and Information Centre, Bristol

Fitzgerald S T, Palmer M H, Kirkland V et al 2002 The impact of urinary incontinence in working women. A study in a production facility. Women and Health 35:1–15

Getliffe K A, Fader M, Cottenden A et al 2007 Absorbent products for incontinence: 'treatment effects' and impact on quality of life. Journal of Clinical Nursing (in press)

Goldsmith R 1992 The queue starts here: a raw deal for women's access by design. Centre for Accessible Environments, London

Hannestad Y, Rortveit G, Sandvik H et al 2000 Community-based epidemiological survey of female urinary incontinence: the Norway EPINCOT study. Journal of Clinical Epidemiology 53:1150–1157

Hu T-W, Wagner T H, Hawthorne G et al 2005 Economics of incontinence. In: Abrams P, Cardozo L, Khoury S, Wein A (eds) Incontinence, vol 1. Health Publication, Paris, p 73–96

Hunskaar S, Lose G, Sykes D, Voss S 2004 The prevalence of urinary incontinence in women in four countries. BJU International 93:324–330

Hunskaar S, Burgio K, Clark A et al 2005 Epidemiology of urinary and faecal incontinence and pelvic organ prolapse. In: Abrams P, Cardozo L, Khoury S, Wein A (eds) Incontinence, vol 1. Health Publication, Paris

Irwin D, Milsom I, Kopp K et al 2006 Impact of overactive bladder symptoms on employment, social interactions and emotional well-being in six European countries. BJU International 97:96–100

Johanson J F, Lafferty J 1996 Epidemiology of faecal incontinence. The silent affliction. American Journal of Gastroenterology 91:33–36

Johnson M 1998 Nocturnal enuresis. Urological Nursing 18:259–273

Kamm M 1994 Obstetric damage and faecal incontinence. Lancet 344:730–733

Kelleher C 2000 Quality of life and urinary incontinence. Clinical Obstetrics and Gynaecology 14(2):363–379

Kinchen K S, Burgio K, Diokno A C et al 2003 Factors associated with women's decisions to seek treatment for incontinence. Journal of Women's Health 12:687–698

King's Fund 1983 Action on incontinence: Paper 43. King's Fund Centre, London

McGrowther C, Donaldson M, Shaw C et al 2004 Storage symptoms of the bladder: prevalence, incidence and need for services in the UK. BJU International 93(6):763–769

Mandelstam D 1990 The Continence Advisory Service in the UK. In: ICS Pre-Congressional Symposium on Ethics and Urodynamics. Aarhus, Denmark

Margalith I, Gillon G, Gordon D 2004 Urinary incontinence in women under 65: quality of life, stress related to incontinence and patterns of seeking health care. Quality of Life Research 13(8):1381–1390

Milne J L, Moore K N 2003 An exploratory study of continence care services worldwide. International Journal of Nursing Studies 40:235–247

National Institute for Health and Clinical Excellence 2006 Urinary incontinence: the management of urinary incontinence in women. Royal College of Obstetricians and Gynaecologists, London (RCOG Press). Online. Available: http://www.nice.org.uk/page.aspx?o=CG40

Naughton M J, Shumaker S A 1996 Assessment of health-related quality of life. In: Furberg C D (ed) Fundamentals of clinical trials. Mosby, St Louis, p 185

Newman D, Denis L, Gruenwald C H et al 2005 Continence promotion: prevention, education and organization. In: Abrams P, Cardozo L, Khoury S, Wein A (eds) Incontinence, vol 1. Health Publication, Paris, p 35–72

O'Donnell M, Lose G, Sykes D et al 2005 Help-seeking behaviour and associated factors amongst women with urinary incontinence in France, Germany, Spain and the United Kingdom. European Urology 47:385–392

O'Neale V 2000 Excellence not excuses: inspection of services for ethnic minority children and families. DH London

Papanicalaou S, Hunskaar S, Lose G et al 2005 Assessment of bothersomeness and impact on quality of life of urinary incontinence in women in France, Germany, Spain and the UK. BJU International 96:831–838

Perry S, Shaw C, Assassa P et al 2000 An epidemiological study to establish the prevalence of urinary symptoms and felt need in the community: the Leicestershire MRC Incontinence Study. Journal of Public Health Medicine 22(3):427–434

Perry S, Shaw C, McGrowther C et al 2002 The prevalence of faecal incontinence in adults aged 40 years or more living in the community. Gut 50:480–484

Rockwood T H, Church J M, Fleshman J W et al 2000 Fecal incontinence quality-of-life scale. Diseases of the Colon and Rectum 43:9–17

Roe B H 1990 Development of continence advisory services in the UK. Scandinavian Journal of Caring Sciences 4(2):51–54

Rortveit G, Daltveit A K, Hannestad Y S et al 2003 Urinary incontinence after vaginal delivery or caesarean section. New England Journal of Medicine 348:900–907

Royal College of Physicians 1986 Physical disability in 1986 and beyond. RCP, London

Royal College of Physicians 1995 Report of a Working Party: incontinence – causes, management and provision of services. RCP, London

Royal College of Physicians 1998 Promoting continence: clinical audit scheme for the management of urinary and faecal incontinence. RCP, London

Rudd A G, Irwin P, Rutledge Z et al 1999 The national sentinel audit for stroke: a tool for raising standards of care. Journal of the Royal College of Physicians 33:460–464

Sampselle C M, Harlow S D, Skurnick J et al 2002 Urinary incontinence predictors and life impact in ethnically diverse perimenopausal women. Obstetrics and Gynecology 100(6):1230–1238

Sandvik H, Hunskaar S, Seim A et al 1993 Validation of a severity index in female urinary incontinence and its implementation in an epidemiological survey. Journal of Epidemiology and Community Health 47:497–499

Shaw C 2001 A review of the psychosocial predictors of help-seeking behavior and impact on quality of life in people with urinary incontinence. Journal of Clinical Nursing 10(1):15–24

Swithinbank L, Brookes S, Shepherd A et al 1998 The natural history of urinary symptoms during adolescence. British Journal of Urology 81:90–93

Thom D 1997 Medically recognised urinary incontinence and risks of hospitalisation, nursing home admission and mortality. Age and Aging 26:367–374

Thom D 1998 Variations in estimates of urinary prevalence in the community: effects of differences in definition, population characteristics and epidemiological literature. Journal of the American Geriatrics Society 46:1411–1417

Thomas S, Billington A, Getliffe K 2004 Improving continence services – a case study in policy influence. Journal of Nursing Management 12(4):252–257

William K S, Assassa R P, Smith N et al 2002 Good practice in continence care: development of a nurse-led service. British Journal of Nursing 11:548–559

Chapter 2

Assessing bladder function

Kathryn Getliffe and Mary Dolman

Knowledge has its starting point in ideas.
Lisbeth Hockey (1918–2004)

INTRODUCTION

A good knowledge of the normal function of the bladder and lower urinary tract is important to help understand the effects of abnormal function and to underpin approaches to the promotion of continence and management of incontinence. Although the physiological processes involved in continence control are complex and some aspects remain poorly understood, new knowledge continues to advance, particularly in areas of neurology and cell biology. This chapter begins by addressing the anatomy and physiology of the normal urinary system, including some discussion of changes that may occur during the normal ageing process. Later sections consider abnormalities that can result in problems of incontinence, providing a basis for the subsequent discussion of assessment of urinary incontinence.

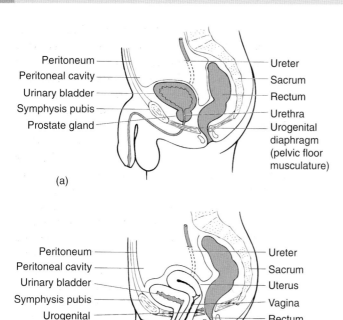

Figure 2.1 Anatomical location of the bladder and pelvic organs: (a) male, (b) female.

NORMAL BLADDER AND LOWER URINARY TRACT FUNCTION

The bladder and lower urinary tract have two main functions: storage of urine at low pressure, and periodic elimination of urine. The major anatomical structures involved in both functions are:

- the bladder and bladder neck
- the urethra and urethral sphincter mechanism
- the prostate gland
- the pelvic floor.

The bladder

The bladder is a hollow muscular organ which lies in the anterior part of the pelvic cavity, behind the symphysis pubis. It is located outside of the peritoneal cavity and extends upwards as it fills, between the peritoneum and the external body wall. In adults the bladder cannot be palpated during normal filling (although in children it is located higher in the abdomen, gradually descending with increasing age). However, if the adult bladder becomes overfilled it can be palpated above the symphysis pubis and may cause observable distension of the lower abdomen. In the male the bladder lies directly in front of the rectum, whereas in the female the vagina is situated between the bladder and the rectum (Fig. 2.1). In both sexes the rectum is separated from the bladder by a tough fascia of fused layers of peritoneum which provides an effective barrier against rectal invasion from tumours of the bladder or prostate. The upper surface of the bladder is covered by the peritoneum, which joins the anterior abdominal wall above the bladder. This anatomical location allows surgical access to the bladder retropubically (e.g. for suprapubic catheterisation) without incising the peritoneal cavity.

The bladder receives urine from the kidneys via the ureters. These are hollow, muscular tubes, approximately 25 cm long and 0.5 cm in diameter, extending from the renal pelvis to the posterior surface of the bladder, near its base (Fig. 2.2). Urine is transported away from the hilum of the kidney towards the bladder by peristaltic-like contractions of the ureters, assisted by gravitational influences. The ureters run obliquely through the

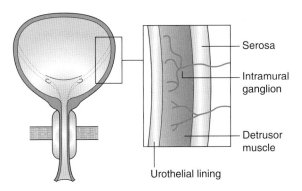

Serosa

Intramural
ganglion

Detrusor
muscle

Urothelial lining

Figure 2.2 Structure of the bladder wall. The bladder
wall is comprised of four layers and has a rich
innervation of cholinergic, adrenergic and non-
adrenergic, non-cholinergic sensorimotor nerves.
Intramural ganglia allow extensive neural interaction.
Reproduced from Chapple & MacDiarmid (2000).

bladder wall for approximately 1–2 cm to open
into the bladder at the left and right ureteric orifices. The oblique angle formed effectively creates
a *valve* mechanism. This mechanism prevents retrograde reflux of urine by compressing the ureter
when pressure inside the bladder increases during
filling, or when muscular contraction of the
bladder occurs, leading to expulsion of urine.

The triangular area formed between the left and
right ureteric orifices and the internal urethral
meatus defines the trigone. This area undergoes
little change in size during bladder filling and is
very sensitive to stretch owing to the large number
of sensory nerve endings it contains.

The bladder wall is generally considered to
have four distinct layers. The innermost *mucosal
layer*, or urothelium, is extensively folded into
rugae when the bladder is not full. It is richly
vascularised and very sensitive to stimuli such as
distension, pain, temperature, etc. (Corcos 2004).
The normal urothelium is composed of three to
seven layers of mucus-secreting, transitional cell
epithelium which facilitates stretching. The urothelial cells which line the luminal surface of the
bladder are described as 'umbrella cells' because
of their shape, being wider at the top. This is an
apt description since one of their functions is to be
impermeable to water and noxious components of
the urine which bathes their surface. In the past it
was thought that the urothelium functioned only

in a passive way as a barrier, but there is now
increasing evidence that it exhibits active sensory
and signalling properties that allow responses to
chemical and physical surroundings, including
bladder volume. This includes the secretion of
factors that can influence muscle contractility
(Drake & Turner 2004).

The second layer, or *submucosa*, is formed of
connective tissue linking the mucosa with the
third layer. The muscle fibres of this third layer
are collectively known as the *detrusor muscle* and
include both circular and longitudinal smooth
muscle fibres, forming an interlacing meshwork.
Contraction of the detrusor therefore causes the
bladder to reduce in length and diameter so that
it is emptied effectively. Individual smooth muscle
cells of the detrusor are able to elongate many
times their resting length during bladder filling,
without increased tension. With this property,
together with the ability of the transitional cells of
the urothelium to change shape and the folds of
urothelium to be smoothed out, the bladder can
accommodate considerable distension as it fills,
without increased pressure on its contents (intravesical pressure). The fourth and outermost layer
of the bladder is the *serosa*, which in some respects
is not strictly a continuation of bladder tissue since
it is composed of peritoneum and covers only the
upper surface of the bladder.

The bladder neck

At the base of the bladder, the bladder neck leads
into the urethra, through which urine is expelled
to the external environment. The male bladder
neck provides a powerful sphincter mechanism
with both urinary and genital roles, since it is of
primary importance in preventing retrograde
ejaculation into the bladder. It consists of an inner
layer of muscle bundles arranged in a circular ori-
entation containing a rich adrenergic, sympathetic
nerve supply. An outer muscle layer is contiguous
with the detrusor muscle and receives both a
cholinergic and adrenergic innervation. In the
female the bladder neck is a far weaker structure
than in males. There is no circular layer of muscle.
The smooth muscle fibres extend longitudinally
into the wall of the urethra and are innervated by
cholinergic parasympathetic nerves.

The bladder neck and proximal part of the urethra are supported by the pubourethral ligaments (attached to the pubic bone) and the *levator ani* muscles of the pelvic floor (see Fig. 2.4). The position of the bladder neck is influenced by the tonic contraction of the pelvic floor. In the female the bladder neck is also partially supported by the anterior vaginal wall since the urethra and anterior vaginal wall are not two separate adjacent structures, but are bound by connective tissue which unites them. Contraction of the levator ani supports the proximal urethra and also pulls the bladder neck anteriorly, compressing it closed against a band of fascia. Relaxation of the muscles allows the bladder neck to descend and facilitates its opening (DeLancey 1990). Therefore the position of the bladder neck is not static but mobile and under voluntary control.

Under normal conditions the location of the bladder neck at rest, during bladder filling, allows transient increases in abdominal pressure to be transmitted equally to the bladder and bladder neck such that continence is maintained. If damage or weaknesses of supporting structures occurs, this can result in 'bladder neck hypermobility', whereby the bladder neck and proximal urethra are allowed to descend to a lower position. Consequently, increases in abdominal pressure will exert pressure on the bladder to empty without a corresponding pressure on the bladder neck keeping it closed. Petros and Ulmsten (1990) suggest a slightly different mechanism in females, termed the 'integral theory'. This proposes that the vagina acts like a hammock with two distinct anatomical segments. The bladder neck is closed off because it is pulled backwards and downwards against an immobilised proximal urethra, by stretching the underlying vagina. Proper function of the pubourethral ligaments, vagina and pubococcygeus muscles is essential to achieve this.

The urethra and the external sphincter

The anatomy of the urethra differs considerably between the sexes. The female urethra is straight and only 3–5 cm long, passing through the muscles of the pelvic floor, with its external meatus opening anteriorly to the vagina, between the clitoris and the vagina. The mucosa is surrounded by a rich, spongy, oestrogen-dependent submucosal plexus encased in fibroelastic and muscular tissue. Its muscle structure comprises an inner longitudinal smooth muscle layer and an outer, circular, striated (voluntary) muscle layer, which forms the *external sphincter* or rhabdosphincter. The urethral sphincter mechanism extends throughout the proximal two-thirds of the urethra, being most developed in the middle one-third of the urethra. Many small mucous glands open into the urethra. By contrast, the male urethra is S-shaped, is approximately 18–22 cm long and can be considered to be composed of four regions (Fig. 2.3):

- The *prostatic urethra* (3–4 cm) is a thin tube of smooth muscle lined by mucosa, passing through the prostate gland which lies below the bladder and is attached to its base. On the posterior wall of the lower part of the prostatic urethra is a pyramid-shaped structure called the *verumontanum* (true mountain). This is an important landmark during surgical resection of the prostate since it is close to the prostate and above the level of the external sphincter. Its identification, therefore, reduces the risk of damage to the external sphincter and subsequent incontinence.

Figure 2.3   Anatomy of the male urethra.

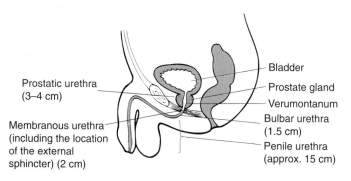

Prostatic urethra
(3–4 cm)

Membranous urethra
(including the location
of the external
sphincter) (2 cm)

Bladder

Prostate gland

Verumontanum

Bulbar urethra
(1.5 cm)

Penile urethra
(approx. 15 cm)

- The *membranous urethra* (2 cm) passes through the pelvic floor musculature and includes the location of the male external sphincter (rhabdosphincter) at the apex of the prostate.
- The *bulbar urethra* (1.5 cm) is surrounded by the 'bulb' of *corpus spongiosum* (part of the erectile tissue extending along the length of the penis) and the contraction of this *bulbospongiosus* muscle assists in emptying of the urethra at the end of voiding.
- The *penile urethra* (15 cm) opens at the urethral meatus. Both the bulbar and penile urethra receive secretions from many periurethral glands via ducts located in the corpus spongiosum.

The external sphincters in both sexes comprise circular striated muscle fibres, which are designed for prolonged contraction – the so-called *slow-twitch fibres*. These fibres are not easily fatigued and are capable of sustained contraction for long periods, with concurrent occlusion of the urethral lumen. Innervation of these fibres is via motor branches of spinal nerves (pudendal nerves) from the level of the sacral vertebrae S2–S4. The cell bodies of these neurones are found predominantly in a specific area of the sacral anterior (ventral) horn of the spinal cord, known as Onuf's nucleus. Urethral pressure exerted by tonic contraction of the urethral smooth muscle plays an important role in the maintenance of continence. However, the vascularity of the closely closed folds of urethral mucosa may also be a contributing factor. Rud et al (1980) have suggested that vascular tissue contributes one-third of urethral closure pressure.

The prostate gland

The prostate is made up of glandular tissue and smooth muscle, which is controlled by the sympathetic nervous system with release of noradrenaline onto the alpha adrenoreceptors on the muscle cells. The proportion of smooth muscle increases in benign prostatic hyperplasia. The prostate secretes lubricant into the seminal fluid.

The pelvic floor

The muscles, ligaments and fascia which form the pelvic floor provide a sling-like support for the organs of the lower pelvis (Fig. 2.4). The pelvic floor is pierced by the rectum posteriorly and by the urethra and vagina anteriorly. In addition to the provision of support, the pelvic floor contributes to the action of the external sphincter in maintaining urethral closure.

Fibres of the *levator ani* and the *pubococcygeus* are particularly important in effective closure during events associated with a sudden increase in abdominal pressure such as coughing or sneezing. The pubococcygeus contains a mixture of both fast- and slow-twitch (70%) muscle fibres, with *fast-twitch fibres* comprising around 30% (Gilpin et al 1989). The fast-twitch fibres, which tire easily, are responsible for the fast reflex response associated with coughing and for providing a strong maximum contraction to suppress an urgent desire to void. The fibres of the pubococcygeus are not attached directly to the walls of the urethra but in females insert into the lateral walls of the vagina. Consequently, digital vaginal examination can be used to evaluate muscle tone and strength of voluntary contraction.

Several reflexes play important roles in the control of micturition. These include the perineodetrusor inhibitory reflex (Mahony et al 1977, 1980) whereby the tone of the pelvic floor musculature promotes reflex inhibition (relaxation) of the detrusor. Reduction in pelvic floor tone can result in an overactive detrusor and contribute to problems in maintaining continence (Mahony et al, 1977). When the detrusor contracts, the detrusosphincteric inhibitory reflex produces reflex inhibition (relaxation) of the pelvic floor and external urethral sphincter.

NEURAL CONTROL OF CONTINENCE

Nervous control of the detrusor and sphincteric mechanisms is coordinated by an intricate series of nervous pathways that are dependent on central, as well as peripheral, autonomic and somatic neural pathways (Fig. 2.5). Although the mechanisms of continence are not fully understood, a complex process of neuromuscular coordination is required to regulate switching between urinary storage and urinary elimination modes (see Box 2.1 for an overview of physiological processes involved in transmission of nerve

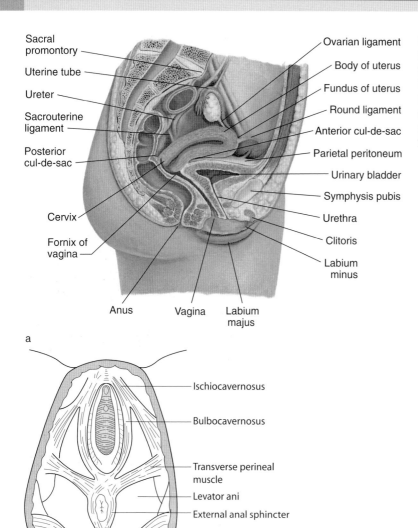

Sacral promontory

Uterine tube

Ureter

Sacrouterine ligament

Posterior cul-de-sac

Cervix

Fornix of vagina

Anus   Vagina   Labium majus

Ovarian ligament

Body of uterus

Fundus of uterus

Round ligament

Anterior cul-de-sac

Parietal peritoneum

Urinary bladder

Symphysis pubis

Urethra

Clitoris

Labium minus

a

Ischiocavernosus

Bulbocavernosus

Transverse perineal muscle

Levator ani

External anal sphincter

Gluteus maximus

b

Figure 2.4 Pelvic floor musculature. (a) Lateral section of the female pelvis. Reproduced from Mosby's Dictionary of Medicine, Nursing and Health Professions, 7th edn, Mosby, St Louis: 2006. (b) The perineal muscles. Reproduced from Sweet (1988).

impulses and muscle contraction). During storage of urine the bladder outlet is closed and the detrusor muscle is relaxed, allowing intravesical pressure to remain low over a wide range of bladder volumes. When voluntary voiding is required, the initial event is relaxation of striated urethral muscles, followed by detrusor muscle contraction. These two different sets of activities are mediated by three sets of peripheral nerves: pelvic nerves (parasympathetic), hypogastric nerves (sympathetic) and pudendal nerves (somatic).

1. *Pelvic nerves* are the important parasympathetic nerves supplying the detrusor smooth muscle and bladder neck sphincter. These nerves originate at the S2–S4 level of the spinal cord and run ventrally to innervate the bladder, urethra and rectum. They provide an excitatory (motor or efferent) input to the bladder (causing muscle contraction) and an inhibitory input to the urethral smooth muscle (promoting relaxation), thereby allowing urine to be eliminated. These nerves are cholinergic, i.e. the neurotransmitter is acetylcholine.

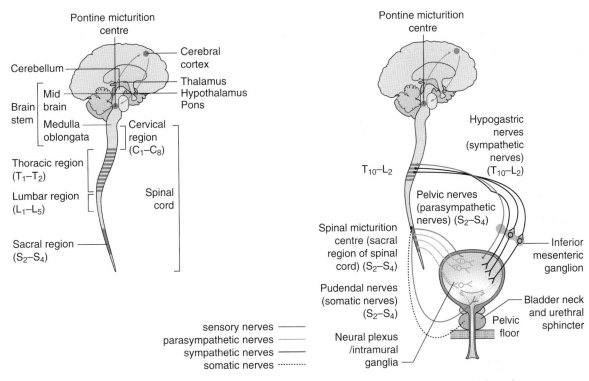

Figure 2.5   Neural control of the lower urinary tract. Reproduced from Chapple & MacDiarmid (2000).

2. *Hypogastric nerves* are sympathetic nerves that arise at a higher level in the spinal cord, the thoracolumbar region, T2–L3. These nerves supply the smooth muscle of the base of the bladder (trigone) and the bladder neck sphincter. Their main function is to inhibit detrusor activity (promote detrusor relaxation) and stimulate the internal sphincter smooth muscle, particularly in men where they prevent retrograde ejaculation. These nerves are adrenergic, i.e. the neurotransmitter is noradrenaline.

3. *Pudendal nerves*, which arise at the S2–S4 sacral level of the spinal cord, innervate the striated muscle of the pelvic floor and external urethral sphincter (rhabdosphincter). These nerves aid voluntary control over elimination of urine and the ability to perform pelvic floor muscle contractions.

The pelvic, hypogastric and pudendal nerves also contain afferent (sensory) axons that transmit information, such as a feeling of bladder fullness, from the lower urinary tract to the spinal cord where it is relayed to higher centres in the brain by spinal tract neurones.

Neurotransmitters

Tissue response to the neurotransmitter acetylcholine is mediated by muscarinic and nicotinic receptors on cell surfaces. Further subclassifications are made on the basis of structure and responses to pharmacological agents. The main contraction of the bladder results from the release of acetylcholine and its action on M_3 muscarinic receptors (see Ch. 9). Adrenergic receptors are sensitive to the neurotransmitter noradrenaline and are classified as alpha or beta receptors, with beta receptors present in the bladder. A number of other receptors have also been identified in bladder tissue although precise roles are less clear.

Micturition centres

Within the spinal cord, between S2 and S4, is an area known as the *spinal micturition centre*. This

Box 2.1   Nerve impulses and muscle contraction

In order for a muscle to contract it must be activated by an impulse which travels down a motor neurone to stimulate muscle fibres. Neurones consist of a cell body and several extensions, which convey the nerve impulses to and from the cell body. The nerve impulse is a wave of electrochemical activity that passes along the nerve fibre using energy already stored as part of the membrane potential. A resting membrane potential is present across the membrane of the cell body and the whole length of the nerve fibres, the longest of which is the axon. The resting membrane potential occurs because there is a small build-up of negative charge just inside the membrane and an equal build-up of positive charge on the outside. Such a separation of positive and negative electrical charges is a form of potential energy, which is measured in volts or millivolts (mV). A cell that exhibits a membrane potential is said to be polarised. When the membrane potential changes from −70 mV (resting potential) to +30 mV it generates an action potential (impulse) and excitation occurs. This involves a process of depolarisation (with reversal of the membrane polarisation from negative to positive) followed by repolarisation and is controlled by sodium (Na^+) and potassium (K^+) pumps which control the permeability to these ions (Tortora & Grabowski 2002).

A nerve impulse is triggered only when depolarisation reaches about −55 mV. Once this threshold is reached, the impulse, or action potential, is generated automatically and spreads along the nerve fibre at a rate characteristic for that particular type of nerve fibre. The speed of travel of the nerve impulse is not related to the stimulus strength. The diameter of the fibre and the presence or absence of an insulating cover (myelin sheath) are important: generally the larger the nerve fibre diameter in myelinated nerves, the lower the electrical resistance and faster conduction. The nerve impulse passes from one node to the next at the nodes of Ranvier where there is interruption to the myelin sheath.

Each muscle is composed of many individual muscle fibres and these are innervated by the motor neurones.

There is only a single axon innervating a given muscle fibre; however, a single motor neurone axon may innervate an average of 150 muscles fibres (Fig. 2.6). At the neuromuscular junction a chemical neurotransmitter (acetylcholine) is released and crosses the synaptic gap to bind with receptors on the muscle fibre membrane and stimulate the muscle fibre to contract. Muscle relaxation occurs passively by the cessation of the transmission – there is no special message from the nerve to induce relaxation. The strength of muscle contraction is controlled by the number of muscle fibres contracting and the diameter of the fibres – large diameter fibres contract more forcefully than smaller ones. Muscle tone is generated by sustained small contractions, which give firmness to a relaxed skeletal muscle. At any instant a few muscle fibres are contracted while most are relaxed. Exercise increases muscle strength by increasing the number of fibres 'recruited' to contract and, over a longer period of time, by an increase in size in the individual muscle fibres. This is the aim of pelvic floor exercises (see later in this chapter and Ch. 3).

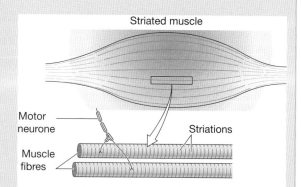

Figure 2.6   Skeletal muscle and a motor neurone innervating more than one muscle fibre with only one axon at a time.

---

acts as a relaying centre for incoming sensory nerve impulses providing information about bladder activity and for outgoing motor nerve impulses (see Fig. 2.5). From the spinal micturition centre, nerve fibres also link to the micturition centres in the brain stem (pons) and cerebral cortex, relaying information to higher centres and allowing voluntary inhibition of the micturition reflex. The *pontine micturition centre* can be considered as a type of 'neural switch' between the storage and voiding functions of the bladder (de Groat 1994). Voluntary control of voiding appears to be dependent on connections between the frontal cortex and regions within the hypothalamus as well as the brain stem. Lesions to the cortex have been associated with increased bladder activity by removing cortical inhibitory control. Brain imaging studies suggest that micturition is controlled predominantly by the right side of the brain (Yoshimura et al 2004).

Because of the very low location of the sacral spinal micturition centre, the control of micturition is very vulnerable to dysfunction resulting from damage to the spinal cord occurring anywhere above this level. Furthermore, since effective function is dependent on complex neural networks extending between the sacral spinal cord and the cerebral cortex, changes in lower urinary tract function are common early signs of a number of neurological diseases (see Ch. 6).

URINE STORAGE AND VOIDING

Bladder filling

Bladder function comprises cycles of filling and emptying (Fig. 2.7). Urine production by the kidneys is continuous and during the bladder filling phase the rugae flatten and bladder volume increases with very little change in internal (intravesical) pressure (Fig. 2.8). This is termed *compliance* and is possible because the lining layers of

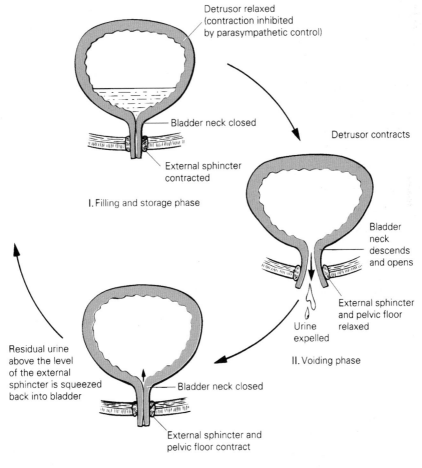

Figure 2.7   Bladder cycle of filling and emptying – muscular contraction and relaxation.

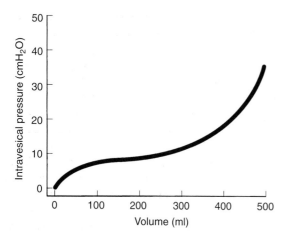

Figure 2.8 Intravesical pressure changes during filling, showing that minimal changes in pressure occur during the initial period of filling.

Box 2.2   Summary of control of micturition: effective storage

- Sustained contraction of the urethral external sphincter and urethral smooth muscle ensures urethral pressure is higher than intravesical pressure – *voluntary control of the sphincter by motor impulses from parasympathetic fibres in the pudendal nerves.*
- Relaxation of the detrusor muscle allows a low intravesical pressure to be maintained during filling (compliance).
- Unimpaired pathways between pontine and sacral centres are necessary to coordinate these activities.
- The bladder is supported by the muscles of the pelvic floor. Transitory increases in abdominal pressure are transmitted equally to the bladder and the urethra so that intravesical and urethral pressure differences are maintained.
- The tone of the pelvic floor musculature promotes reflex relaxation of the detrusor through the perineodetrusor inhibitory reflex.
- The bladder neck is closed at rest, but an effective watertight seal depends on a number of factors including competence of the external sphincter and pelvic floor muscles, the tone of the bladder neck and urethral smooth muscle component, and the vascularity of the closely closed folds of urethral mucosa.

transitional epithelial cells can overlap and slip over each other as the volume increases and because of the intrinsic ability of the smooth muscle to maintain constant tension over a wide range of stretch (Chapple & MacDiarmid 2000). As the bladder fills it first becomes spherical and then 'pear-shaped' as it rises up out of the pelvic cavity. However, the normal pressure rise on filling from around 10 ml of urine to 400 ml is only about 5–10 cmH$_2$O (Berne & Levy 1990). During filling the detrusor muscle is relaxed but urinary leakage is prevented by contraction of the bladder neck and external sphincter. At approximately 150–250 ml capacity, an awareness of distension and a mild desire to void is usually experienced which can be suppressed by conscious inhibitory control from the cerebral cortex until a suitable time and place for voiding occurs.

Voiding

The voiding phase is initiated voluntarily and can normally be delayed until appropriate circumstances are recognised. The simultaneous relaxation of the external sphincter and the bladder neck, and the contraction of the detrusor muscle, is coordinated via the 'spinal–pontine–spinal' reflex which involves the micturition centre in the pons. Relaxation of the external sphincter initially leads to a reduction in pressure within the urethra, and relaxation of the pelvic floor muscles allows the bladder neck to descend and to open (often described as funnelling) (Chapple & MacDiarmid 2000). Simultaneous parasympathetic stimulation of the detrusor muscle results in its contraction, producing a rise in intravesical pressure (typically around 100 cmH$_2$O) and expulsion of urine under pressure. As emptying is completed and the urinary flow ceases, the external sphincter closes under voluntary control and the proximal urethra also contracts, forcing any urine above the level of the external sphincter back into the bladder. Finally, the higher centre inhibition is again enforced, allowing the filling cycle to recommence. The control of micturition is summarised in Boxes 2.2 and 2.3.

> **Box 2.3 Summary of control of micturition: effective emptying**
>
> - Emptying of the bladder is initiated voluntarily, but relies also on involuntary contraction of the detrusor muscle – *response to sensory impulses from nerve endings in the bladder wall and trigone area providing conscious awareness of bladder filling.*
> - Relaxation of the voluntary muscles of the pelvic floor allows the bladder neck to descend and open – *mediated by inhibition of motor impulses via pudendal nerves.*
> - Sustained detrusor contraction increases intravesical pressure and is maintained to ensure the bladder empties fully – *inhibition mediated via cortical, pontine and sacral centres is removed and muscle contraction is stimulated via parasympathetic motor fibres in pelvic nerves.*
> - Concurrent relaxation of the urethral sphincter results in a lower urethral pressure compared with intravesical pressure – *mediated by inhibition of motor impulses via pudendal nerves.*
> - The detrusosphincteric inhibitory reflex produces reflex relaxation of the pelvic floor and external urethral sphincter on detrusor contraction.
> - Unimpaired pathways between pontine and sacral centres are necessary to coordinate these activities.

ACHIEVING AND MAINTAINING CONTINENCE

Control of micturition depends on maturation of the nervous system to provide the complex coordination processes needed and to allow voluntary control mechanisms to 'mask' the more primitive reflex activity which predominates in infants. Control is also dependent on learned behaviour and this is commonly achieved by the age of 3–4 years (see Ch. 5).

In early infant life the development of the central nervous system is incomplete and bladder (and bowel) emptying occurs involuntarily via spinal reflexes. However, by about 2 years of age conscious inhibition becomes possible with development of the cerebral cortex. The child learns to interpret sensations of bladder fullness and to briefly inhibit the desire to void. As bladder capac-

ity increases, successful control develops with practice and continence becomes subconscious and automatic for most individuals.

Normal bladder function has been defined as 'the ability to store and void urine at will in suitable places and at convenient times' (Feneley 1986). However, from a clinical viewpoint, bladder function should always be considered in the context of what is 'normal' for that particular individual, including what is *perceived* as 'normal' by the client or patient, since this may not necessarily be the same as the perception of a healthcare professional.

There are a variety of causes or circumstances that may contribute to failure to achieve or maintain continence. Whilst physiological difficulties or abnormalities are apparent in the majority of cases, psychological, environmental and social factors may also play an important part in determining continence or lack of it. For example, some patients with congenital abnormalities, including neurological problems or learning disabilities, may never achieve continence. Others experience deterioration in their ability to control their bladders owing to indirectly related factors such as poor mobility or manual dexterity, or mental illness such as severe depression. For some individuals (often elderly) or victims of disease such as stroke, symptoms of incontinence are likely to be multifactorial (e.g. limited mobility, physiological impairment of bladder control, cognitive disability, communication difficulties). Any or all of these factors may be compounded by multiple medications prescribed.

Box 2.4 summarises the basic skills required to achieve urinary continence. If one or more of the foregoing basic skills is lacking, for whatever cause, urinary incontinence is a likely consequence.

'Normal patterns of micturition'

Normal patterns of micturition are difficult to define, particularly as the majority of studies that have considered frequency of micturition have been conducted on patients attending clinics for investigation of urinary dysfunction. Patterns of diurnal voiding vary from individual to individual and may change within the lifespan of each

Box 2.4   Basic skills required to achieve urinary continence

- The ability to initiate micturition voluntarily at an appropriate time
- The ability to delay voluntarily the onset of micturition temporarily
- The ability to recognise socially acceptable places and/or circumstances to micturate
- The ability to communicate needs and interpret oral/written signs necessary to get assistance or locate a toilet
- Possession of sufficient physical mobility and manual dexterity to reach a toilet, adjust clothing, maintain an appropriate body position during micturition, manage doors, flushing systems, seats and washing facilities

individual. However, two studies of healthy female populations (151 women and 33 women, respectively) both demonstrated very similar mean frequencies of voiding during 24 h (5.8 ± 1.4 and 5.6 ± 1.26, respectively) (Kassis & Schick 1993, Larson & Victor 1988), with no identifiable age-related changes in pattern in either study. It is generally accepted that most adults will usually void at 3–5-h intervals during the day and will have no need to void at night, but when undertaking an assessment it is important to recognise that individual habits may vary.

Under normal circumstances:

- bladder capacity is approximately 500 ml and the bladder empties, leaving no residual urine
- males void at a pressure of 40–50 cmH$_2$O and a maximum flow rate of 30–40 ml/s
- females void at a pressure of 30–40 cmH$_2$O and a maximum flow rate of 40–50 ml/s.

ALTERATIONS IN PATTERNS OF URINARY ELIMINATION

When alterations in patterns of urinary elimination occur, the characteristics of the symptoms expressed are often indicative of the type of underlying problem. The most commonly occurring symptoms are presented below.

- *Frequency* describes an abnormally frequent desire to void, often of only small quantities (e.g. less than 200 ml). Frequency is often defined as emptying the bladder more than eight times a day (Wein 2000).
- *Urgency* describes an intense desire to void immediately. It often accompanies frequency.
- *Dysuria* is abdominal discomfort or pain, and a burning or smarting sensation accompanying voiding.
- *Residual urine* is urine retained in the bladder after micturition due to incomplete emptying. This stagnant urine can provide a focus for infection and for the formation of bladder stones or calculi. The actual amount can be measured by passing a catheter to withdraw the urine or by ultrasound scan. If the amount retained is 100 ml or more some action should be taken (see bladder scanning below).
- *Nocturia* is disturbance of sleep by the need to void. Some degree of nocturia is accepted as 'normal' by many individuals. It is important to distinguish between being woken by the need to void and waking for some other reason and then deciding to void.
- *Nocturnal enuresis* is urinary incontinence while asleep. It occurs most often in children but may continue into adulthood.
- *Alterations in urinary stream* (e.g. hesitancy) are usually due to some obstruction in the bladder outlet region or in the urethra. Hesitancy occurs because more pressure within the bladder is required to force the urine past the obstruction, the muscles tiring before the bladder is empty. After a few moments the bladder contracts again and voiding is resumed.
- *Retention of urine* describes an inability to void. It is not uncommon after surgical procedures or childbirth but is usually temporary. It also occurs as a result of obstruction and in neurological disease such as multiple sclerosis. Acute distension of the bladder can be very painful, although chronic retention which develops more slowly over a period of time may not be. In any situation where retention is prolonged, including in those patients with lack of sensation due to neurological disease or injury, there is a risk of increased back pressure on the upper urinary tract and reflux of urine into ureters and kidneys, with

further risk of upper urinary tract infection and/ or stone formation.

- *Retention with overflow* is characterised by frequent voiding of small amounts (e.g. 25–50 ml). It may be possible to palpate a distended bladder.

These alterations in patterns of urinary elimination are considered in further detail during the discussion of assessment of patients with urinary incontinence, and in subsequent chapters.

PHYSIOLOGICAL BLADDER DYSFUNCTION

Bladder dysfunction can be classified into three main types:

- overactive bladder with or without incontinence
- genuine stress incontinence
- voiding difficulties caused by outflow obstruction, detrusor hypoactivity or failure to coordinate detrusor contraction and urethral relaxation (dyssynergia).

Overactive bladder

Overactive bladder (OAB) is the term given to a clinical condition characterised by the symptoms of frequency, urgency and/or urge incontinence where these occur in the absence of any identifiable local pathology (such as a urinary tract infection). Under normal circumstances the detrusor muscle is relaxed during bladder filling and contracts only when voluntary voiding is initiated. In OAB the irritative symptoms are caused by uncontrollable contractions of the detrusor while the bladder is filling (detrusor instability). The contractions may occur spontaneously or on provocation (e.g. with coughing or vigorous exercise), or while the patient is attempting to inhibit micturition. Whilst the contractions may be sufficiently strong to cause incontinence, the bladder may not be emptied effectively and large residual volumes of urine (greater than 100 ml) are common. The bladder's capacity also decreases since it no longer has the opportunity to fill completely.

Patients with OAB usually complain of urgency with little or no warning of the need to void, and may be incontinent of urine before reaching the toilet. In addition, they commonly experience persistent frequency and nocturnal enuresis. Overactivity can be objectively demonstrated by urodynamic studies, which measure pressure changes as they occur within the bladder and urethra during filling of the bladder. (This assessment technique is discussed in detail later in the chapter.)

Most prevalence studies have focused on urinary leakage (urge incontinence) but this is only one of the symptoms of OAB and occurs in only about one-third of cases (Chapple & MacDiarmid 2000). Even without urinary leakage, 'dry OAB' with its symptoms of frequency and urgency can severely disrupt people's lifestyles.

Causes of overactive bladder contractions

Causes of overactive bladder contractions are varied. Neurological lesions resulting from conditions such as strokes, Alzheimer's disease, Parkinson's disease, multiple sclerosis, tumours and spinal cord lesions, may cause loss of inhibitory impulses from the brain, allowing inappropriate activation of the sacral reflex arc so that the bladder begins to contract before micturition is voluntarily initiated. Alternatively, symptoms may arise from increased sensory input from the bladder arising from local causes such as acute urinary tract infection (UTI), stones, local tumours, faecal impaction or prostatic enlargement. Increased fluid intake, particularly of alcohol or drinks containing caffeine, can also cause local irritation. However, in a majority of cases OAB is *idiopathic*, where no detectable pathological cause can be identified.

Genuine stress incontinence

Genuine stress incontinence is characterised by a loss of a small amount of urine if there is any increase in abdominal pressure (exerted on the bladder) from physical exertion, such as coughing, sneezing, running or jumping. It is defined by the International Continence Society as the complaint of involuntary leakage on effort or exertion, or on sneezing or coughing (Abrams et al 2005).

It is important to distinguish between genuine stress incontinence and OAB since both can result in leakage with coughing, but a distinction can usually be made by urodynamic investigation. However, mixed incontinence can occur with symptoms of both stress and urge incontinence, and is most common in postmenopausal women. Stress incontinence is predominantly a female problem, although it can occur in males (e.g. after prostatectomy). It is usually associated with bladder outlet incompetence which can occur at the level of the bladder neck, the urethral sphincter, or both, and is exacerbated by weakness of the supporting pelvic floor muscles. It is particularly common in multiparous women who have had traumatic or prolonged vaginal deliveries.

Voiding difficulties

Outflow obstruction

Outflow obstruction is more common in males than in females (where it is often a missed diagnosis; see Ch. 3). It is most frequently associated with prostatic enlargement (which increases with age in men over 45 years), urethral stricture and chronic constipation. The bladder is emptied by frequent voiding of small amounts and micturition is associated with hesitancy, poor urine flow and postmicturition dribble. Frequency, urgency and nocturia or constant dribbling can occur if there is a large residual volume of urine.

Detrusor hypoactivity

In detrusor hypoactivity the muscle is underactive and fails to provide a sustained or adequate contraction. This condition is usually caused by damage to peripheral nerves to the bladder, or by damage to the lower spinal cord, in conditions such as diabetic neuropathy, pelvic injury and multiple sclerosis. The sensation of bladder filling may be absent or reduced and the bladder often increases in capacity by overstretching. Large residual volumes (500–2000 ml) may accumulate, with overflow incontinence. This condition is considered more fully in Chapter 6.

AGE-RELATED CHANGES AND RISKS FACTORS FOR INCONTINENCE

Although urinary incontinence is certainly not an inevitable part of the ageing process, older people have the highest known prevalence of urinary or faecal incontinence of any group, with the exception of those with neurological dysfunction or spinal cord injury. Incontinence may be associated with ageing because elderly people are perhaps more susceptible to physiological, pharmacological and psychological risk factors which may influence their ability to maintain continence (see Ch. 6). The main physiological age-related changes that may predispose to incontinence are summarised in Box 2.5.

Comorbid conditions and medications

Numerous medical conditions which may impact on continence status are more common in older people. These often result in multiple medications which may also influence continence. These issues are considered further in Chapters 6 and 9.

Transient incontinence

Older adults can also experience transient incontinence as a side effect of some other difficulty. For example, transient incontinence may occur as a result of a change of environment, which may include difficulty in finding the toilet. An illness such as a chest infection, accompanied by a severe cough, can raise intra-abdominal pressure, resulting in stress incontinence, or a urinary tract infection may result in urgency leading to incontinence (see Ch. 6).

ASSESSMENT OF INCONTINENCE

A thorough assessment is the most crucial component of effective continence care provision and the importance of developing good assessment skills, learned through experience, should never be underestimated. In recent years a wide range of continence assessment tools have been developed. These can be useful in assisting practitioners and promoting equity for patients, in relation to quality of assessment and subsequent decision making.

Developing assessment skills

Good interviewing skills develop with experience and include some important components, which

Box 2.5   Physiological age-related changes that may predispose to incontinence

Age-related changes	Potential effects on continence
Bladder function • Decreased capacity (smaller voided volume) • Increased involuntary detrusor contractions • Decreased contractility during voiding (associated with slower flow rate and small increases in postvoid residual volume) • Increased residual urine	• Increased likelihood of urinary symptoms and incontinence • Frail older people may have a combination of detrusor overactivity on filling and poor contractility during voiding, which may result in a large postvoid residual leading to leakage
Urethra • Decreased closure pressure in women	• Increased likelihood of stress and urge incontinence
Prostate • Increased incidence of benign prostatic obstruction	• Increased likelihood of urinary symptoms and incontinence
Decreased oestrogen (women)	• Increased incidence of atrophic vaginitis and related symptoms • Increased incidence of recurrent urinary tract infections • Decreased urethral closure pressure
Increased nighttime urine production	Increased likelihood of nocturia and nighttime incontinence
Altered neurotransmitter concentrations and actions	Increased likelihood of lower urinary tract dysfunction
Altered immune function	Increased likelihood of recurrent urinary tract infection

Adapted from Fonda et al (2005).

will be well known to experienced interviewers. They start with preparing an appropriate interview environment, with due regard for space, comfort and privacy. By observing the patient/client's behaviour from the moment they enter the interview room, the assessor can gain an idea of the individual's attitude, feelings and possible coping mechanisms. The way in which questions are asked can evoke different answers, so finding the 'right' language and asking questions clearly is essential. Recognising body language (posture, eye contact, tone of voice) is part of the interviewing process as often the signals are non-verbal, particularly when talking about sensitive subjects such as continence. Patients usually want empathy, not sympathy, and conveying understanding of the problems stems from a sound knowledge base.

The assessor also needs patience and good listening skills, commodities which are sometimes difficult to demonstrate in busy clinical settings. An assessment, done properly, takes time and at least an hour may be required at an initial assessment. Most patients/clients need time to feel relaxed, comfortable in the presence of the assessor and not embarrassed. It is unlikely that all the information needed will be obtained at the first meeting and ongoing data collection may include laboratory tests, radiography, etc., as well as further verbal information from the patient or carers.

Data collection

The key points to be included in an initial assessment are summarised in Box 2.6.

This section provides general guidance on components of the assessment process and readers are encouraged to review the quality of forms currently in use in their own clinical areas and, if

---

Box 2.6 Key points for initial assessment

HISTORY TAKING AND RECORDING
- Relevant medical, surgical and obstetric history
- Urinary/bowel symptoms and how they differ from normal patterns
- Onset of symptoms and whether related to specific activities
- List prescribed medications and over-the-counter (OTC) medicines
- Attitude to problem, how symptoms affect daily living and desire for treatment
- Support services available
- Environmental/living conditions/mental awareness
- Aids and appliances used/needed/mobility/dexterity

CLINICAL ASSESSMENT
- Urinary/bowel diary recorded over 3–7 days
- Assess impact on quality of life using an appropriate measure/scale
- Fluid intake
- Urinalysis
- Constipation

PHYSICAL EXAMINATIONS AND TESTS
- Abdominal palpations
- Vaginal (for details, see Ch. 3) or rectal examination (for details, see Ch. 8)
- Flow rate (for details, see Ch. 4)
- Assess postvoiding residual with bladder scanning/ultrasonography
- Pad test

---

necessary, to design a form relevant to their own workplace that conforms to their organisation's philosophy.

There are many assessment 'forms' available to collect patient data in relation to bladder and/or bowel dysfunction. Indeed, most organisations will have developed their own unique assessment forms and/or care guidelines or patient pathways. In today's context of clinical governance, assessment records provide a source of data for audit of services and are used to compare clinical baseline information with intervention and outcome measures (subjective and objective) at discharge (see Ch. 11). Auditable parameters which are likely to be important to a continence service include:

- waiting time to first appointment
- appropriate and inappropriate referrals
- waiting time in clinic
- total numbers seen for type of incontinence.

Frequency/volume chart

A frequency/volume chart is an extremely valuable way of determining a patient's usual pattern of voiding. Many patients find a relatively simple chart such as that illustrated in Figure 2.9a easy to use and it can also be used as a bladder retraining chart. However, it is a matter of personal preference as all charts achieve the same objective of recording the frequency and volume of voiding per day. Another example is given in Figure 2.9b. Five days of baseline charting is usually requested although there is evidence that even 3 days is sufficient to provide a reliable indication of the patient's voiding pattern.

The charting can be repeated at a later stage during treatment and used as feedback to demonstrate improvement in both frequency (reduced) and voiding volume (increased). Frequency/volume charts can also be used where prompted voiding strategies are employed in the care of patients with cognitive impairment. Charting facilitates the identification of the patient's normal pattern of voiding so that they can be prompted to go at the most appropriate times to aid success (see Chs 6 and 7). Whatever information is required, it is essential to include clear, simple instructions at the top of the chart, especially if it is to be used in a ward situation where multidisciplinary carers will be doing the recording.

The inclusion of some form of quality of life (QoL) measure as part of the assessment is an important way of determining how living with incontinence symptoms is affecting the patient's daily life (see Ch. 1). The patient's perception of how much bother is caused by their incontinence is likely to have a strong association with the incontinence-related goals they wish to achieve (Williams et al 2002) and their motivation to achieve them. In many ways this subjective measure is at least as important as more objective measures. A simple example of a QoL question is 'How bothersome is your bladder on a daily/weekly basis?' with answers expressed on a scale

DAY	DAYTIME Time/volume (millilitres)	NIGHTTIME	Number of pads used in 24-hour period
1	Example: *7 am/200* *1 pm/at work* *6 pm/400* *11 pm/300*	*3 am/200* *6 am wet*	
2			
3			
4			
5			
6			
7			

AVERAGE DAILY INTAKE (in cups) ....

a

Frequency/Volume chart

Week Commencing: /   /

	Monday		Tuesday		Wednesday		Thursday		Friday		Saturday		Sunday	
	In	Out	In	Out	In	Out	In	Out	In	Out	In	Out	In	Out
6am	300				350						200		190	
7am			200				250		350		100			170
8am		50			150					250		190		
9am	250	150	100				150							
10am					150			200					100	
11am	175	100			175				200		180			
12.00			250		100							150		130
1pm								200		200				
2pm	190	W		130	150			175					270	
3pm						W		W	100	W	270			
4pm								W						
5pm	300	200				150	250			150		W		W
6pm				190	200									
7pm		75		W				150			100		180	
8pm					100				200	175				
9pm	150	100											120	
10pm				150						175	190			175
11pm								100	100					
12.00				50		W	100				100			
1am													100	120
2am		W								W		W		
3am						120								
4am														
5am			150											
Waking	6am		7.45am		7.30am		7.00am		6.30am		7.45am		7.40am	
Retiring	12.30am		11.30pm		12.51am		Midnight		Midnight		12.30am		11.30am	
Pad usage	3		1		2		4		3		5		2	

b

Figure 2.9   (a) A typical frequency/volume chart to be filled in by a patient (day 1 completed: note that the patient could not measure urinary output at work). (b) An example of a completed frequency/volume chart. (b) Reproduced from Chapple & MacDiarmid (2000).

of 1–5, where 1 = not at all and 5 = intolerable. There are a large number of QoL instruments in the published literature, many of which have been designed for use in comparative research trials of different treatments for incontinence (see Ch. 1). Where a QoL measure is to be used regularly in clinical practice it is sensible to choose one which is relatively simple and quick for patients to complete.

The use of an evidence-based care pathway (Bayliss et al 2000) provides a process to enhance consistent quality of assessment, appropriate referrals, investigations and subsequent treatments. In the model developed by Bayliss et al, a colour-coded questionnaire can be used by patients to identify symptoms which are indicative of one of the three main bladder problems: stress incontinence, OAB (urgency with or without incontinence) and voiding dysfunction. Standard statements on the assessment form represent normal parameters for continence and any variance from the 'normal' has to be recorded with reasons and comments. The initial assessment findings may result in giving advice or basic treatments but will indicate if onward referral is necessary.

INTERPRETATION OF THE ASSESSMENT

Duration of symptoms

If the onset of incontinence is recent it may be due to a transitory state such as urinary tract infection, anxiety, stress, bereavement or depression. If the symptoms have existed for a number of years, the underlying cause must be investigated. Many patients delay seeking help for months or even years. Even if cure cannot be achieved, symptoms can be improved in 70% of cases and strategies for management of incontinence can be enhanced (DH 2000). It is never too late to improve the situation.

Medical history

Many medical conditions can affect the normal functioning of both the bladder and bowel, and these underlying causes need appropriate treatment, preferably by clinical teams which include

expertise in continence. Examples are neurological conditions, multiple sclerosis, diabetes (type 1 and type 2), spinal injuries, learning disabilities, stroke, dementia and back pain. Conditions which exacerbate incontinence include asthma and chronic chest conditions, because continual strain is exerted on the urethral sphincter mechanism by coughing, which increases abdominal pressure.

Surgical history

Previous surgical interventions need to be noted. Gynaecological and urological surgery are particularly important, but notice should be taken of any surgery where a Foley catheter was inserted because this may have initiated a long-term problem of outflow obstruction, caused by possible scarring or necrosis of the urethral lining. Retention of urine following surgery can be another cause of subsequent bladder dysfunction. Prostatectomy may leave a man with a postmicturition dribble, possibly due to a weak detrusor contraction or a weak sphincter; 'milking' the urethra (see Ch. 4) and pelvic floor exercises are conservative treatments for this problem.

Urological history

The key information to consider includes the following:

- *Incontinence*
  - Onset: When did it start?
  - Duration: How long has the problem existed?
  - Degree: Mild, moderate, severe?
  - Type: Stress, urge, overflow, enuresis?
- *Irritative symptoms*
  - Frequency: How often in 24 hours?
  - Urgency: Able to reach toilet in time?
  - Nocturia: Need to get up for toilet at night?
  - Dysuria: Does it hurt to pass urine?
- *Voiding difficulties*
  - Poor stream: Is the urine flow slow/intermittent?
  - Hesitancy: Trouble starting urine flow?
  - Straining: Straining to empty the bladder?
  - Residual: Is the bladder emptying completely?

- *Urinary tract infection*
  - Urinalysis/midstream specimen of urine: Confirmed or suspected?
- *Suprapubic pain*
  - Interstitial cystitis: Pain, discomfort remains after emptying bladder, frequency?

Urinary symptoms and possible causes

- *Frequency*: overactive bladder, sensory urgency, UTI, cystocele, urinary residual.
- *Urgency*: all the above, plus pregnancy, small bladder capacity, menopause, pelvic mass, radiation, lesions, obstructions, habit, excess fluid intake, anxiety.
- *Stress incontinence*: weak pelvic floor, bladder neck open, overactive bladder, retention.

Mobility and dexterity

An individual who has difficulty with mobility often fails to reach the toilet in time, and so regular, timed toileting may be useful to try to maintain continence. Similarly, reduced manual dexterity may prevent someone from managing their clothing or performing intermittent self-catheterisation (ISC) (see Ch. 10), so alternative techniques need to be considered.

Medications

Many drugs can disturb bladder and bowel function (see Ch. 9). A constant review of medications is necessary to see whether dosages can be reduced, stopped or taken at different times of the day. Polypharmacy often occurs in the elderly when medications are not reviewed regularly in this way.

Physical examination

Pelvic floor muscle assessment and vaginal assessment are discussed in detail in Chapter 3. Other physical examinations include observation of the abdomen for surgical scars, and palpating the abdomen for bladder distension and constipation. A rectal examination may be used for palpating a prostate or to feel for a faecally loaded rectum but this is considered an invasive procedure and

appropriate permission needs to be sought from the patient (RCN 2000). Observation of skin condition around the symphysis pubis and groin may reveal soreness from urinary incontinence or the wearing of pads. Vaginal dryness or atrophic vaginitis can be observed by parting the labia and observing for signs of redness, inflammation and tissue atrophy. It is essential that physical examinations which include digital palpation of the pelvic floor and digital rectal examinations are carried out by a fully trained assessor.

Social and environmental factors

This is a most important part of assessment. The impact of incontinence on working life, sexual relationships, family and friends may be dramatic. Embarrassment may lead to someone becoming virtually housebound and unable to continue working. Attitudes towards incontinence will often determine a person's motivation to comply with treatment or management. The workplace, home or institutional setting may contribute to difficulties in maintaining continence, particularly in older people (Box 2.7). Chapter 6 covers some of the psychological, environmental and social factors influencing continence in frail older people, but some factors may be equally applicable to younger people, particularly those with physical or learning disabilities.

Objective measures

An objective measure of continence improvement can be made by a pad weighing test. A dry pad is weighed and then weighed again after a set time of wearing. The increased weight is an indication of urine loss. From the initial assessment to the discharge date, it is hoped that the loss will be reduced. Urodynamic investigations before and after intervention can also provide an objective measure of outcome as well as an initial determination of diagnosis (see later in this chapter). If the assessor is familiar with the use of a biofeedback device or a perineometer for measuring pelvic floor muscle strength, then the reading at discharge would again be expected to be higher than that at initial assessment, demonstrating an increase in pelvic floor strength.

Box 2.7 Psychological, environmental and social factors that may influence continence in older people, at home or in care facilities

Unhelpful	Helpful
TOILETS	
Too far away	Close to bedrooms and living areas
Too few	Enough for 'peak demand' times
Too narrow for a wheelchair	Easy wheelchair access
Difficult to use	Raised toilet set and rails available
Difficult to identify	Good signposting
Unpleasant to use – cold, smelly, dirty, with lack of soft toilet paper	Easy to identify (e.g. doors colour coded)
	Warm and clean with spare toilet rolls in view
CLOTHING	
Difficult to adjust	Elasticated tracksuit bottoms
	Use of Velcro in place of zips and buttons
Unattractive and undignified clothing (e.g. no pants, or dress open up the back) can reduce motivation to be continent	Attractive but practical
	Special adaptations and gadgets may be available to help physically disabled people
CARERS AND OTHER PEOPLE	
Being rushed (e.g. by carers)	Sufficient time to make a leisurely and relaxed visit to the toilet
Lack of privacy (e.g. commode in a shared bedroom, door of toilet left open)	Neither overlooked, nor overheard
Lack of security (e.g. fear of being forgotten and left in the toilet)	Convenient means of summoning help
Carer's attitude is either: very critical of incontinence	Carer's attitude is one of support and encouragement to achieve continence
or	
continually gives permission for incontinence (e.g. 'It doesn't matter, we will clean it up')	

PATIENT PSYCHOLOGICAL PROBLEMS

Depression amongst elderly people is not always recognised, but can be a major factor in impaired self-care. Alternatively, continence problems can cause anxiety and feelings of shame, making the individual feel that the problem is untreatable and therefore exacerbating feelings of low self-esteem.

DIAGNOSTIC INVESTIGATIONS

Diagnostic investigations include urodynamics, ultrasound, X-ray of kidneys, ureter and bladder (KUB), cystoscopy or biopsy. These are usually ordered by the medical team but may also be ordered by other members of the integrated continence team (DH 2000).

Urinalysis

A simple reagent strip can detect abnormalities in the urine, and this test should be done for every patient at the initial assessment. Only if abnor-malities are detected should a specimen of urine be sent for culture and sensitivity. Urine analysis has three principal applications:

- screening – for disease, both systemic and renal
- diagnosis – to confirm or refute a suspected condition
- management – to monitor the progress of an established disease.

Reading a reagent strip

- *Specific gravity*. The normal range is 1.002–1.035. Very low values represent water diuresis and very high values indicate dehydration.

- *pH*. This represents the acidity/alkaline balance. The normal range varies between 4.5 and 8.0. At low values the urine is more acidic, which may predispose to formation of calculi in the kidney or bladder.
- *Appearance and odour*. The colour of urine is normally yellow, but the intensity of colour varies inversely with the rate of urine formation. 'Concentrated' urine has a relatively strong yellow colour while 'dilute' urine is pale. Colour can change due to food pigments, colouring agents and drugs. Urine is normally odourless, but in patients with a urinary tract infection it may smell foul or of ammonia.
- *Protein*. This indicates possible renal disease. Further investigations, including urine culture, should be carried out.
- *Nitrites and leucocytes*. A positive nitrite test on a reagent strip indicates bacterial infection. Raised leucocytes (pyuria) also indicate infection. (This test is not included on all reagent strips.) If the patient is asymptomatic, antibiotics are not normally required. If systemic symptoms are present, full microbiological analysis is needed to establish sensitivity and to aid prescription of antibiotics.
- *Glycosuria and ketones*. A positive reagent strip indicates possible type 1 diabetes. Blood tests should also be taken for diagnosis of other conditions, such as thyrotoxicosis.
- *Blood*. Further investigations are essential if blood is detected in the urine. It can indicate impaired renal function or bladder papillomas. However, it may also be detected in the urine of female patients during menstruation.

A simple urine test performed with reagent strips can reveal conditions that would remain undetected if not included as part of an assessment for urinary incontinence. It is an essential part of a nurse's assessment.

BLADDER SCANNING

When a voiding dysfunction is suspected, or when there is no clear diagnosis, a diagnosis which is often missed is a postvoiding residual volume (PVR). Wherever possible, all patients attending a continence clinic should have a routine pre- and postvoiding bladder scan as part of standard care

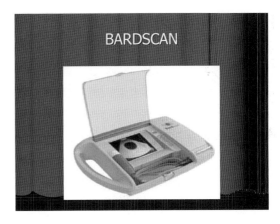

Figure 2.10 Picture of a portable ultrasound scanner (Bard Ltd).

practice. Clinical studies have shown that there is a ±20% accuracy when measuring a PVR using a portable ultrasound bladder scanner (Fig. 2.10) and the results provide strong evidence to support diagnostic decisions (Goode et al 2000, Dudley et al 2003). The advantages over using a urethral intermittent catheter to measure a residual volume are a non-invasive procedure with no risk of infection for patients.

A PVR is the amount of urine left in the bladder within 10–15 min after voiding and urinary retention is the inability or failure to empty the bladder completely with voiding. Elevated PVRs lead to an increased risk of urinary retention, urinary tract infections, hydronephrosis, pyelonephritis and renal insufficiency. Chronic urinary retention is characterised by an ongoing inability to completely empty the bladder during voiding. A PVR volume greater than 100 ml is generally accepted as the criterion to define a bladder voiding dysfunction. The causes of incomplete emptying are an obstruction (anything that obstructs the bladder outlet) or a hypotonic contraction of the detrusor muscle (age-related, neurological or resulting from an overdistended bladder). Box 2.8 indicates those patients most likely to be at risk of urinary retention who should have a bladder scan and the bladder scan procedure is presented in Box 2.9.

There are some practical tips/guidance to be considered when using a bladder scanner. Beware of artefacts which can give the wrong image or readings. Patients who are obese may make your

> **Box 2.8   Patients at risk: clinical indications for bladder scanning**
>
> - Diabetes
> - Spinal injuries
> - Neurological conditions such as multiple sclerosis, Parkinson's disease, dementia
> - Patients taking multiple medications, particularly antidepressants and anticholinergics
> - Postoperative procedures following general anaesthetic (incidence 16% according to Rosseland et al 2002)
> - After gynaecological surgery (prevalence 9.2% according to Bodker & Lose 2003)
> - After removal of Foley catheter
> - Pregnancy, pelvic organ prolapse in women
> - Suprapubic pain and distension
> - Reduced urinary output (dehydration or blocked catheter)
> - Elderly and children

> **Box 2.9   Bladder scanning procedure**
>
> 1. Patient in supine position with clothing adjusted down to suprapubic area.
> 2. Squeeze scanning gel onto skin above symphysis pubis and a small amount onto head of scan probe.
> 3. Position probe over pubic bone and work in gel, angle head at 45–90° and move gently until bladder image seen. Bladders come in different shapes and sizes so do not rely on first reading.
> 4. Keep probe head still for scanning and do at least three scans for accuracy or until you are satisfied with your scan.
> 5. Ask patient to go and empty the bladder and then repeat scan within 10–15 min.
> 6. Results are calculated by scanner in millilitres and an outline displayed. The largest volume is always recorded.
> 7. Print results for patient's notes or manually record results.
> 8. If persistently high postvoiding residual volume, consider intermittent catheterisation or indwelling catheter.

scanning difficult or impossible and constipation or bowel gas can blur the image. Even though the procedure is non-invasive, some patients can still have tension in the abdominal muscles and a clear explanation of the procedure can help with relaxation. The position of the patient or the scan probe may be incorrect but bladders are not always where you expect them to be so move the probe around and alter the angle. A hairy pubic area may prevent the gel from making good contact with the skin and so the gel needs to be 'worked' into the skin gently to avoid trapping air. Training is required before performing any bladder scan, followed by at least three scans supervised by a senior or consultant nurse specialist.

URODYNAMICS

Urodynamic investigations study the dynamics of the lower urinary tract – the bladder and urethra (Chapple & MacDiarmid 2000). They comprise uroflowmetry, cystometry and urethral pressure profile (UPP). Some patients will require a video-cystometrogram, whereby the filling and voiding phases can be observed on a screen and the information stored on videotape.

The purpose of urodynamic studies is to define the pathophysiology of the bladder and urethra, and the investigations provide information about the way the bladder accommodates to increasing volumes, central nervous system control over the detrusor reflex and sensory qualities. There are now many urodynamic centres throughout the UK and a few satellite community centres run by specially trained nurses. These investigations are not appropriate for all patients because of their invasive nature, but they are essential for both men and women prior to any surgical intervention. These studies form just one part of a range of investigations required for diagnosis.

Uroflowmetry

Uroflowmetry measures the rate at which the urine is voided, in millilitres passed per second (peak flow rate should be at least 15 ml/s for a volume of at least 150 ml). The patient sits on a commode or, if male, can void directly into a funnel of the machine.

The most common method for measuring the flow rate is by a rotating disc at the bottom of the funnel, which spins continuously as urine is voided onto it. As this happens, the motor demands more power in order to keep the disc rotating at a constant speed. The change in power required is then used to calculate the flow rate (Laker 1994). The patient is asked to attend the clinic with a full bladder, so this investigation can take place prior to cystometry. Ideally, a series of flow rates should be taken, but this is not always possible. It is essential, therefore, to ask the patient whether the flow and volume were 'normal'. If not normal for the patient, this should be noted on the recording. Privacy is important for this test as hesitancy and slow urine stream may be due to the embarrassment of someone else being in the room. Figure 2.11 shows some simplified flow rate profiles.

Cystometrogram (CMG)

The patient may be investigated in the supine, sitting or standing position, and various provocative manoeuvres may be applied. Here the bladder pressure is recorded both during filling and when voiding. Figure 2.12 shows an example of a cystometric recorder. A straightforward CMG does not outline the bladder neck; this is where videocystometry is required to see whether the bladder neck stays closed or opens inappropriately. As this is a highly invasive procedure, patients need information which is provided in a sensitive, non-threatening way prior to an appointment (there is quite a high non-attendance rate). A suggested patient handout explaining the procedure is provided in Box 2.10.

The procedure

After the patient has emptied the bladder for the flowmetry test, the next part of the investigation is cystometry. With the patient in a supine position and using a strictly aseptic technique, a Nelaton urethral catheter is inserted into the bladder. This is for filling the bladder with saline, water or radiopaque contrast. An intravesical pressure catheter – a polythene cannula 1 mm external diameter – is inserted at the same time.

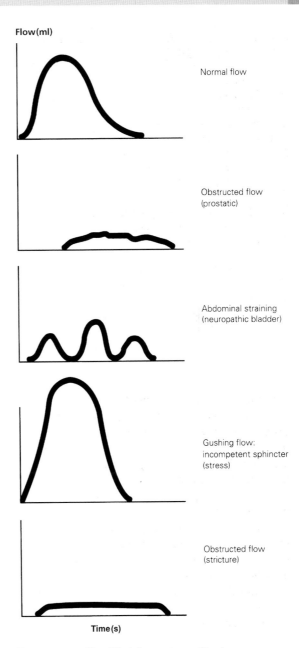

Figure 2.11   Simplified flow rate profiles in uroflowmetry.

Any residual urine will be noted and measured and if necessary a specimen taken for culture. Next, a rectal plug is inserted into the rectum, using a 2 mm external diameter water-filled polythene cannula, protected by a finger cot against faecal contamination. This measures the intra-abdominal pressure. The computer will subtract

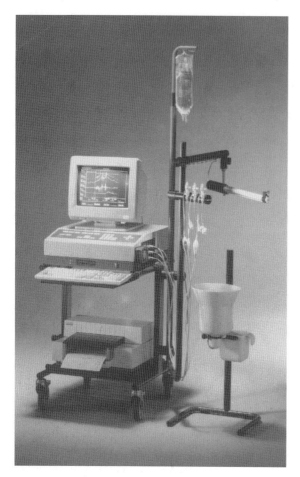

Figure 2.12   Dantec cystometry recorder. Courtesy: Dantec Electronics Ltd.

Box 2.10   Urodynamic investigations: a patient's guide

1. Urodynamics investigates the functioning of your bladder.
2. The test takes about 40–60 min.
3. Try to drink 500 ml (1 pint) of water prior to the test so that you arrive with a fairly full bladder. You will not have to wait long for the test to begin.
4. You will undress and put on a gown which is provided.
5. You will be asked to empty your bladder into a commode-like toilet which is electronically connected to a recording machine. This measures the rate of the flow of urine.
6. You will then lie on a couch (or X-ray table, if pictures are to be taken) so that two small catheters can be put into the bladder. One fine catheter measures the pressure inside the bladder, the other is for filling the bladder with water.
7. A small rubber balloon is placed just inside the rectum. This measures the pressure in your abdomen.
8. Water enters your bladder slowly and any bladder activity is recorded on the machine.
9. When you feel full the water flow is switched off and the filling catheter is removed. You will be asked to cough while still lying down so that any leakage can be noted.
10. When you stand up you will be asked to give a series of coughs and/or gentle movements to see whether leakage occurs.
11. Finally, you empty your bladder again on the commode-like toilet before the pressure catheters are removed.
12. The way your bladder is functioning will have been recorded and a diagnosis of the problem can be made.

the intra-abdominal pressure from the intravesical pressure, thus giving the intrinsic intravesical pressure or detrusor pressure. The two pressure lines are connected to the cystometer and flushed with water to allow the recordings to take place.

The patient is asked to cough; this raises the abdominal pressure and therefore the total bladder pressure, but the detrusor pressure should show no rise. Bladder filling can then commence while the patient remains in the supine position or moves to a standing position with the pressure lines securely fastened to the leg with micropore tape.

Normal physiological filling of the bladder occurs at approximately 1 ml/min, but this is too slow for practical cystometry. A 'medium-fill' rate of between 10 and 100 ml/min is generally used. In patients with a suspected neuropathic bladder the filling rate is reduced to 10–20 ml/min because filling too quickly may give an abnormal rise in bladder pressure. 'Rapid-fill' rates (above 100 ml/min) are rarely used as they may initiate spurious detrusor contractions.

Cystometric recording

1. The infusion is started via an intravenous giving-set. Saline should be at body temperature.
2. The patient is instructed to report the first sensation of bladder filling. This is marked FS (first sensation) on the cystometrogram.
3. The patient is asked to suppress the desire to void and report when the urge is so strong that the bladder feels entirely filled. This volume is marked on the recording (maximum cystometric bladder capacity) and the infusion is stopped. The filling Nelaton catheter is then removed.
4. For provocative tests for detrusor instability or stress incontinence, the patient may now be asked to cough repeatedly and strongly, and to do on-the-spot star jumps or walking.
5. The patient then empties the bladder as for uroflowmetry, but the pressure transducers are brought in line with the symphysis pubis to prevent artificial pressure rise. During the voiding phase the patient is asked to try to stop the urine flow, thus suppressing detrusor contraction. Voiding then continues to completion. The voided volume should equal the infused volume.
6. The pressure catheters are removed and the patient can dress before discussing the results.

Interpretation of cystometry recordings

Residual urine

Normally the bladder empties completely. In cases with residual urine, the amount may vary considerably from day to day in the same patient. A normal urinary residual is less than 50 ml.

Bladder resting pressure

The bladder resting pressure is often 5–15 cmH$_2$O in the supine position and 20–50 cmH$_2$O in the standing position, depending primarily on the weight of the intra-abdominal organs. Normally the detrusor pressure on filling is less than 10 cmH$_2$O for 300 ml or 15 cmH$_2$O for 500 ml.

First sensation to void

The first sensation (FS) reflects the functioning of the sensory pathways from the bladder. In a normal bladder, the first desire to void occurs at volumes between 150 and 250 ml, depending on the filling rate. If the detrusor is decompensated or the sensory nerve function is deficient, the first sensation to void occurs at larger volumes, and it may even be difficult for the patient to report any desire to void.

Maximal cystometric bladder capacity

The maximal cystometric bladder capacity depends on the filling rate, the sensory nerve function and the detrusor function. Normal capacity is 400–600 ml. In patients with an overactive detrusor or contracted bladder the capacity may vary from 50 to 250 ml. In hypotonic or 'floppy' bladders the capacity may be 500–1000 ml. A cystometric recorded maximal bladder capacity differs from the functional capacity as measured by voided volumes in micturition diaries or charts.

Bladder pressure during filling

The normal bladder accommodates to rapid changes in volume, from empty to maximal cystometric capacity, with a pressure increase of less than 10 cmH$_2$O for 300 ml or 15 cmH$_2$O for 500 ml. Abnormal increases in bladder pressure during filling may be due to fibrosis in the bladder wall (contracted bladder, low compliance), to detrusor contractions, or to movements during the investigation (e.g. talking, laughing or coughing). Straining causes abrupt pressure variations, with steep pressure increases and steep decreases. Detrusor contractions are seen as more gradual, bell-shaped increases in the bladder pressure. An overactive detrusor function is characterised by involuntary detrusor contractions during filling of the bladder, either spontaneous or after provocative manoeuvres, which cannot be suppressed by the patient.

Summary

Detrusor functioning reflects the integrated functioning of the central and peripheral neuromuscular control of the lower urinary tract. Peripheral efferent and afferent neuronal pathways connect the muscular and sensory structures in the bladder

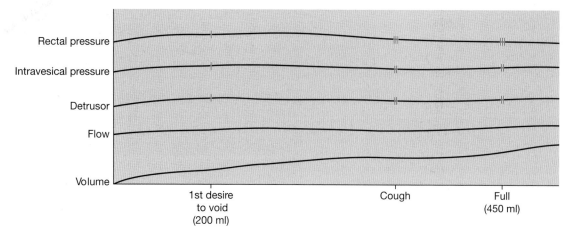

Figure 2.13   Normal filling cystometry.

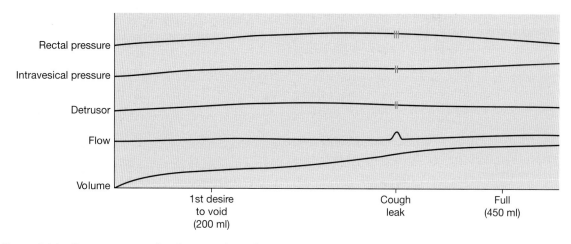

Figure 2.14   Cystometry recording for stress incontinence.

and urethra with the central nervous system (CNS).

An overactive detrusor function may be due to lesions in the CNS or to disease in the bladder or the urethra. An overactive detrusor function may also be diagnosed in normal, asymptomatic patients. This reflects the fact that all diagnostic investigations have a certain proportion of false-positive and false-negative test results in relation to a given symptom or diagnosis. Hence there is a need for more than one diagnostic approach: cystometry is often done in conjunction with bladder ultrasound.

Figures 2.13–2.17 show some urodynamic line graphs to illustrate normal filling cystometry, stress incontinence, sensory urge, detrusor instability and an underactive (hypotonic) bladder.

Videocystometry

The procedure is essentially the same as a plain CMG, except that it needs to be carried out in an X-ray department and a radiopaque contrast is used for the filling medium. Radiographs can be taken intermittently throughout the procedure as requested by the investigator while viewing on a

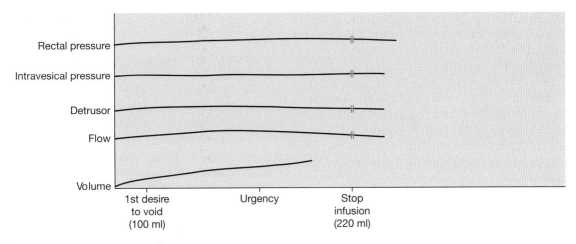

Figure 2.15   Cystometry recording sensory urge.

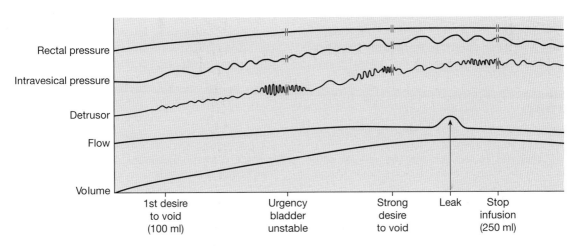

Figure 2.16   Cystometry recording for detrusor instability.

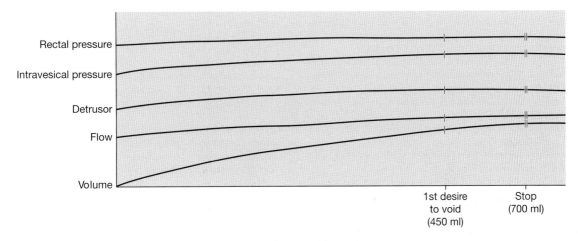

Figure 2.17   Cystometry recording for an underactive (hypotonic) bladder.

screen monitor. On the monitor the bladder neck and urethra can be observed during filling and voiding. The information is stored on a videotape. This method is preferable in the male if an outflow obstruction is suspected as it can be seen where the obstruction is located (i.e. prostatic, bladder neck or urethral stricture). A video screening also shows evidence of bladder trabeculation, diverticulae and/or ureteric reflux, and this significantly enhances the diagnostic capability of the procedure.

Urethral pressure profile (UPP)

This is the measurement of the intraurethral pressure from the bladder neck to the external meatus. It involves passing a catheter along the urethra into the bladder, and then mechanically withdrawing it at a constant rate so that the pressure along the urethra can be recorded. This test needs to be repeated three times to reach an accurate recording.

KEY POINTS FOR PRACTICE

- Clear understanding of the normal function of the bladder is important in order to recognise and understand abnormal function and to underpin care strategies
- Careful and thorough patient assessment takes time and empathy (not sympathy). It may require more than one session to complete
- Symptoms can provide good indications of underlying problems but further diagnostic investigations may be needed and clear protocols and pathways for referral should be established
- Not all symptoms of incontinence are due to abnormal bladder and lower urinary tract function. Coexisting problems can affect capacity to achieve and maintain continence

References

Abrams, P, Cardozo L, Khoury S and Wein A 2005 Incontinence, vol 1. Health Publication, Paris

Bayliss V, Cherry M, Locke R et al 2000 Pathways for continence care: development of the pathways. British Journal of Nursing 9(17):1165–1172

Berne M R, Levy M N 1990 Principles of physiology. Wolfe, St Louis

Bodker B, Lose G 2003 Postoperative urinary retention in gynecologic patients. International Urogynecology Journal Pelvic Floor Dysfunction 14(2):94–97

Chapple C R, MacDiarmid S A 2000 Urodynamics made easy, 2nd edn. Churchill Livingstone, London

Corcos J 2004 Simplified anatomy of the vesico-urethral functional unit. In: Corcos J, Schick E (eds) Textbook of the neurogenic bladder. Martin Dunitz, London

De Groat W C 1994 Neurophysiology of the pelvic organs. In: Rushton D N (ed) Handbook of neuro-urology. Marcel Dekker, New York

DeLancey J O 1990 Functional anatomy of the female lower urinary tract and pelvic floor. In: The neurobiology of incontinence (Ciba Foundation Symposium). John Wiley, Chichester, p 57–76

Department of Health 2000 Good practice in continence services. DH, London

Drake M J, Turner W H 2004 Physiology of the smooth muscles of the bladder and urethra. In: Corcos J, Schick E (eds) Textbook of the neurogenic bladder. Martin Dunitz, London

Dudley N J, Kirkland M, Lovett J, Watson A R 2003 Clinical agreement between automated and calculated ultrasound measurements of bladder volume. British Journal of Radiology 76:832–834

Feneley R C L 1986 Normal micturition and its control. In: Mandelstam D (ed) Incontinence and its management, 2nd edn. Croom Helm, London

Fonda D, DuBeau C E, Harari D et al 2005 Incontinence in the frail elderly. In: Abrams P, Cardozo L, Khoury S, Wein A (eds) Incontinence, vol 2. Health Publication, Paris

Gilpin S A, Gosling J A, Smith A R B, Warrell D 1989 The pathogenesis of genito-urinary prolapse and stress incontinence of urine: a histological and histochemical study. British Journal of Obstetrics and Gynaecology 96:15–23

Goode P S, Locher J L, Bryant R L et al 2000 Measurement of postvoid residual urine with portable transabdominal bladder ultrasound scanner and urethral catheterization. International Urogynecology Journal 11(5):36–46

Kassis A, Schick E 1993 Frequency-volume chart pattern in a healthy female population. British Journal of Urology 72:708–710

Laker C 1994 Urological nursing. Scutari Press, London

Larson G, Victor A 1988 Micturition patterns in a healthy female population studied with a frequency/volume chart. Journal of Urology and Nephrology Supplement 114:53–57

Mahony D T, Laferte R O, Blais D J 1977 Integral storage and voiding reflexes. Urology 1:95–105

Mahony D T, Laferte R O, Blais D J 1980 Incontinence of urine due to instability of micturition reflexes (Parts 1 and 2). Urology 3:229–239, 379–388

Petros P E, Ulmsten U I 1990 An integral theory of female urinary incontinence. Experimental and clinical considerations. Acta Obstetrica et Gynecologica Scandinavica Supplement 153:7–31

Rosseland L A, Stughaug A, Breivik H 2002 Detecting postoperative urinary retention with an ultrasound scanner. Acta Anaesthesiologica Scandinavica 46(3):279–282

Royal College of Nursing 2000 Digital rectal examination and manual removal of faeces. Guidance for nurses. RCN, London

Rud T, Andersson K E, Asmussen M 1980 Factors maintaining the intraurethral pressure in women. Investigative Urology 17:343–347

Sweet B R 1988 Mayes midwifery, 11th edn. Baillière Tindall, Edinburgh

Tortora G, Grabowski S 2002 Principles of anatomy and physiology. Harper Collins, New York

Wein A 2000 Overactive bladder: defining the disease. American Journal of Managed Care 6(11):S559–S564

Williams K S, Assassa R P, Smith N et al 2002 Good practice in continence care: development of a nurse-led service. British Journal of Nursing 11:548–559

Yoshimura N, Seki S, Chancellor M B 2004 Integrated physiology of the lower urinary tract. In: Corcos J, Schick E (eds) Textbook of the neurogenic bladder. Martin Dunitz, London

Chapter 3

Mainly women

Mary Dolman

Having once decided to achieve a certain task, achieve at all costs of tedium and distaste. The gain in self-confidence of having accomplished a tiresome labour is immense.

T.A. Bennett

INTRODUCTION

Urinary incontinence (UI) is a distressing symptom which can lead to a profound deterioration in quality of life, including sexuality, and many women adopt avoidance behaviours rather than seek professional advice or treatment, at least until symptoms become intolerable. However, as knowledge about the control of micturition and the function of the pelvic floor muscles increases (see Ch. 2), healthcare professionals with expertise in continence care have an increasing range of strategies available to prevent and treat incontinence. Women are more prone to UI than men because of the influence of female hormones on the lower urinary tract and because the pelvic floor muscles are stretched and can be damaged during childbirth. Other factors such as use of epidural anaesthesia, obesity and some changes associated with normal ageing (see Chs 2 and 6) can also play a part.

The most common type of UI in younger and middle-aged women is stress urinary incontinence (SUI) (Hannestad et al 2000) and this represents a major focus within this chapter. Overactive bladder symptoms with or without incontinence (urge incontinence) are more common in middle and older age groups and will be discussed later in the chapter, together with treatment options for mixed symptoms and difficulties in emptying the bladder.

Risks of UI in women can be reduced if education about the function and use of the pelvic floor muscles is given during adolescence in school, college and universities, but certainly before the first pregnancy. Teaching girls the importance of doing pelvic floor exercises before pregnancy offers a proactive strategy towards incontinence prevention.

UI is a common condition which is more prevalent in women than diabetes, hypertension or depression (see Ch. 1) but many women find it difficult to approach their doctor to discuss their symptoms and are unaware of other help, such as self-referral to a continence advisor, helplines or user-group support such as *In*contact (UK). UI is not a disease but a symptom and clinicians should approach incontinence with the same enthusiasm as any other symptom such as chest pain or haematuria. Unless incontinence is properly addressed it will not go away and the patient will be drawn into a downward spiral towards isolation and depression. This chapter, in discussing UI in women, will include prevention, assessment, treatment options, surgical procedures, management devices and the impact such symptoms have on sexuality and quality of life.

PREVALENCE OF UI IN WOMEN – A GLOBAL PERSPECTIVE

It is not the number of episodes of urine leakage per day, week or month that determines the impact of incontinence on women's lives but rather 'when is it a problem to the patient?'. However, this can be much more difficult to research and most prevalence studies on incontinence are based on the presence of symptoms within a given period of time, such as the number of incontinence episodes in the last 30 days, 3 months or 6 months.

Hunskaar et al (2004) presented a European prevalence study on UI in women in four countries using a definition of 'incontinence beyond their control in the last 30 days' (Fig. 3.1). Data were collected using a postal survey sent to 29 500 community-dwelling women aged over 18 years; the prevalence rates reported were: UK (32%), Germany (34%), France (32%) and Spain (15%). Stress urinary incontinence was the most prevalent type. Hunskaar (1999) compared the prevalence of incontinence in Asia and Japan with rates in Europe and the USA (Box 3.1). Data published by the Asian Society for Female Urology, using a survey population total of 5506, give a further breakdown of prevalence rates (Box 3.2).

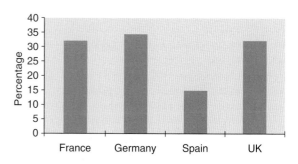

Figure 3.1 Percentage of female incontinence in Europe. After Hunskaar et al (2004).

Box 3.1   Prevalence of urinary incontinence in women (after Hunskaar 1999)

Asia:	14.6%	Europe:	26%
Japan:	32%	USA:	37%

Box 3.2   Breakdown of prevalence rates in Asia (Asian Society for Female Urology)

Thailand:	17%	Korea:	8%
Philippines:	13%	Malaysia:	6%
India:	12%	Indonesia:	5%
Taiwan:	12%	Singapore:	4%
Pakistan:	11%	*Overall*:	
Hong Kong:	8%	14.6%	

Box 3.3   Prevalence of urinary incontinence in American women (National Family Opinion Survey 2002)

Last 30 days:	37%	Last 3–4 years:	26.3%
<1 year:	26.3%	>4 years:	33.5%
Last 1–2 years:	13.8%		

The variation in results is probably due to the type of questions asked and their interpretation. In Asia the question was: 'Did you lose urine before you made it to the bathroom?' This indicates the problem was due to urgency. In Europe and the USA the question used was: 'Have you lost urine beyond your control within the last 30 days?' This gives a more comprehensive view of urinary incontinence in general. Other differences are obviously cultural and relate to degrees of embarrassment. In the USA a survey conducted by the National Family Opinion Survey Company (sponsored by Eli Lily, 2002) showed the overall results on the prevalence of UI in American women to be 37% (Box 3.3).

It is clear that urinary incontinence is a common problem for many women throughout the world, with high costs to individuals and services. In many countries incontinence is receiving greater recognition and it is becoming easier to talk about this sensitive subject. However, services are variable and very poor in some places, leaving many women with limited opportunities for treatment.

EMBRYOLOGICAL DEVELOPMENT OF THE VAGINA AND URETHRA

To have a better understanding of some of the possible causes of female continence problems it is necessary to be aware of the embryological development of the bladder, urethra and vagina and their sensitivity to hormonal effects. As early as the sixth week of gestation a primitive bladder and the anorectal canal are developing from the urorectal septum. Between the eighth and twelfth week of intrauterine life, the urogenital membrane forms the distal part of the urethra, the upper bladder and the vagina. Meanwhile, the fallopian tubes, uterus and trigone muscle of the bladder develop from the paramesonephric ducts (Cardozo et al 1993).

These early structures have common embryological origins which can be influenced by hormones after puberty (Fig. 3.2). The submucosal folds along the urethra are sensitive to oestrogen and when fully oestrogenised help to provide a 'watertight' seal. When there is a decrease in oestrogen prior to menstruation or after the menopause the watertight seal is less efficient and urinary leakage can occur.

TYPES OF FEMALE URINARY DYSFUNCTION

- Stress urinary incontinence
- Overactive bladder (OAB) (urgency to void with or without urinary leakage)
- Mixed urinary symptoms (stress and urgency)
- Overflow incontinence/voiding dysfunction.

The characteristics of each of these types of urinary dysfunction are discussed in Chapter 2. Stress urinary incontinence (SUI) is considered in detail here since it occurs almost exclusively in women.

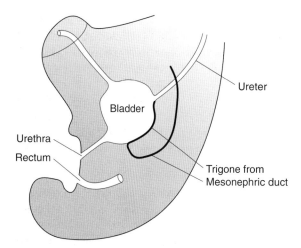

Figure 3.2 Diagram of embryological development at about the eighth week.

Stress urinary incontinence

The International Continence Society (ICS) (Abrams et al 2005) has defined SUI at three levels: as a symptom, as a sign and as a condition.

- *Symptom*. Stress urinary incontinence is the complaint of involuntary leakage on effort or exertion, or on sneezing/coughing (Fig. 3.3)
- *Sign*. Stress urinary incontinence is the observation of involuntary leakage from the urethra, synchronous with exertion/effort, or sneezing/coughing
- *Condition*. Urodynamic diagnosis of stress incontinence is noted during filling cystometry and is defined as the involuntary leakage of urine during increased abdominal pressure, in the absence of a detrusor contraction.

Risk factors for SUI in women

The risk factors for SUI have been investigated in a number of studies but the evidence is at times conflicting. There are extensive data to suggest that pregnancy and childbirth are precipitating events which can influence the occurrence of SUI (Foldspang et al 1999) (see also Box 3.4). During the course of pregnancy the pelvic floor muscles become relaxed and softened due to the release of the hormone relaxin, to allow for the tremendous stretching that will occur during labour and the

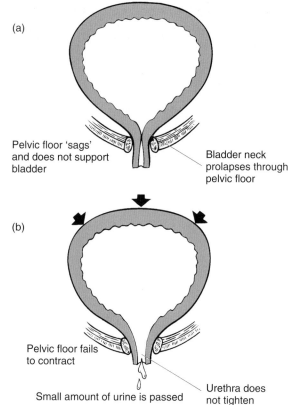

Figure 3.3 (a) Stress incontinence caused by weakness of pelvic floor muscles. (b) Coughing, laughing, running, etc. cause a rise in intra-abdominal pressure which results in leakage of urine.

birth of the fetus (Sweet 1988). Relaxin is released each month prior to ovulation and if fertilisation does not occur the hormone ceases production until the next cycle. This could be an explanation for the stress incontinence experienced by some young women in the period immediately prior to menstruation. Half of all women pregnant for the first time experience SUI during the last trimester (Eason et al 2004) while the incidence of incontinence 9 weeks postpartum has been reported as 21% following spontaneous delivery and 36% following forceps delivery. If incontinence occurs immediately postpartum it is often transient and continence is restored within 6 months.

Bladder dysfunction may become more severe with each additional pregnancy due to additional trauma and there appears to be a potential further

Box 3.4   Research study 1: The prevalence of pelvic floor disorders and their relationship to gender, age, parity and mode of delivery

This study by MacLennan et al (2000) set out to define the prevalence of pelvic floor disorders in a community setting in relation to gender, age, parity and mode of delivery using a survey by random selection of 4400 households: 3010 interviews were conducted in the respondents' homes, some men were included and the women were aged 15–97 years. The results revealed the prevalence of all types of self-reported urinary incontinence in men to be 4.4% and in women 35.3%. Nulliparous women reported urinary incontinence and this increased after pregnancy according to parity and age. The highest prevalence (51.9%) was reported in women aged 70–74 years. Pregnancy, >20 weeks, regardless of the mode of delivery, greatly increased the prevalence of major pelvic floor dysfunction; this was defined as any type of incontinence, symptoms of prolapse or previous pelvic floor surgery. Using a multivariate logistic regression, pelvic floor dysfunction was significantly associated with caesarean section, spontaneous vaginal delivery and instrumental delivery. Other associations with pelvic floor morbidity were age, body mass index, coughing, osteoporosis, arthritis and reduced quality of life scores.

This study concluded that pelvic floor disorders are very common and strongly associated with female gender, ageing, pregnancy, parity and forceps delivery. Caesarean delivery is not associated with a significant reduction in long-term pelvic floor morbidity compared with spontaneous vaginal delivery.

incontinence. Labour causes a decrease in bladder sensation and if an epidural analgesia has also been administered, this can result in bladder over-distension if urinary output is not carefully monitored postpartum (Dolman 1992). It has been shown by Weil et al (1983) that a single overdistension of the detrusor muscle can result in long-term voiding difficulties because once the detrusor has been overstretched its ability to contract long enough and strong enough to empty a bladder fully is impaired.

Some authors have questioned the impact of vaginal birth; however, Buchsbaum (2005) reported that urinary incontinence is not linked to a vaginal birth delivery but rather that familial factors seem to play an important role. Buchsbaum used a comprehensive questionnaire to assess pelvic floor disorders in pairs of nulliparous/parous postmenopausal sisters in 143 pairs and a clinical evaluation of urinary incontinence and genital prolapse was also carried out in 101 of the pairs. The incidence of urinary incontinence in the parous group was 49.7% which was not significantly higher than 47.6% in the nulliparous group, nor did the severity differ significantly between the groups. The same urinary status seen in one sister was often seen in the other, thus suggesting a familial disposition. If this should be the case, then further studies are needed to explore if there is a genetic link as this would have great implications for basic research, treatment options, prevention strategies and risk management. Hannestad et al (2004) also reported evidence of a familial risk of urinary incontinence in women in their large scale cross-sectional survey.

Menopause and SUI

Although the relationship between menopause and SUI remains unclear, clinicians still quote menopause as a major risk factor for both SUI and urge incontinence. The theory is that the lack of circulating oestrogen after menopause can result in bladder muscle weakness and atrophy of the mucosal tissue which lines the urethra. This atrophy, together with a decline in mucus production within the urethra, weakens its ability to maintain a watertight seal when intra-abdominal pressure is increased (e.g. coughing, sneezing,

decline in bladder control with ageing and reduced oestrogen levels at the menopause. The mechanism of SUI following delivery is thought to be pressure, stretch and shearing stress to the muscles and nerves of the pelvic floor, especially when the baby is over 4 kg (8.5 lbs) or if there is a prolonged second stage of labour. Episiotomy, forceps and ventouse (vacuum) assisted deliveries compound the risk of neuromuscular damage to the pelvic floor muscles (Klein et al 1997).

Poor bladder management during labour can result in voiding difficulties such as overflow jumping, Valsalva manoeuvre). Until recently oestrogen treatment (orally or vaginally), used either alone or in combination with other treatments for postmenopausal women, has been thought to improve incontinent episodes. The urethra and the trigone muscle of the bladder are covered by squamous epithelium similar to the vagina and, as these tissues contain oestrogen receptors, oestrogen replacement should increase the urethral closure pressure. There have been many uncontrolled trials of oestrogen therapy as a treatment for incontinence which have shown a subjective improvement. However, other trials found no objective improvement measures of urine loss (Thom et al 1997, Jackson et al 1999, Sherburn et al 2001). Jackson et al (1999), in a controlled trial, found no significant difference between treatment with oestrogen and control groups in the number of incontinent episodes at follow-up at 3 and 6 months. A large observational study by Thom et al (1997) showed an increased risk of urinary incontinence in older women who were taking hormone therapy. The question arises: 'Should hormone therapy be a recommended treatment for urinary incontinence in postmenopausal women?' A newer theory emerging from research studies is that pelvic connective tissue resilience decreases in later life and this is more noticeable in women who have had a hysterectomy, pelvic floor surgery, chronic constipation and repeated urinary tract infections (Sherburn et al 2001). Hence mechanical factors are more likely to contribute to urinary incontinence after the menopause and not depletion of oestrogen alone (Box 3.5).

Lack of oestrogen after the menopause can cause urethritis and trigonitis, often associated with atrophic vaginitis. This is easily recognised during a digital pelvic floor assessment by parting the labia and looking at the vulva and vaginal introitus which will appear red, inflamed and very dry. Vaginal dryness means there is a loss of sexual lubrication and intercourse will be painful and uncomfortable. Treatment for this condition is oestrogen replacement directly into the vagina with topical oestrogen cream, oral systemic oestrogen or Estraderm patches (best for women who have had a hysterectomy). Oestrogen replacement should improve the condition of the vaginal, ure-

---

Box 3.5   Research study 2: Pelvic connective tissue resilience decreases with vaginal delivery, menopause and uterine prolapse

This study by Reay-Jones et al (2003) looked at the onset of pelvic visceral prolapse and incontinence in women who had delivered vaginally to ascertain if menopausal-associated connective tissue weakening was causing their problems ($n = 85$). The uterosacral ligament resilience was assessed to determine whether it influenced uterine or pelvic floor mobility, or varied with age, vaginal delivery, menopause or histological variations in the ligament. It was found that uterosacral ligament resilience was significantly reduced with vaginal delivery, menopause and symptomatic uterovaginal prolapse.

The study concluded that when pelvic floor muscles are weakened, the decrease in pelvic connective tissue resilience related to the menopause can lead to symptomatic visceral prolapse.

These results lead to further questions and the need for more in-depth research.

---

thral and trigonal epithelium, and restore the premenopausal vaginal flora (Cardozo et al 1993). It is clear that oestrogen replacement is necessary if the above symptoms are present but its efficacy as a treatment for incontinence requires further robust research. Current conclusions based on reviews of the literature suggest there is little benefit from oestrogen therapy in the management of urodynamically diagnosed SUI (Al-Badr et al 2003, NICE 2006).

Hysterectomy

'I was alright until I had my hysterectomy' is a very common statement heard in the continence clinic. In effect, a hysterectomy can be considered as a surgical menopause, especially if accompanied by bilateral salpingo-oophorectomy. Oestrogen therapy is usually commenced immediately to prevent common menopause symptoms, osteoarthritis and cardiovascular disease (Abernethy 2005). In addition to oestrogen depletion, postoperative scarring and infection have been suggested by Smith et al (1970) as aetiological factors for urinary symptoms following a hysterectomy. Urethral obstruction due to periurethral fibrosis and damage to the bladder base and proximal urethra during a total hysterectomy can result in scar formation. Women experience frequency and difficulty with emptying the bladder and feel the need to 'go again' only a few minutes later. Frequency of micturition may be caused by a urinary tract infection resulting from incomplete bladder emptying or urethritis. A recent report from a postal survey of 25 000 women to determine if they had bladder problems 5 years after a hysterectomy, found that women who had had laparoscopic-assisted vaginal hysterectomy reported severe UI but not severe urgency or frequency. However, the symptoms of UI, frequency and nocturia were greater in women after a hysterectomy than those who had endometrial ablation (McPherson et al 2005). There is an increased risk of bladder problems when a hysterectomy is performed for cervical cancer or the patient has had radiotherapy treatment prior to surgery (Behtash et al 2005).

Other risk factors for SUI

Ethnic origins   The prevalence of SUI is thought to be significantly lower in African–American women than in Asian, Hispanic and white women (Duong & Korn 2001). It has been suggested that white women have a shorter urethra, weaker pelvic floor muscles and a lower bladder neck than women in other racial groups, thus making them more likely to have SUI. This difference may be related to greater urethral volume and higher urethral closure pressures during pelvic floor muscle contractions in African–American women. It must also be remembered that pelvic floor muscle exercises are part of normal culture in these women, hence stronger muscles.

Age   Pelvic floor muscle weakness accelerates after the menopause (see above) and progresses with general ageing. Prolapse of pelvic organs may occur due to weakened visceral ligaments.

Obesity and chronic cough   An increased body mass index (BMI) has been shown in cross-sectional and case-controlled studies to be a risk factor for SUI (Elia et al 2001). It is thought that the extra weight impairs the blood flow and nerve innervation to the bladder, and there is constant pressure on the bladder with greater urethral mobility, thus predisposing to SUI. A 'smoker's' cough is more violent than in a non-smoker and frequent coughing puts strain on the pelvic floor muscles. Coughing may also stimulate a detrusor contraction, resulting in urinary leakage.

Pelvic surgery   Pelvic organ prolapse can occur due to weakened pelvic floor muscles and degeneration of fascia and ligaments in general. Thus a prolapse of the bladder (cystocele) (Fig. 3.4), rectum (rectocele) (Fig. 3.5) or the uterus (enterocele) can descend from the normal anatomical position and either lie below the support of the pelvic floor muscles or protrude into the vaginal walls. If the pelvic floor muscles are weak, the proximal urethra will lie below the pelvic floor muscles; therefore, when there is any increased intra-abdominal pressure, such as coughing, it is not transmitted equally to the bladder (promoting emptying) and external sphincter (promoting closure) and SUI will occur (see Fig. 3.3). Surgical repair of any prolapse (discussed later in this chapter) may lead to urinary dysfunction after a period of time.

Physical exercise   It is commonly claimed that physical exercise is important for health, but what if urinary leakage occurs? It is thought that as many as 50% of women who exercise regularly have some degree of SUI and often have to wear a tampon or pad. Some stop exercising altogether in order to cope with the incontinence, others change to a sport which does not increase intra-abdominal pressure to avoid the problem. High risk sports which put pressure on the bladder include gymnastics, netball, martial arts, horse riding, weight lifting, running, etc.; lower risk activities include swimming, walking, rowing and low impact aerobics.

The overactive bladder in women

The International Continence Society changed the older terminology for unstable bladder/bladder instability to overactive bladder (OAB) in 1997. This complex syndrome includes urinary urgency with or without incontinence, usually accompanied by urinary frequency and nocturia and sometimes nocturnal enuresis. Other symptoms can include incontinence associated with giggling, handwashing, 'key in the door' and sexual activity. Although there may be a discernable physiological cause in some cases, more often the symptoms are idiopathic with no pathological or metabolic explanation. In some women the symptoms may be due to long-term bad toileting habits, such as going to the toilet 'in case' when there is no need to void or voiding at the first sensation while the bladder is still filling. This behaviour can result in reduced bladder capacity because the bladder is not allowed to fill fully and eventually its ability to hold a 'normal' volume is greatly decreased. Stewart et al (2003) conducted a national overactive bladder evaluation (the NOBLE study) and found the likelihood of urge incontinence in women significantly increased between the ages of 35 and 44 years, with an even greater probability after age 55 years.

While the symptoms of urgency and frequency alone have a significant negative impact on patients' quality of life, urge incontinence is even more disruptive since it gives the individual very little to time to take avoiding action (Milsom et al 2001). Despite this, women often do not seek medical advice and rely on their own coping strategies; for example, knowing exactly where all the toilets are when they are out! Cardozo (1991) found an increase in the incidence of OAB following surgery for stress incontinence, but as OAB and stress incontinence symptoms often coexist, a differential diagnosis is commonly made on evidence during urodynamic investigation when there is failure to inhibit detrusor contractions. This is particularly important if surgery is being considered for stress incontinence but urodynamics is not necessarily required before treating symptoms of urgency or urge incontinence (Radley et al 2001).

OAB has been found to have a greater impact on quality of life than stress incontinence because of the predominant symptoms of frequency and urgency which produce a sudden and overwhelming desire to pass urine which cannot be suppressed or delayed. Sexual and relationship problems are common (Kizilkaya Beji et al 2005). In a study of 106 women with OAB attending a urogynaecology clinic, 72% of those who were sexually active (58 women) felt their bladder symptoms adversely affected their sex life and

47% reported incontinence during coitus (Rosario et al 2000). People with OAB easily become isolated and depressed, refuse to socialise and tend to withdraw from sexual activity. Such findings are not restricted to the elderly population. Van der Vaart et al (2002) evaluated the impact of OAB and urge incontinence on the quality of life in women aged 20–45 years using the Incontinence Impact Questionnaire (IIQ). The researchers found diminished social and physical function, emotional and embarrassment domains associated with OAB. Reduced mobility was also noted in this age group which is particularly distressing for young and active women.

In older age groups there is a tendency towards urinary tract infections in association with OAB and this is likely to be due to failure to completely empty the bladder due to frequent but inefficient bladder contractions. Frequency and urgency are also associated with an increased risk of falls in older people (Brown et al 2000) (see Chs 1, 2 and 6). In the UK it is thought that OAB affects approximately six million people with a cost to the NHS of more than £350 million per year (Hussain & Nethercliffe 2004). Treatment options for OAB are discussed later in the chapter.

Voiding dysfunction

As the symptoms of urgency, frequency and passing small amounts of urine may mean overflow incontinence and not an overactive bladder, it is most important to determine the correct type of incontinence prior to commencing any treatment intervention. To treat the wrong type of incontinence can have a disastrous effect on the patient (Box 3.6). Retention of urine is due to an obstruction (common in men because of an enlarged prostate; see Ch. 4), a hypotonic detrusor contraction, as in the elderly, or a completely flaccid bladder (neurogenic origins). Women do suffer from voiding difficulties but this is often poorly recognised. A urethral obstruction in women may result from scarring or fibrosis when catheterisation has been used or as a consequence of postsurgical procedures for stress incontinence. Diabetic neuropathy, spinal cord lesions and neurological conditions, side effects of drugs, postepidural anaesthesia, excessive pelvic floor muscle

Box 3.6   Case study 1

Joan, aged 67 years, had been an insulin dependent diabetic for 30 years and found it very hard to lose weight so she was clinically obese; she was also on the waiting list for a hysterectomy for fibroids. She went to her GP because she often wet the bed at night and also complained of daytime urgency and frequency of micturition. Joan was prescribed oxybutynin 15 mg nocte. She was referred to the continence service because after 3 months on oxybutynin the symptom of nocturnal enuresis had worsened and she was gaining weight around her waist despite a strict diet.

Verbal history and abdominal palpation alone indicated a hypotonic bladder and the oxybutynin was stopped immediately. A postvoiding bladder scan revealed 100 ml voided, with 1.5 litres residual. Urinalysis showed a urinary infection and glucose. Joan had her insulin reassessed and was prescribed antibiotics for the UTI. An intermittent catheter was used to drain the residual urine and she tried to learn this technique herself with the specialist nurse at home. Unfortunately, due to her size and failing eyesight she never mastered intermittent catheterisation and a long-term catheter was inserted.

She lived with an indwelling catheter which was changed every 3 months by the district nurse. Her bladder was completely flaccid and no detrusor contractility ever returned. She used a catheter valve during the day and emptied 4-hourly; she used continuous drainage at night when she went to bed. She only had one catheter-related infection in 8 years and finally died aged 75 of heart problems in a nursing home.

activity (see below), chronic constipation, pelvic tumours and prolapses can all affect the bladder's ability to empty properly. The only way to diagnose incomplete emptying and to measure postvoiding residuals of urine is to take an ultrasound scan of the bladder (see Ch. 2).

ASSESSMENT FOR CONTINENCE PROMOTION

A detailed assessment can take as long as an hour to do on a new patient who may then require further investigations. However, nurse-led clinics (see Ch. 11) in continence care can offer a wide range of investigations and treatment can be commenced immediately once the clinician is sure of the diagnosis. Box 3.7 outlines a series of lifestyle measures to aid promotion of continence.

There are four key areas to consider when assessing women for UI:

- dealing with any reversible, underlying condition which may be causing the incontinence
- identifying special problems that may need to be referred to a urogynaecologist
- eliminating overflow incontinence due to voiding dysfunction
- distinguishing between stress and urge incontinence and, if there are mixed symptoms, determining which is the most dominant symptom causing distress.

Potentially reversible causes of urinary incontinence

Symptomatic urinary tract infections (UTIs)

UTIs cause inflammation of the bladder and are characterised by painful micturition, with frequency and urgency. A simple urinalysis check will indicate if an infection is present but often the UTI will clear up on its own within a few days (avoiding unnecessary use of antibiotics). Where symptoms persist, antibiotics may be required and a midstream urine specimen should be sent for microbiological testing to identify the infecting organism and its antibiotic sensitivity. For women who experience recurrent UTIs further investigations may be needed, including checks for residual urine.

Atrophic vaginitis

Women who have inflamed and atrophic vaginal mucosa may also have similar inflammatory changes in the urethra and trigone muscle in the bladder. This again can present with symptoms of urgency and may give a burning sensation when passing urine. Oestrogen replacement can cure this problem. The clinician must examine the area by parting the labia and noting the red inflamed area at the entrance to the vagina.

Box 3.7 Proactive lifestyle and other measures to promote continence

1. Diet
   - Eat balanced nutritional foods for general good health
   - Eat 20–30 g fibre daily to avoid constipation
   - Do not exceed recommended body mass for height/age
   - Drink semi-skimmed milk for calcium intake to help prevent osteoporosis

2. Fluid intake
   - Daily water intake should be approximately 1–2 litres
   - Avoid drinking excess alcohol, caffeinated drinks (tea and coffee) or carbonated drinks as these may influence bladder behaviour (although further evidence from well-designed clinical trials is still needed); try alternative drinks such as herbal infusions

3. Toileting habits
   - Do not empty bladder too soon; aim to allow the bladder to fill and to hold a good quantity (e.g. 350–500 ml) before going to the toilet
   - Try to remember the bladder capacity is 'normally' sufficient for 4–5-hourly emptying
   - Try to make sure the bladder is emptied completely when visiting the toilet. Residual urine can increase the risk of urinary tract infection
   - Sit comfortably and always give yourself enough time on the toilet to empty the bladder

4. Chronic cough
   - Treat underlying chest conditions to reduce coughing episodes as severe coughing puts added strain on the pelvic floor muscles and weakens them

   - Stop smoking as this causes coughing and increased pressure is transmitted to the pelvic floor muscles

5. Medications
   - Review all medications that can affect the bladder/bowel directly or indirectly
   - Some nurses are trained to prescribe and will know the side effects of common medications which can be stopped, the dosage reduced or an alternative prescribed
   - Review the times at which medications are taken as this may also influence the effect on the bladder

6. Before pregnancy and during labour
   - Learn how to carry out regular pelvic floor exercises correctly and exercise regularly to provide strong, healthy and flexible muscle to assist in labour and thus reduce risks of trauma
   - Carry out regular pelvic floor exercises to reduce the risk of incontinence during pregnancy

7. After childbirth
   - Commence pelvic floor exercises again about 6 weeks after delivery

8. Professional advice
   - At the 6–8 week postnatal check-up, mention any bladder or pelvic floor muscle problems and discuss any symptoms of incontinence early
   - Make sure the pelvic floor exercises are being carried out correctly
   - Ask for a continence assessment. Early treatment usually means a cure!

Impacted faeces

A rectum impacted with faeces will put extrinsic pressure on the bladder neck, thus causing an obstruction to the urinary flow, and retention with overflow incontinence can occur. Removal of constipated faeces and ongoing bowel management will cure this problem (see Ch. 8).

Medications

A number of medications taken for long-term conditions can influence incontinence and/or urinary retention and all medications should be reviewed on a regular basis (see Ch. 9). Some symptoms of incontinence can be resolved on stopping the drug or changing to an alternative.

Endocrine problems

Poor glucose control in diabetes can lead to osmotic diuresis with increased urine flow and bladder filling (Weiss & Newman 2002). This may cause incontinence in patients predisposed to OAB contractions but symptoms should improve when glucose levels are under control.

Restricted mobility

When patients have restricted mobility, as with arthritis or injury, the urgency symptom may become urge incontinence if they are unable to reach a toilet in time. Wherever possible, try to improve mobility and provide easy access to a commode or bathroom.

Identifying special problems

By collating the verbal history from the patient, the results of the urinalysis and observations from the physical examination it should be possible to determine whether additional investigations are necessary or if the patient should be referred to a urogynaecologist. Conditions needing specialised consultation would include:

- haematuria without urinary infection as there may be renal damage causing this problem
- severe prolapse of the bladder, rectum or uterus where surgical intervention is inevitable (these patients must be referred to a surgical consultant)
- women who have had previous pelvic/incontinence surgery or radiation for cancer (these patients need assessment with a specialist nurse and consultant).

Eliminating overflow incontinence due to voiding dysfunction

Overflow incontinence due to voiding dysfunction is not as common in women as in men but it is most certainly underreported and frequently overlooked. Once the neurological or drug-induced causes of an underactive bladder have been eliminated, a postvoiding residual urine test should be a routine investigation. This non-invasive procedure is done using a bladder scanner. A normal, acceptable, residual urine in women is 50–100 ml but a larger volume may lead to identification of a previously undiagnosed condition.

Distinguishing between stress and urge incontinence

When all the above possibilities have been discussed with the patient and test results are nega-

Table 3.1 Distinguishing between SUI and urge incontinence

Symptom	SUI	Urge incontinence
Urine leakage with coughing, sneezing, etc.	Yes	No (sometimes)
Nocturia	No	Yes
Frequency > 8 times in 24 h	No	Yes
Uncontrollable urge to go to toilet	No	Yes
Volume of urine loss with incontinence	Small	Small/moderate/ large

tive, the verbal symptom profile is now assessed. The key symptom factors are listed in Table 3.1.

Some women will give a history that suggests both problems, i.e. mixed incontinence, in which case treatment should be started for whichever is the most troublesome symptom first. Some treatments will help both problems at the same time, i.e. pelvic floor exercises, biofeedback and electromuscular stimulation (discussed later in the chapter).

PHYSICAL EXAMINATION

Stage one

The physical examination is an integral part of patient assessment for female continence problems. The procedure needs to be explained in detail and the patient's consent obtained as vaginal examination is an invasive course of action. Women are often anxious and tense about an examination so the first thing to do is to try to put the woman at ease and encourage relaxation. Some women think a vaginal examination can take place with pants still being worn!

With the woman resting comfortably in the crooked supine position, with a small sheet or blanket providing a modesty cover, first observe for abdominal or perineal scarring, vaginal discharge or skin excoriation (incontinence dermatitis). Gloves must be worn for the next part of the examination which is to part the labia and note skin colour in the vagina for dryness, redness and atrophic vaginitis or if there is a severe prolapse.

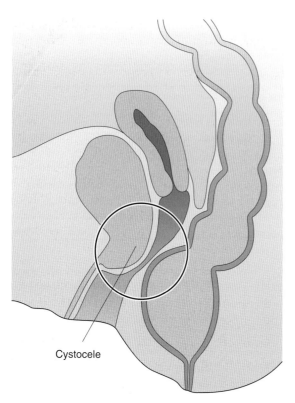

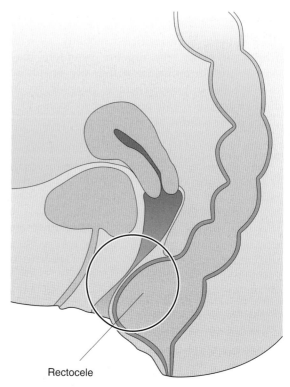

Figure 3.4 The bladder bulging into the vagina is a cystocele.

Figure 3.5 The rectum bulging into the vagina is a rectocele.

Sometimes a cystocele can appear as large as a tennis ball at the introitus! Ask the woman to cough repeatedly and note if there is any urine loss and then ask her to tighten the pelvic floor muscles. Observe if there is any movement at all: if the perineum descends (bulging), this means the woman is bearing down with the muscles; if the anal sphincter 'winks' at you, the pelvic floor muscles are contracting correctly.

Stage two

Insert a gloved and lubricated index finger gently into the vagina and if you easily feel the cervix then there is decent of the uterus. Note also if the woman mentions any painful areas from within the vagina when palpating 360° about 2.5 cm (1") inside the introitus. Palpate for cystocele (Fig. 3.4) or rectocele (Fig. 3.5). If there is mild prolapse, record this in the notes; however, if moderate or severe prolapse is found you must refer to a urog-

ynaecologist. Support the bladder neck with the tip of the index finger and ask the woman to cough; note if there is palpable descent of the bladder, bladder neck hypermobility or a bulging urethral meatus.

Stage three – palpating pelvic floor function

The function of the pelvic floor musculature is a critical factor to most bladder dysfunction as the pelvic floor supports the bladder neck and urethra. In addition, the perineal–detrusor reflex can inhibit unwanted detrusor contractions. To evaluate the strength of the pelvic floor muscles, insert gloved and lubricated index and middle fingers into the vagina and part the fingers slightly (up and down or left to right, whichever feels comfortable to the clinician) to stimulate the muscles and to improve awareness for muscle isolation. Ask the woman to contract the muscle around the fingers with as much force as possible and for as long as possible. The clinician should observe if other muscles are being used, such as the abdominal, gluteal and thigh muscle groups. Having established that the pelvic floor muscle is contracting, a few seconds rest between each contraction will be needed so the muscle does not fatigue but at the same time the clinician must assess its full potential. Four criteria of muscle activity should be noted:

- intensity of contraction
- duration of contraction
- number of contractions achieved before the muscle fatigues
- alteration in muscle movement.

The intensity of contraction can range from barely perceptible to a firm squeeze. Duration involves the number of seconds the clinician feels the muscle contraction and how many times the contraction can be repeated. Between each contraction there must be a rest period which should be least as long as, if not longer than, the contraction itself. Alteration in muscle movement refers to the fact that in women with a well-supported and well-functioning pelvic floor muscle, the contraction should lift the base of the clinician's fingers upwards. With experience, clinicians will gauge the range of pelvic floor muscle ability and activity. Although this is only a subjective assessment (objective assessment can be obtained through biofeedback equipment), this information can be utilised to help determine an individualised exercise programme.

Palpation of the pelvic floor at a glance

1. With the patient in the crooked supine position, observe skin condition, abdominal/perineal scars or vaginal discharge.
2. Ask the woman to contract the pelvic floor and note anus 'winking' or perineum bulging.
3. Part the labia and note atrophic vaginitis or severe prolapse.
4. Insert a gloved and lubricated index finger into the vagina and palpate the rim of the muscle for indentations, pain, muscle bulk and mild prolapses.
5. Insert gloved and lubricated index and middle fingers into the vagina, part slightly and ask for

a forceful muscle contraction around the fingers. Note intensity of contraction – barely moving or forceful.

6. Ask the patient to rest the muscle before the next contraction. Count, in seconds, the duration of the contraction.
7. Ask the patient to rest the muscle. Determine the number of repetitions that can be achieved before the muscle fatigues.
8. Ask the patient to rest the muscle and then perform 2–5 quick contractions.
9. Set an individual exercise programme which is achievable by the patient (to help sustain motivation) and which may include gradually increasing the amount of exercise.

PELVIC FLOOR EXERCISES

The anatomy of the pelvic floor and its innervation are discussed in Chapter 2.

Exercises should not be generic (i.e. the same regime for all) but based on each patient's pelvic floor functional ability. Bø and Finckenhagen (2001) tested the Oxford Grading Scale (commonly used to grade pelvic floor muscle function) for interrater reproducibility and found it was not reproducible; hence the current thinking on pelvic floor muscle squeeze pressure remains subjective to the assessor. However, the mnemonic PERFECT suggested by Laycock (1994) will help a clinician in recording the findings of pelvic floor muscle activity (Box 3.8).

Once patients have been taught to identify and isolate the pelvic floor muscles their exercise programme can be set for them. This must include

---

Box 3.8   P.E.R.F.E.C.T.

P = Power is the force of the contraction
E = Endurance is the time in seconds the contraction is held (slow-twitch fibres)
R = Repetitions is how many contractions can be achieved before fatigued
F = Fast is quick contractions without holding
E = Every
C = Contraction
T = Timed

quick, 1–2 s holding contractions, often referred to as 'quick flicks' which work on the fast-twitch fibres required for rapid, involuntary action when coughing, sneezing, lifting, etc. This is followed by a series of sustained endurance contractions with a target length of duration which is achievable by the patient; for example, hold 2, 3, 4, 5 s or longer. In between each contraction there must be a resting period of the same duration or longer. The number of repetitions per day will depend on compliance and memory (Dolman & Chase 1996), but it is highly recommended to do a series of exercises with a regular daily activity such as cleaning one's teeth or having a drink. The exercises can be performed sitting, lying down or standing. To make the exercises meaningful the woman should use them functionally. Whenever leakage is likely to occur for an individual, on sneezing, coughing, lifting or carrying heavy objects, they should learn to tighten the pelvic floor muscles before doing the activity. When a woman fully complies with an exercise programme, results can be noticed as early as 4–6 weeks, but for most women the reality is that a reduction in leakage symptoms can take 3 months to achieve. It is better to aim to increase the duration of each contraction at a submaximal force rather than increase the number of contractions. Repeated exercises increase muscle bulk and this will help support the bladder neck. *The quality of the exercise is more important than the quantity.*

Two research studies on the long-term effects of pelvic floor exercises are cited below. One study (Box 3.9) demonstrates the long-term effects of pelvic floor exercises after 4 years and the other (Box 3.10) demonstrates adherence to exercises after 15 years.

Compliance with pelvic floor exercises

If women are able to contract their pelvic floor they may gain almost immediate control in certain situations using the method known as 'The Knack' (Miller et al 1996). This requires a voluntary contraction before and during an anticipated stressful event to stop or reduce urine leakage. However, it is clear from Bø et al's work (2005) (Box 3.10) that in the long term women rarely continue with pelvic floor exercises. Dolman and Chase (1996)

Box 3.9   Research study 3: Long-term effects of pelvic floor exercises

The long-term effects of pelvic floor exercises and bladder retraining were evaluated by O'Brien and Long (1995) on 229 women, 4 years after their first randomised controlled trial of the management of incontinence in primary care. Using a similar questionnaire they asked the women about their continence status in respect of pad usage, exercises or other treatments in the intervening 4 years. The results showed 69% of the women had either maintained their original improvement or cure, or had improved further, although 16% had deteriorated and a further 15% neither benefited from the original programme nor had further change. They noted that only 27% of women did their exercises for more than a year and 61% exercised for less than a year, while 12% stopped exercises immediately.

In conclusion, it was felt that continuation of pelvic floor exercises for 1 year or more was strongly associated with improvement or maintenance (56/61) of benefit compared with exercises for less than a year (102/168).

---

suggested that in order to maximise compliance with pelvic floor exercises, health professionals need to provide women with appropriate information and to develop techniques that help them to remember to perform their exercises. Education for women on pelvic floor exercises must include the reasons why the exercises need to be done, not only during and after childbirth, but as a life-long activity.

Compliance is more likely to be maintained and/or improved if women know they are contracting, and therefore exercising, the correct muscles. It is not unusual for women to think they have been doing the right exercises, only to find out years later they have been tightening their abdominals and buttocks. Chiarelli et al (2003) found that, in a sample of 720 postpartum women, although they knew how often pelvic floor exercises should be done (at least every other day) few did the exercises over their lifetime as it was perceived that they were only relevant during childbirth years. This raises issues for healthcare professionals to provide the educational gaps on

Box 3.10   Research study 4: Lower urinary tract symptoms and pelvic floor muscle exercise adherence after 15 years

Bø et al (2005) assessed lower urinary tract symptoms and adherence to exercises 15 years after ending an organised training programme. This was a small study of only 52 women who were originally diagnosed with SUI on urodynamic investigation and were assigned to either an intensive exercise group or to exercises at home. Six months later, 60% in the intensive exercise group were almost cured compared to 17% in the home exercise group. Fifteen years later, the original participants were invited to complete a postal questionnaire on current urinary symptoms and pelvic floor muscle training.

There was a 90.4% response and no difference was found between the two groups in their urinary outcomes or satisfaction, even with those who had had incontinence surgery during those years. Interestingly, half the number in each group had had surgery! Despite the fact that 28% of all women were doing pelvic floor exercises (PFE) at least once a week, those who had had surgery reported more severe incontinence and leakage which interfered with daily life than those who had not had surgery.

This study concluded that the marked benefit of PFE in the short term was not maintained 15 years later and that adherence to continuing exercises is low once original treatment and contact had ceased.

pelvic floor exercises throughout a woman's lifespan. Perhaps the gap needs to be filled by promoting the sexual benefits of pelvic floor exercises as many women will listen to that advice!

Sexual benefits of pelvic floor exercises

The pubococcygeus has often been referred to as the 'love muscle'. Women with strong pelvic floor muscles seem to enjoy the bonus of good sexual response, as found in a study of orgasm by Graber and Kline-Graber (1979). They reported that orgasm was significantly related to maximum pubococcygeal squeeze pressure. The pelvic floor muscles are directly responsible for the amount of sensation that women feel during intercourse (Chiarelli 1991). The vaginal mucosa is not well endowed with sensory nerves and most vaginal

sensations come from the pelvic floor muscles that loop around and behind the vagina. The pubococcygeus also directly affects the amount of sexual sensation male partners feel – by tightening these muscles the woman is able to exert a firmer grip.

The nerve endings in the muscles respond to being stretched, so the firmer and stronger the muscle is, the more it responds to the erect penis. As the glans of the penis moves back and forth during intercourse, the firm muscles rhythmically stretch and relax, thus heightening vaginal sensations. The pubococcygeus is also responsible for helping to lubricate the vaginal walls during foreplay and intercourse, so, sexually speaking, these muscles play a vital role.

To summarise, a strong pelvic floor muscle will:

- increase vaginal lubrication during foreplay and intercourse
- enhance sexual sensation vaginally
- increase orgasmic response
- enhance the maintenance of urinary continence.

EXCESSIVE PELVIC FLOOR MUSCLE TENSION: RELATED DISORDERS

So much emphasis is given to pelvic floor muscle weakness and the need for positive exercises that disorders presenting with excessive pelvic floor activity are not often recognised and are overlooked. The muscles need to relax to allow the bladder neck to open and initiate voiding and relax the anal canal for defecation to take place without effort. Conversely, when the pelvic floor muscles are contracted this inhibits the smooth muscle of the bladder, rectum and colon from contracting so that voiding and defecation cannot take place and continence is maintained. This coordinated interaction between smooth and voluntary muscle is essential for normal bladder and bowel control.

Disorders displaying excessive muscle tension are characterised by failure to relax at rest or when urination/defecation is required. Neurological causes are often associated with this condition but even in the absence of this, muscle tension can still exist. Causes can be obscure but women with a highly anxious disposition, experiencing high levels of stress or in pain may have tense muscles. Trauma to the pelvic floor muscles, which might have subtle nerve damage leading to pain or muscle spasms, can cause muscle overactivity because, in response to pain, the muscles contract as a protective reaction (Tries 2004). Pain or discomfort during sexual intercourse (dyspareunia) may be due to muscle tension and conditions such as vaginismus/anismus are not uncommon. A rare, but nevertheless painful, condition known as vulvodynia has shown a higher tonic resting tone of the pelvic floor muscle when measured by electromyography biofeedback (Glazer et al 1998). Although biofeedback can be used to diagnose pelvic floor tension and instability, the technique is still in its infancy as a relaxation treatment tool for vulvodynia. Further research studies are in progress. Pelvic floor muscle tension is also associated with voiding dysfunction where symptoms of hesitancy, interrupted and slow stream, urinary urgency and painful urination can be reported.

The use of biofeedback is described in detail later in this chapter but it is appropriate to mention here that it can be helpful as a behavioural approach to changing pelvic floor muscle from overactivity to a relaxed tonic activity. There is some evidence that biofeedback is proving beneficial for reducing pain and overcoming constipation and voiding dysfunction; however, it must only be used by a qualified and knowledgeable clinician, and is not readily available in all clinics. Table 3.2 provides a summary of treatments for female urinary incontinence.

PRINCIPLES OF BIOFEEDBACK FOR ASSESSING AND TREATING PELVIC FLOOR MUSCLE DYSFUNCTION

Although the literature does not support the use of biofeedback alone in treating lower urinary tract dysfunction (Schiotz et al 2003), it is a very useful adjunct to other modalities. Biofeedback represents a growing field in health care for both diagnostic and treatment purposes. Manufacturers not only sell equipment for use in clinical departments but also for patients to use in their own homes. The increasing demand by women to overcome urinary dysfunction using non-surgical interventions means that all those who specialise in treating urinary or faecal problems should be aware of biofeedback techniques and be proficient in using them.

Biofeedback is a process which provides a person with visual/auditory information about physiological functions of the body which are autonomic (under involuntary control). Diagnostic biofeedback includes procedures such as electrocardiography (ECG), electroencephalography (EEG) and the relatively new process for nurses, electromyography (EMG), which measures the electrical activity of skeletal muscle. The intrinsic electrical activity of skeletal muscle is measured in microvolts (μV) at rest and also measures the electrical potentials induced by a voluntary muscle contraction (Vodušek 1994). The bioelectrical activity reveals the muscle's pattern of contractility which demonstrates whether a muscle is normal, myopathic (weak) or reinnervated (improved function following treatment).

There is improved proprioception, which is sensation pertaining to stimuli originating from within the body regarding spatial position and muscular activity. In other words, the patient has a better awareness of where the pelvic floor muscle is and learns to control its contraction and relaxation voluntarily.

Biofeedback using specialised equipment provides an objective assessment of pelvic floor muscle function which the patient can also see or hear (depending on the equipment used), whereas the digital assessment is subjective (as described earlier in this chapter). By having the means to record a patient's progress (or not), the therapist can tailor a treatment programme to suit each individual.

Aims of biofeedback for continence

1. To improve coordination and control of the pelvic floor muscle to treat bladder dysfunction, faecal incontinence or soiling.
2. For constipation, biofeedback aims to increase the patient's control of the defecatory muscles so that the use of laxatives, suppositories or enemas can be reduced or stopped.

Table 3.2 Treatments for female urinary incontinence at a glance

Treatment	Advantages	Disadvantages	Suitable for:
PFE	Safe	Time consuming; low compliance	SUI and urge incontinence in motivated, cognitively intact women with weak muscles but ability to contract
PFE with biofeedback	Safe	Requires specialist trained clinician	Assessment of pelvic floor function; isolates muscle and motivates exercise programme
Bladder reeducation	Safe	Difficult to achieve; needs time and encouragement	Cognitive, compliant and patient women with urgency ± incontinence
Medications	Requires minimal effort	Potential for adverse effects	OAB for short-term use. SUI for short-term use when unwilling to do PFE
Electrical stimulation	Requires commitment	Time-consuming on a daily basis	Difficulty in doing PFE; symptoms not improving; try before surgery
Injection bulking agents	High short-term cure rates	Effectiveness diminishes over time	Women with sphincter deficiency
Surgery	Effective treatment in competent hands	Surgical risk; may cause other problems such as voiding difficulties	Mainly for SUI and prolapses; surgical options available (including tension-free vaginal tape)

OAB, overactive bladder; PFE, pelvic floor exercises; SUI, stress urinary incontinence.

Devices and methods for measuring biofeedback

1. Manometric: A manometer is a device that measures pressure using a graded scale with a vaginal probe, e.g. Bourne Perineometer, PFX (Mediwatch).
2. Weighted vaginal cones and similar devices: BeContent, Educator, Periform with indicator.
3. Digital examination by nurse or therapist with verbal feedback or self-examination.
4. EMG using a single needle into perineal muscle is used in research and detects signals from one motor unit.
5. sEMG uses sensor electrodes attached to the skin, intravaginal probes or intra-anal probes.
6. Ultrasonography of pelvic floor muscle (specialist physiotherapists).

Assessing pelvic floor muscle contractility using sEMG

It is important to have the patient in a relaxed and quiet environment. An explanation of the technique will assist relaxation along with some soothing background music, if possible. The surface sensors are put in place (vagina/rectum or perianal) with the patient lying comfortably in the

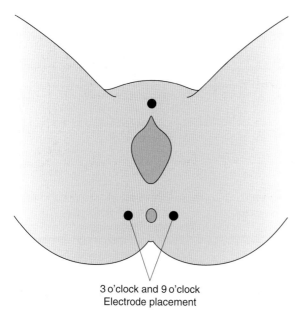

Figure 3.6   Diagram to show electrode placement either side of anal sphincter, at 3 o'clock and 9 o'clock.

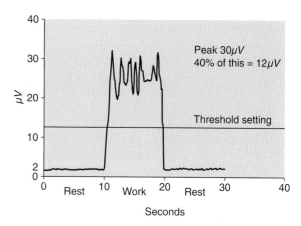

Figure 3.7   Example of contraction and calculation of threshold (e.g. average peak reading 30 μV and 40% of this value = 12 μV, the threshold setting).

supine or left lateral position. The woman may wish to insert the probe herself, but the skin sensors will need to be applied by the nurse. Special adhesive skin sensors can be placed at 3 o'clock and 9 o'clock either side of the anal sphincter (Fig. 3.6).

If the pelvic floor muscle alone is being assessed a single channel device is used and a reference lead must be attached to the skin (thigh) or hip bone to complete the circuit. If extraneous muscle groups are to be monitored (abdominals, gluteus maximus), then a dual channel device will be used and the electrodes placed accordingly on the abdominal muscle or gluteals, plus the reference electrode, usually on the thigh. The leads are then attached to the measuring device and the assessment can begin.

Without tiring the pelvic floor muscle, the woman should practise contracting and relaxing it to get the idea of what to look for on the computer screen in the form of a graph or numbers shown on the screen. The visual/auditory signal will provide feedback and act as a motivator to continue working.

Setting the threshold

As each individual's threshold level will vary, this must be established for each patient. The threshold is the goal or target point which can be achieved using maximal muscular contractions which are held for approximately 5 s, then relaxed for 5–10 s, and repeated four times. The threshold level is calculated as 40–50% of the average of the two highest peaks achieved during the contractions and this will be the patient's starting threshold or goal. Measured in microvolts, the threshold level should increase as the pelvic floor muscle improves its endurance and strength (Fig. 3.7).

Work/rest cycle

A weak pelvic floor muscle needs to build up endurance and strength gradually and to do this a series of contractions/relaxation is performed to work on the slow-twitch muscle fibres. The contraction is at maximal strength, held 4–5 s, then relaxed at least 4–5 s, and repeated five times. It is important to have the muscle relaxed at least the same length of time, if not longer, than the contraction, so that the muscle does not fatigue. The baseline resting activity of the pelvic floor muscle is usually 3 μV or less and after each contraction the muscle should return to its resting measurement (Fig. 3.8). If it does not do this, there will be

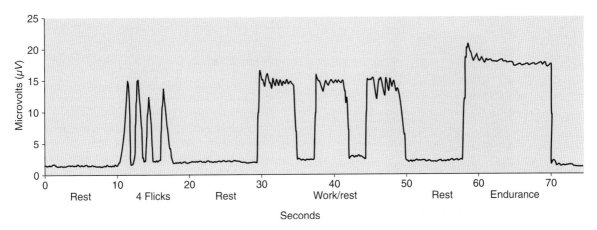

Figure 3.8   EMG line graph.

a 'staircasing' baseline. The average of the peaks may rise or fall (according to the muscle status). The average muscle deviation is calculated by the instrument being used; below 20% is considered adequate but below 12% is considered good. The onset of the contraction and the onset of the relaxation are measured in seconds and anything under 1 s is considered a normal response. As the muscle's strength improves, a longer period of time for a contraction/relaxation can be used at submaximal contraction, held for longer periods of time so muscle endurance becomes proficient. It is encouraging to have a patient work/rest the muscle for 10 or 20 s for, say, two cycles. By this stage the patient should have a healthy muscle and be symptom free.

The power of the muscle is developed by working on the fast-twitch muscle fibres. Before commencing any endurance programme, it is useful to do five quick maximal muscle contractions within 10 s, lasting only 1 s each. These exercises are essential for the muscle to automatically contract (subconsciously) during activities such as coughing, bending down, etc.

Progressive biofeedback training

- Increase work/rest ratio
- Increase threshold
- Increase percentage of maximal contraction
- Change patient position from lying/sitting to standing

- Use in functional situations – while coughing, bending, lifting.

Phases of development using biofeedback

1. Gives an awareness, identification and coordination of the pelvic floor muscle.
2. Transition – muscle control where development and strengthening begin.
3. Muscle strengthening complete and pelvic innervation improves with symptoms decreasing.
4. Muscle tone good. Digital palpation finds a firmer, bulkier and broader muscle.

The advantages of biofeedback for pelvic floor muscle control are numerous but importantly there are no side effects to this therapy. There is immediate information of the functional ability of the pelvic floor muscle so that the nurse/therapist can set an exercise or treatment programme for each individual. It stimulates motivation and compliance with exercises from the visual/auditory reinforcement and provides an objective progress report of pelvic floor muscle rehabilitation. The data on each patient should be kept in the history notes and reviewed alongside other treatments.

Before 'home' biofeedback units (Fig. 3.9) were available for patients to purchase and thus use daily at home, a patient would visit a specialist department once a week for several weeks for a 20–30 min appointment – a process that is both

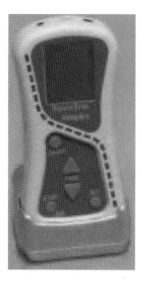

Figure 3.9 'Simplex' biofeedback unit for home use. Reproduced by kind permission of de Smit Medical Ltd.

time-consuming and expensive. It should be borne in mind, however, that while using biofeedback 'at home', progress must still be monitored at monthly intervals in a specialist clinic until the patient is discharged.

There are several patient groups that can benefit from using biofeedback. Having conscious control of the pelvic floor muscle both for contraction and relaxation will alleviate many symptoms and therefore give the individual a greater degree of control over their condition (Box 3.11). Urinary symptoms such as stress incontinence (Mørkved et al 2002), overactive bladder (urgency and urge incontinence; Wang et al 2004) and bladder outlet problems due to failure of muscles to relax can be overcome using biofeedback. For faecal urgency/incontinence (Ilnyckyj et al 2005), soiling, constipation and anismus, biofeedback has proven excellent results (Norton & Chelvanayagam 2004) (see also Ch. 8).

Contraindications to using biofeedback

Although biofeedback is a safe technique, no studies have been reported on its use during pregnancy and therefore it is usually not recommended. Women who have had a miscarriage or have been advised to avoid sexual intercourse should also avoid biofeedback if a vaginal probe is to be used. Women who suffer from vulval or vaginal inflammation or infection should not try biofeedback until the infection has been treated. However, studies using biofeedback for vulvovaginal pain (vulvodynia and vulvar vestibulitis) by Glazer et al (1998) reported 50% of patients became asymptomatic following biofeedback treatment. (*Note*: This is a very specialised area for pelvic floor muscle dysfunction and has only been mentioned here for interest.) Biofeedback is not recommended if a patient has had pelvic surgery within the last 3 months or for patients with psychosexual problems.

Training in the use of biofeedback equipment and clinical applications of use are available and nurses should always adhere to the NMC Professional Practice Guidelines (2003).

NEUROMUSCULAR ELECTRICAL STIMULATION (NMES)

The precise mechanism of electrical stimulation in the treatment of stress incontinence is unclear (Goode et al 2003); however, it has also been used in treating an overactive bladder with results which indicate a greater subjective improvement rate (Wang et al 2004). Like all conservative approaches for urinary/faecal incontinence or symptoms of overactive bladder, treatments given in isolation may not be as beneficial as in combination with other modalities; for example, NMES with biofeedback, pelvic floor exercises and bladder re-education.

Figure 3.10 (a) Electrical stimulator unit. (b) Periform probe. (c) Veriprobe. Both types of probe can be inserted into the vagina. (a, b) Reproduced by kind permission of de Smit Medical Ltd.

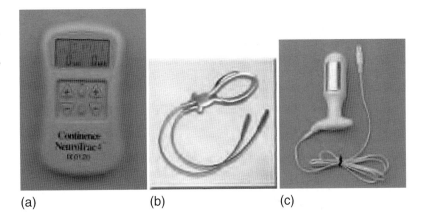

(a)   (b)   (c)

Neuromuscular electrical stimulation is used to stimulate nerves and muscles to produce a therapeutic response (Fig 3.10a). Although there are units which can be bought by individuals direct from companies, their use should first be recommended and under supervision from a trained nurse or therapist. Professional training is provided by experts in the field and, in the UK, through de Smit Medical Ltd.[1]

Before using NMES some questions should be considered:

- *What effect is intended and can this be achieved?* Sometimes this is not known until treatment is tried and often any effect will take a number of weeks to be recognised. However, an experienced clinician can usually judge effectiveness following the assessment.
- *Can this treatment complement other modalities from which the patient will benefit and be cost-effective?* Sometimes a referral to a physiotherapist is required to achieve this.
- *Is it safe for this patient?* There are some contraindications to NMES (see below).

Contraindications for use of NMES

Contraindications are listed in Box 3.12. This is quite an extensive list of contraindications and

> **Box 3.12   Contraindications for use of NMES**
>
> - Patients with a cardiac pacemaker
> - Pregnancy (no evidence but do not put woman at risk)
> - Atrophic vaginitis
> - Retention of urine
> - Pelvic masses and fistulae
> - Local inflammation
> - Immediately postpartum
> - Sexually abused
> - Umbilical/body piercing
> - Urinary tract infections
> - Vaginal discharge/menstruation
> - Inability to understand treatment
> - Severe prolapse
> - Recent surgery
> - Recent radiotherapy
> - Sensory deficit in vagina/anus
> - Unstable epilepsy
> - Haemophiliac

careful assessment will be necessary to make sure this mode of treatment is safe for the patient.

Understanding the terminology for electrical stimulation

Before detailed use of NMES is described, some terminology needs to be explained. Chapter 2 provides an overview of the physiological process involved in nerve impulses and muscle contraction.

- *Current.* A current is the flow of electrons along a conductor in a closed circuit. This is measured

---

[1]   De Smit Medical Ltd, 118A Station Road, Yate, Bristol BS37 4PQ

in amperes (amps). The electrical force is measured in volts (V) and produced by mains electricity or a battery creating an electrical potential difference between two points. An electrical current when flowing in one direction is known as a direct current (DC); when it changes direction repeatedly it is known as an alternating current (AC). Herbert (2003) states that: 'Most electrotherapy equipment gives a biphasic current, which is a direct current that has two phases during each impulse (positive and negative), thus giving the effect of a net zero direct current. This protects the tissues from a build up of electrochemicals, while still allowing effective stimulation of the tissues.'

- *Intensity/amplitude.* This is the strength of the pulse being delivered which is closely related to the current. Measured in milliamps (mA), the intensity is affected by the resistance it encounters from the tissues (e.g. skin, vaginal secretions). Sufficient intensity is required to recruit and increase contractible tissue.
- *Frequency.* This is the number of times electrical impulses per second are delivered and is measured in Hertz (Hz). The frequency chosen depends on the type of tissue being stimulated as in slow-twitch muscle fibres requiring a frequency between 10 and 20 Hz and fast-twitch fibres responding to 30–60 Hz (Fall & Lindstrom 1991).
- *Pulse duration.* This is the time factor in microseconds (μs) or milliseconds (ms) and refers to the length of time each electrical impulse lasts. The pulse duration can be altered to the patient's tolerance of discomfort but must reach a desired therapeutic effect.
- *Resistance.* As the name suggests, there is resistance or hindrance to the flow of the electrical impulses. The unit of measurement for resistance is the Ohm (Ω) and Ohm's Law states that the strength or intensity of an unvarying electrical current is directly proportional to the electromotive force (EMF) and inversely proportional to the resistance of the circuit. The skin has high resistance and can cause a problem between the electrode and the skin. It is also supplied with sensory nerve endings which makes the need for sufficient input of electrical stimulation uncomfortable for the patient. To overcome this, a water-based lubricant can help to reduce the resistance and the discomfort.
- *Duty cycle.* This is the relationship between the electrical stimulation being 'on' and being 'off'. The time stimulation 'off' must equal or be longer than the 'on' stimulation so that the muscle does not become fatigued and gives a period of time for recovery. Very weak muscles will need at least twice as long a rest time as the stimulation 'on' time. This programme can be customised according to the assessment findings.
- *Electrode.* Simply, the device by which the electrical current is delivered. In clinical practice there is a choice between a Periform probe and a Veriprobe which are used in the vagina (Fig. 3.10b,c); an Anuform probe is used in the anus and surface skin electrodes with special adhesive lubricants can reduce resistance.

Electrical stimulation parameters

Gibson et al (1988) showed that nerves control muscle by transmitting a neurological code. This code occurs in two frequency bands according to the type of muscle fibres being stimulated. Postural fibres – slow-twitch fibres – require a tonic feeding at the rate of 10 pulses per second (pps) if given for periods of 1 h or more each day. Using this technique, it is possible to maintain a baseline muscle tone until voluntary contraction can be controlled. Muscles treated this way are able to preserve bulk, capillary bed density and their essential ability to utilise oxygen (Fall 1984). Using a stimulation frequency of 10 Hz for 20 min/day is believed to reduce overactive bladder contractions (Lewey 1999) by direct inhibition of the micturition centre in the sacral part of the spinal cord at level S2–S4. A reduction in symptoms can often be seen after 2 weeks of treatment but up to 6 weeks of daily treatment can produce better results when the woman has regained better bladder control. This treatment is often used prior to the use of medications or in conjunction with an anticholinergic medication (see Ch. 9) and bladder re-education techniques.

The second frequency band occurs at 30 pps, and feeds information to the fast-twitch muscle fibres which give power to a movement. This feeding occurs naturally in a phasic way and therefore treatment to promote these fibres is given for shorter periods of time. This physiological approach to stimulating the muscles also requires pulses that are shaped like the naturally occurring nerve signals, and with very brief pulse widths. By mimicking nature as accurately as possible, electrical stimulation has been used for prolonged periods without causing any undesirable side effects. Its use for the overactive bladder over 6 weeks has produced reduction in symptoms; however, in clinical practice, its effectiveness is short lived and needs to be repeated after a period of 12–18 months (see Box 3.13). With this treatment for stress incontinence, the repeated muscle contraction by stimulation produces muscle bulk and therefore a reduction in stress incontinence symptoms. Again, however, if the woman does not continue with pelvic floor exercises she is likely to return to the clinic after a year asking for further treatment with electrical stimulation!

Effective application

For electrical stimulation to be effective the pulse duration and the intensity must be sufficient to overcome the excitation threshold of nerve fibres to be stimulated (Haslam 1998) for a contraction to take place. Pulse widths of too long a duration stimulate sensory nerves and will be uncomfortable and painful; too low an output will be comfortable but will have no therapeutic effect. The degree of movement by any muscle is controlled by two factors:

1. the muscle fibres contracting
2. the intensity of the contraction in each.

As the total impetus for muscle contraction increases, a larger number of motor neurones are 'recruited', thus activating more muscle fibres. Electrical stimulation to a muscle via a motor nerve has the specific purpose of influencing its metabolic pathway, thus preventing or reversing the changes of atrophy.

Recommended applications

- *Urgency*. Frequency at 10 Hz with a pulse duration of 200–250 ms. The duty cycle can be 4/2 s or 4/4 s and the treatment should be for 20–

> **Box 3.13   Case study 2**
>
> Chris had been urodynamically diagnosed with an overactive bladder 2 years ago and prescribed anticholinergics. At 35 years old she did not want to be on medication for the rest of her life and stopped taking the tablets although her symptoms were under control. When her urgency with incontinence returned she self-referred to the continence clinic. She was very depressed because she had had to stop her fitness class and many social activities, including dancing, because she was afraid of 'accidents'.
>
> She had one child aged 5 years. The vaginal delivery was easy and the baby weighed 7 lbs. Chris has not had any gynaecological surgery. She works part-time as a secretary which fits in with the family commitments. Chris had not been told of bladder re-education and so had almost stopped drinking in an attempt to reduce her continence problem. Chris was given a chart to keep for a week and had to record the volume of drinks, toilet visits and episodes of incontinence. She was given full instructions on bladder re-education and taught to contract the pelvic floor muscle whenever she felt the 'urge' to urinate. Her pelvic floor muscle squeeze was good.
>
> She was seen 2 weeks later with her chart at which time her frequency per day was 10–14 times and nocturia 2–3 times. The above education was continued and she was asked to increase her daily fluid intake to 2 litres. She was also commenced on electrical stimulation for urgency (described above) for 20 min each day. A further 2 weeks later her frequency was 8–10 times during the day and nocturia 1–2 times. Her self-confidence was returning. She did not take further medication and continued with bladder re-education and electrical stimulation for a further 4 weeks when her symptoms were back to normal values: 4–8 times daily and no nocturia. She had control of her urgency and used her pelvic floor muscles functionally. Her intake of fluids was no longer restricted and she was back in the social world. She was discharged from the clinic.
>
> One year later Chris was back in the clinic asking for electrical stimulation as frequency symptoms had returned which she was unable to control. She decided to buy her own unit for use when required as she felt confident using one and liked the idea of no medication. She has not needed to return to the clinic again.

25 min/day. The outcome objective here is to strengthen the perineal–detrusor inhibitory reflex and suppress the parasympathetic detrusor activity. Fast-twitch fibre recruitment is avoided but there is trophic strengthening of deep, slow-twitch postural muscle fibres. This application increases energy levels and enhances the ability to utilise oxygen; protein synthesis also improves.

- *Stress incontinence.* Frequency at 30–40 Hz with a pulse duration of 200–250 ms. The duty cycle is 4/4 s on and off but can be customised to avoid fatigue. A tetanic contraction is required at maximum tolerable intensity. The clinical outcome expected is an improvement in muscle bulk and tone and women are encouraged to work with the stimulation to improve awareness and start their own contractions of the pelvic floor muscle. A daily treatment of 25 min is recommended.

Stimulation units can be used at home but a clinician should have prescribed the treatment for the symptoms and should monitor progress.

Other approaches to strengthening pelvic floor function

Weighted vaginal cones and similar systems

Another method used to improve the performance of pelvic floor muscle exercises is to supplement the exercises with weighted vaginal cones. A cone is inserted into the vagina and if the muscles are contracted correctly the cone is prevented from slipping out of the vagina. The weight of the cone is selected so that it can just be retained but the pelvic floor muscles have to be exercised to keep the cone in position. As pelvic floor muscle strength increases, the weight of the cone can be increased. Although the method seems intuitively as if it should work, there is little research evidence to show that cones work and their use has declined. Other products such as the *BeContent Pelvic Floor Toning System* and *The Educator* (http://www.desmitmedical.com) are designed to work on similar principles except that an indicator tip is attached to the cone/probe which should move downwards when the pelvic floor muscles are contracted correctly. The aim is to improve awareness of contraction for some women.

BEHAVIOURAL THERAPIES FOR OAB

The mainstay of treatment for OAB is behavioural therapy, often combined with pharmacotherapy with anticholinergic agents such as oxybutynin (see Ch. 9). The therapeutic value of time spent with a knowledgeable and caring practitioner should not be underestimated and reassurance that this is a common, treatable condition can have significant benefits.

Bladder re-education programmes

The purpose of re-educating a bladder is to achieve effective control of micturition at a level which is satisfactory for the patient. This behavioural technique is used primarily to control and reduce symptoms of urgency and frequency, and a variety of distraction techniques can be used to help to suppress urgency and gradually extend toileting intervals. When trying to retrain a bladder to hold a 'normal' volume the approach should be to increase the time between each void by teaching the patient to 'hold on' when the bladder sensations are noticed and to tighten the pelvic floor muscle as forcefully as possible for 5 s. Allowing the bladder to fill to capacity and then to empty completely is the goal, but this takes time and patience so the patient must be mentally and physically capable and also well motivated. Intervals between voids may increase by only 10–15 min at first. A weekly chart can help some patients to see their own progress (but it can also depress others who fail to respond to this therapeutic approach). Bladder re-education is often done in combination with anticholinergic drugs (see Ch. 9) and/or electrical stimulation as mentioned earlier in the chapter.

Other forms of behavioural bladder training include prompted voiding and timed voiding which may be appropriate in patients with cognitive and/or physical deficits (see Chs 6 and 7). Systematic reviews of bladder re-education strategies have been carried out for bladder training (Wallace et al 2004), prompted voiding (Eustice et al 2002), timed voiding (Ostaszkiewicz et al 2005) and habit training (Ostaszkiewicz et al 2004).

CYSTITIS AND URINARY TRACT INFECTION (UTI)

This subject requires a book of its own so it will only be mentioned briefly here. Nurses deal with catheter-related UTIs very frequently and this is covered in Chapter 10. Many women experience a UTI during their lifetime; most are asymptomatic and clear up spontaneously. However, some women will have recurrent symptomatic infections which affect the quality of their life, including sexual relationships.

Indigenous intestinal bacterial flora are the primary source of urinary pathogens. These organisms contaminate the vagina and perineum and ascend into the bladder via the short urethra in the female (males are much less prone to UTIs). The most common organism is *Escherichia coli,* which accounts for up to 85% of acute infections. Less common organisms are *Proteus mirabilis, Klebsiella pneumoniae, Aerobacter aerogenes* and, rarely, Gram-positive cocci.

A UTI can affect any part of the urinary tract, but it is the 'adherence' of the bacteria that is an important factor in the pathogenesis of infections. The urinary tract has a natural ability to resist bacterial colonisation and the intruding bacteria are efficiently eliminated by the interaction of multiple mechanisms, including the flushing action of voiding, urine acidity, osmolality, organic acids and high concentrations of urea, which have a role in inhibiting bacterial adherence and growth. The bladder mucosa has intrinsic antibacterial properties and destroys those bacteria remaining on its surface after micturition. Self-help remedies include increasing fluid intake of water and cranberry juice (see Ch. 10). If women do not empty their bladder completely and leave a residual urine, it reduces the host defence and makes them more susceptible to UTIs (Iravani 1988).

Symptomology

The woman complains of frequency of micturition, but dysuria may be absent or only minor with a UTI. If *cystitis* is the problem (inflammation of the bladder tissue), the woman complains of frequency of micturition, urgency, dysuria and suprapubic discomfort. Between 20 and 30% of women presenting with classic symptoms of cystitis will *not* have a urinary tract infection.

Investigations

A midstream specimen of urine (MSU) is essential for diagnosis, and antibiotic treatment should be commenced only according to the results of the culture and sensitivity. It is unsound practice to treat a woman with a presumptive diagnosis as many cultures are negative and antibiotics will not be required.

Upper tract pathology may be adequately investigated by renal ultrasound and X-ray of kidneys, ureters and bladder (KUB). Cystourethroscopy may be performed and a bladder biopsy may show evidence of chronic inflammation. Cystourethroscopy is more relevant in the elderly, as recurrent UTI could be the presenting symptom of a transitional cell carcinoma.

Women under 40 years of age should have a urodynamic investigation to eliminate the diagnosis of detrusor instability as this condition also gives rise to urgency symptoms. Urodynamic studies will also reveal mechanical outflow obstruction which may have resulted from previous bladder neck surgery. These women may not be emptying the bladder completely, thus suffering from symptoms of cystitis, but will have negative urine cultures.

Interstitial cystitis

Frequent episodes of cystitis do not inevitably lead to interstitial cystitis (IC) but if a condition becomes chronic it must be investigated further. Women are affected more commonly than men but IC can occur at any age. The cause of IC is still unknown, hence the difficulty in treating the condition. The main symptoms present as frequency (which may be up to 60 times a day in severe cases), urgency and pain. Pain can be in the abdomen, urethra or vaginal area, thus pain is also associated with sexual intercourse. Differences between IC and bacterial cystitis are shown in Box 3.14.

Symptoms vary between patients and many self-help coping mechanisms are learned from other sufferers via the Interstitial Cystitis Support Group or on http://www.interstitialcystitis.co.uk. The International Painful Bladder Foundation (http://www.painful-bladder.org) is another source of information and support. Because of the time it takes to get a diagnosis and then explore the different approaches to treatment, support groups play an important role and offer educational literature and information.

Box 3.14 Differences between IC and bacterial cystitis

Interstitial cystitis	Bacterial cystitis
Long-term frequency	Frequency during attacks
Clear urine specimen	Urine cloudy and odorous
No bacteria present in urine	Bacteria shown in urine
Symptoms not relieved by antibiotics	Symptoms relieved by antibiotics
Temporary relief when voiding	Pain during voiding
Pain/discomfort with bladder filling	No symptoms with bladder filling
Continuous/permanent symptoms	Attacks last a few days

A urologist is likely to include some or all of the following investigations which are essential for any urological problem: urine and blood tests; cystoscopy usually followed by a cystodistension; urodynamic studies; ultrasound; bladder biopsy; voiding cystourethrogram; X-ray of kidneys, urethra and bladder and, of course, a full physical examination.

Treatments offered

There is not one effective treatment to suit all patients but the most common approaches which aim to alleviate the symptoms include:

- *Bladder distension.* This is stretching the bladder with water while the person is under general anaesthetic.
- *Oral medications.* These include anti-inflammatories, antispasmodics, antihistamines, muscle relaxants and antidepressants (amitriptyline appears to have anti-pain properties).
- *DMSO (dimethyl sulfoxide).* A medication which is instilled into the bladder and is believed to have an anti-inflammatory effect, thus reducing pain.
- *Cystostat.* A bladder instillation to restore defective bladder lining and barrier function.
- *TENS unit.* A unit which supplies a low electrical current via surface electrodes attached over the

bladder to relieve pain. Can be administered continuously or intermittently.
- *Diet and nutrition.* Eliminating certain foods may decrease the severity of the symptoms.

The long-term debilitating effect of IC cannot be understated as quality of life is seriously eroded. People become isolated and fear going out in public, the pain is often too great for socialising. Repeatedly getting up at night to go to the toilet results in severe tiredness and going to work is difficult. Research continues to seek effective treatments but until the cause is known this is difficult. Patients with this condition require a lot of support and should be given the contact number of the support group in their area.

Cranberry juice

Several studies have focused on the antimicrobial adherence activity of cranberry juice and its alteration of the urinary pH (Schmidt & Sobata 1988). Cranberry juice contains substantial quantities of alpha-D-mannopyranoside, a derivative of the sugar D-mannose. This compound attaches to the lectins of bacteria and inhibits 'adherence' to the bladder wall. Pure cranberry juice with no added sugar is best and can even be taken by diabetics, but monitor carefully. A recommended dose at the first sign of a burning sensation on micturition is to drink 250 ml and repeat 4-hourly. Capsules are also available and the recommended dose is to take two twice a day or one every 3 h.

SURGICAL PROCEDURES FOR BLADDER DYSFUNCTION

It is not within the remit of this book to look at surgical options in detail but an indication of the range of interventions is provided below.

Prolapse

- *Anterior colporrhaphy*: to correct a cystocele
- *Posterior colporrhaphy*: to correct a rectocele
- *Manchester repair* (not common): amputation of cervix in addition to anterior repair
- *Sacrospinous fixation*: to correct vaginal vault prolapse via the vagina

- *Sacrocolpopexy*: as above but performed through an abdominal incision.

Stress urinary incontinence

- *Marshall–Marchetti–Krantz*. Retropubic procedure to elevate and stabilise the urethra and bladder neck.
- *Burch colposuspension*. Similar to above.
- *Laparoscopic colposuspension*. Smaller incisions and longer to perform than above procedure but an increased rate of surgical complications.
- *Tension-free vaginal tape (TVT) colposuspension*. The tape rests without tension under the urethra like a hammock which gives support during increased intra-abdominal pressure. (A more detailed explanation of the above surgical interventions with pre- and postoperative nursing care can be found in Lee (2005).)
- *Transobturator sling (TOT)*. Recently introduced as an alternative to TVT as fewer complications are reported (Miklos 2004). Rather than the TVT sling through the abdominal wall, the TOT is introduced by a needle through the obturator foramen.
- *Periurethral injection*. Injecting a bulking agent, usually collagen, either side of the urethra. Short-term cure rate is high but efficiency deteriorates over time.

Overactive bladder

- *Cystodistension*. To increase bladder capacity by overstretching the bladder with water while the patient is under anaesthetic. This procedure has not been shown to have a lasting effect.
- *Intravesical Botox*. Botulinum A toxin (Botox) injected into the detrusor muscle blocks the release of acetylcholine from presynaptic cholinergic nerve terminals, resulting in neuronal blockade. It lasts about 9 months and the patient may need to do intermittent self-catheterisation (ISC). This relatively new approach still needs further investigation of effects (Hussain & Nethercliffe 2004).
- *Augmentation cystoplasty*. Increasing bladder capacity by augmenting it down the trigone with a segment of ileum. Not without complications and ISC may be necessary.

- *Urinary diversion*. A last resort for intractable incontinence for those unable to do ISC. The bladder is bypassed and a stoma created on the abdomen where urine is collected into a urostomy bag.

SUMMARY

This chapter has highlighted bladder problems in women and their effect on quality of life and sexuality. Although education via healthcare professionals, the media, the Internet and women's magazines has increased over the years, there remains reluctance by the majority of women to seek advice when symptoms are first noticed. It can be seen from this chapter that cure is frequently possible with conservative treatments if started early enough and surgery can be avoided. Promoting compliance with a lifetime programme of pelvic floor exercises is still a challenge to healthcare professionals as is, indeed, the approach to continence promotion in women. Specialist nurses and therapists can offer a wide range of non-invasive treatments and offer education to support staff in the community and in hospital environments. In October 2006 the National Institute for Health and Clinical Excellence (NICE) published a guideline for the management of urinary incontinence in women, in conjunction with the National Collaborating Centre for Women's and Children's Health. Key priorities for implementation are summarised in Box 3.15.

KEY POINTS FOR PRACTICE

UNDERSTAND
- the effects of childbirth on the prevalence of urinary incontinence and the role of female hormones in the incidence of bladder dysfunction
- the special issues surrounding the menopause and bladder dysfunction
- the effects of incontinence on quality of life and sexuality
- the value of performing a pelvic floor examination and be trained in the techniques

SKILLS
- Be proficient in treatment skills for biofeedback and electrical stimulation

> **Box 3.15** Summary of some of the key priorities for implementation from the NICE guidelines on the management of urinary incontinence (UI) in women (2006)
>
> **ASSESSMENT AND INVESTIGATION**
> - At the initial clinical assessment the woman's UI should be categorised as stress UI, mixed UI or urge UI/overactive bladder syndrome (OAB). Initial treatment should be started on this basis. In mixed UI treatment should be directed towards the predominant symptom
> - Bladder diaries should be used in the initial assessment of women with UI or OAB. Women should be encouraged to complete a minimum of 3 days of the diary covering variations in their usual activities, such as working and leisure days
> - The use of multichannel cystometry, ambulatory urodynamics or videourodynamics is not recommended before starting conservative treatment
>
> **CONSERVATIVE MANAGEMENT**
> - A trial of supervised pelvic floor muscle training of at least 3 months' duration should be offered
>
> as a first line treatment to women with stress or mixed UI
> - Bladder training for a minimum of 6 weeks should be offered as a first line treatment to women with urge or mixed UI
> - Immediate release, non-proprietary oxybutynin should be offered to women with OAB or mixed UI as a first line drug treatment if bladder training has been ineffective. If immediate release oxybutynin is not well tolerated, other formulations should be considered. Women should be counselled about the adverse effects of antimuscarinic drugs
> - Pelvic floor muscle training should be offered to women in their first pregnancy as a preventative strategy for UI

- Improve your skills in bladder scanning and do not forget voiding difficulties in women – an often missed diagnosis

BE PROACTIVE

- Find out about support groups for interstitial cystitis, menopause, Urostomy Association, *In*contact and other self-help groups for your patients
- Design your own leaflets for patients for pelvic floor exercises and bladder re-education, or any useful charts to encourage compliance

Useful websites

http://www.bloomex.com
http://www.desmitmedical.com
http://www.dxu.com/primarycare

http://www.fpnotebook.com
http://www.greenjournal.org
http://www.hsc.mb.ca/nursing
http://www.icsoffice.org
http://www.medscape.com
http://www.ncbi.nlm.nih.gov/entrez
http://www.neenpelvichealth.com
http://www.nice.org.uk
http://www.obgyn.net
http://www.pelvicfloor.com
http://www.promocon.co.uk
http://www.SUI.com
http://www.thewomenshealthsite.org
http://www.thoughttechnology.com/biofeed.htm
http://www.uagbi.org
http://www.universityobgyn.com

References

Abernethy K 2005 The menopause. In: Andrews G (ed) Women's sexual health, 3rd edn. Baillière Tindall, London, p 453

Abrams P, Cardozo L, Khoury S, Wein A 2005 Incontinence, vol 1. Health Publication, Paris

Al-Badr A, Ross S, Soroka D et al 2003 What is the available evidence for hormone replacement therapy in women with stress urinary incontinence? Journal of Obstetrics and Gynaecology Canada 25(7):567

Aukee P, Immonen P, Laaksonen D E et al 2004 The effect of home biofeedback training on stress incontinence. Acta Obstetrica et Gynecologica Scandinavica 83(10):973–977

Behtash N, Ghaemmaghami F, Ayatollahi H et al 2005 A case-control study to evaluate urinary tract complications in radical hysterectomy. World Journal of Surgical Oncology 3(1):12

Bø K, Finckenhagen B 2001 Vaginal palpation of pelvic floor muscle strength: inter-test reproducibility and comparison between palpation and vaginal squeeze pressure. Acta Obstetrica et Gynecologica Scandinavica 80(10): 883

Bø K, Kvarstein B, Nygaard I 2005 Lower urinary tract symptoms and pelvic floor muscle exercise adherence after 15 years. Obstetrics and Gynecology 105:999–1005

Brown J, Vittinghoff E, Wyman J et al 2000 Urinary incontinence: does it increase risk for fall and fractures? Journal of the American Geriatric Society 48:721–725

Buchsbaum G M 2005 Vaginal birth not linked to urinary incontinence. Obstetrics and Gynecology 106:1253–1258

Cardozo L 1991 Urinary incontinence in women: have we anything new to offer? British Medical Journal 303:1453–1457

Cardozo L, Cutner A, Wise B 1993 Basic urogynaecology. Oxford Medical Publications, Oxford

Chiarelli P 1991 Women's waterworks: curing incontinence. de Smit Medical, Bristol

Chiarelli P, Murphy B, Cockburn J 2003 Women's knowledge, practices, and intentions regarding correct pelvic floor exercises. Neurourology and Urodynamics 22(3):246–249

Dolman M 1992 Midwives' recording of urinary output. Nursing Standard 6(27):25–27

Dolman M, Chase J 1996 Comparison between the health belief model and subjective expected utility theory: predicting incontinence behaviour in post-partum women. Journal of Evaluation in Clinical Practice 2(3):217–222

Duong T H, Korn A P 2001 A comparison of urinary incontinence among African American, Asian, Hispanic and white women. American Journal of Obstetrics and Gynecology 184:1083–1086

Eason E, Labrecque M, Marcoux S et al 2004 Effects of carrying a pregnancy and of method of delivery on urinary incontinence: a prospective cohort study. BMC Pregnancy and Childbirth 19:4

Elia G, Dye T D, Scariati P D 2001 Body mass index and urinary symptoms in women. International Urogynecology Journal 12:366–369

Eustice S, Roe B, Paterson J 2002 Prompted voiding for the management of urinary incontinence in adults (Cochrane Review). Cochrane Library Issue 2. Update Software. John Wiley, Chichester

Fall M 1984 Does electricostimulation cure urinary incontinence? Journal of Urology 131(4):664–667

Fall M, Lindstrom S 1991 Electrical stimulation: a physiologic approach to the treatment of urinary incontinence. Urologic Clinics of North America 18(2):393–407

Foldspang A, Mommsen S, Djurhuus J C 1999 Prevalent urinary incontinence as a correlate of pregnancy, vaginal childbirth and obstetric techniques. American Journal of Public Health 89(2):209

Gibson J, Smith K, Rennie M 1988 Prevention of disuse muscle atrophy by means of electrical stimulation: maintenance of protein synthesis. Lancet 2(8614):767–770

Glazer H I, Jantos M, Hartmann E H et al 1998 Electromyographic comparisons of pelvic floor in women with dysesthetic vulvodynia and asymptomatic women. Journal of Reproductive Medicine 43:959–962

Goode P, Burgio K, Locher J L et al 2003 Effect of behavioural training with or without pelvic floor electrical stimulation on stress incontinence in women. Journal of the American Medical Association 290(3):345

Graber B, Kline-Graber G 1979 Female orgasm: role of the pubococcygeus muscle. Journal of Clinical Psychiatry 40:348–351

Hannestad Y, Rortveit G, Sandvik H, Hunskaar S 2000 A community-based epidemiological survey of female urinary incontinence: the Norway EPINCOT study. Journal of Clinical Epidemiology 53:1150–1157

Hannestad Y, Lie R, Rortveit G, Hunskaar S 2004 Familial risk of urinary incontinence in women: population based cross-sectional study. British Medical Journal 329:889

Haslam J 1998 Treating urinary incontinence using biofeedback and neuromuscular stimulation. Journal of Community Nursing 12(2):23–25

Herbert J 2003 The principles of neuromuscular electrical stimulation. Nursing Times 19(99):13th May Supplement

Hunskaar S 1999 Prevalence study on urinary incontinence in Asia. Asia Pacific Continence Advisory Board. In: Abrams P, Khoury S, Wein A (eds) Incontinence. Health Publication, Plymouth

Hunskaar S, Lose G, Sykes D et al 2004 The prevalence of urinary incontinence in women in four European countries. British Journal of Urology 93(3):324–330

Hussain M, Nethercliffe J 2004 Update on the non-medical management of overactive bladder. Urology News 6(8):6–8

Ilnyckyj A, Fachnie E, Tougas G 2005 A randomised-controlled trial comparing an educational intervention alone vs education and biofeedback in the management of faecal incontinence in women. Neurogastroenterology and Motility 17(1):58

Iravani A 1988 Causes, diagnosis and treatment of bacterial infections of the urinary tract. Comprehensive Therapy 14(11):49–53

Jackson S, Shepherd A, Brookes S et al 1999 The effect of oestrogen supplementation on post-menopausal urinary stress incontinence: a double-blind placebo-controlled trial. British Journal of Obstetrics and Gynaecology 106:711–718

Kizilkaya Beji N, Yalcin O, Ayyildiz E H 2005 Effects of urinary leakage on sexual function during sexual intercourse. Urologia Internationalis 74:250–255

Klein M C, Janssen P A, MacWilliam L et al 1997 Determinants of vaginal–perineal integrity and pelvic floor functioning in childbirth. American Journal of Obstetrics and Gynecology 176:403–410

Laycock J 1994 Clinical evaluation of the pelvic floor. In: Schüssler J, Laycock J, Norton P, Stanton S (eds) Pelvic floor re-education: principles and practice. Springer-Verlag, Berlin, Chapter 2.2

Lee L 2005 Gynaecological investigations and surgery. In: Andrews G (ed) Women's sexual health. Baillière Tindall, London, p 568–571

Lewey J 1999 Electrical stimulation of the overactive bladder. Professional Nurse 15(3):211–214

MacLennan A H, Taylor A W, Wilson D H et al 2000 The prevalence of pelvic floor disorders and their relationship to gender, age, parity, and mode of delivery. British Journal of Obstetrics and Gynaecology 107(12):1460–1470

McPherson K, Herbert A, Judge A et al 2005 Self-reported bladder function five years post-hysterectomy. Journal of Obstetrics and Gynaecology 25(5):469–475

Miklos J R, Moore R D, Kohli N 2004 Laparoscopic pelvic floor repair. Obstetrics and Gynecology Clinics of North America 31:551–565

Miller J, Ashton-Miller J A, DeLancey J O L 1996 The Knack: use of precisely timed pelvic floor muscle contraction can reduce leakage in SUI. Neurourology and Urodynamics 15(4):392–393

Milsom I, Abrams P, Cardozo L et al 2001 How widespread are the symptoms of an overactive bladder and how are they managed? A population-based prevalence study. BJU International 87:760–766

Mørkved S, Bø K, Fjørtoft T 2002 Effect of adding biofeedback to pelvic floor muscle training to treat urodynamic stress incontinence. Obstetrics and Gynecology 100:730–739

National Institute for Health and Clinical Excellence 2006 Urinary incontinence: the management of urinary incontinence in women. Royal College of Obstetricians and Gynaecologists, London (RCOG Press). Online. Available: http://www.nice.org.uk/page.aspx?o=CG40

Norton C, Chelvanayagam S (eds) 2004 Bowel continence nursing. Beaconsfield Publishers, Beaconsfield

Nursing and Midwifery Council 2003 Professional practice guidelines. NMC, London

O'Brien J, Long H 1995 Urinary incontinence: long-term effectiveness of nursing intervention in primary care. British Medical Journal 311:1208

Ostaszkiewicz J, Johnson L, Roe B 2004 Habit training for urinary incontinence in adults: systematic review (Cochrane Review). Cochrane Library Issue 2. Update Software. John Wiley, Chichester. Online. Available: http://www.update-software.com/Abstracts/AB002801. htm

Ostaszkiewicz J, Roe B, Johnston L 2005 Effects of timed voiding for the management of urinary incontinence in adults: systematic review. Journal of Advanced Nursing 52(4):420–431

Radley S, Rosario D, Chapple C et al 2001 Conventional and ambulatory urodynamic findings in women with symptoms suggestive of bladder overactivity. Journal of Urology 166:2253–2258

Reay-Jones N H, Healy J C, King L J et al 2003 Pelvic connective tissue resilience decreases with vaginal delivery, menopause and uterine prolapse. British Journal of Surgery 90(4):466–472

Rosario D J, Chapple C R, Bradshaw H D, Radley S C 2000 Urinary leakage during coitus is a sign of instability in women with urinary urgency. Abstract, International Continence Society, Tampere, Finland

Schiotz H, Mørkved S, Bo K et al 2003 Effect of adding biofeedback to pelvic floor muscle training to treat urodynamic stress incontinence. Obstetrics and Gynecology 101(5):1024–1025

Schmidt R D, Sobata A E 1988 An examination of the anti-adherence activity of cranberry juice on urinary and non-urinary bacterial isolates. Microbias 55:173–181

Sherburn M, Guthrie J R, Dudley E C et al 2001 Is incontinence associated with menopause? Obstetrics and Gynecology 98(4):628–633

Smith P, Roberts M, Slade N 1970 Urinary symptoms following a hysterectomy. British Journal of Urology 42:3–9

Stewart W F, Van Rooyen J B, Cundiff G W et al 2003 Prevalence and burden of overactive bladder in the United States. World Journal of Urology 20:327–336

Sweet B R 1988 Mayes' midwifery: a textbook for midwives. Baillière Tindall, Edinburgh, p 234

Thom D H, van den Eeden S K, Brown J S 1997 Evaluation of parturition and other reproductive variables as risk factors for urinary incontinence in later life. Obstetrics and Gynecology 90:983–989

Tries J 2004 Disorders related to excessive pelvic floor muscle tension. Online. Available: http://www.aboutincontinence.org/PelvicFloor.html

Van der Vaart C H, de Leeuw J R, Roovers J P et al 2002 The effect of urinary incontinence and overactive bladder symptoms on quality of life in young women. BJU International 90:544–549

Vodušek D 1994 Electrophysiology. In: Schüssler J, Laycock J, Norton P, Stanton S (eds) Pelvic floor re-education: principles and practice. Springer-Verlag, Berlin, Chapter 2.8

Wallace S, Roe B, Williams K et al 2004 Bladder training for urinary incontinence in adults (Cochrane Review). Cochrane Library Issue 1. Update Software. John Wiley, Chichester

Wang A C, Wang Y Y, Chen M C 2004 Single-blind, randomised trial of pelvic floor muscle training, biofeedback-assisted pelvic floor muscle training, and electrical stimulation in the management of overactive bladder. Urology 63(1):61–66

Weil A, Reyes H, Rottenburg R D et al 1983 Effect of lumbar epidural anaesthesia on lower urinary tract function in the immediate postpartum period. British Journal of Obstetrics and Gynaecology 90:428–432

Weiss B D, Newman D K 2002 New insights into urinary stress incontinence: advice for the primary care clinician. http://www.medscape.com/viewprogram/1961

Chapter 4

Mainly men

Angela Billington

All we are, is the result of what we have thought. The mind is everything. What we think . . . we become.

> Buddha (563–483 BC)

INTRODUCTION

There are limited data about the incidence, spontaneous remission rates and risk factors for urinary incontinence (UI) in men. It is estimated that between 2.5 and 4 million adults experience continence problems in the UK (Continence Foundation 2000). In almost all community-based studies to date, the reported prevalence rates are less in men than in women by a 1:2 ratio; however, after the age of 65, prevalence rates are similar (Malmstein 1997, Stenzelius et al 2004). This said, the issue of incontinence in the younger male population cannot and should not be ignored.

The type and age distribution are also different between the sexes, and the risk factors, although less investigated in men, seem to be different. Incontinence should not be considered an isolated problem in men, but rather as a component of a multifactorial problem. These are often referred to as LUTS (lower urinary tract symptoms) which include storage symptoms such as frequency, urgency and nocturia and voiding symptoms such as poor flow, hesitancy, intermittent flow and terminal dribbling.

Whilst many of the causes of incontinence are not specific to either sex and the principles of continence promotion and incontinence management are generally common to both, the male urinary tract and associated structures do present some very specific issues of causality and management. An increasing focus and interest in men's health should result in further research being undertaken in this area. The potential impact of UI on the life of an individual, male or female, should not be underestimated and much can be done to assist men who are experiencing continence problems. This chapter builds upon the principles covered throughout the book and focuses specifically upon those aspects of care that are considered to be 'mostly pertinent to men' – the causes of LUTS and prostate disease.

PREVALENCE

Prevalence of incontinence in men ranges from 3 to 39% depending on the population studied, the definition of incontinence used and the survey methods (Wilson et al 2005). A recent survey of men in four different cities in France, England, Korea and the Netherlands identified an incontinence prevalence rate in men over 65 years ranging from 8% in Seoul to 23% in Birmingham (Boyle et al 2003) but the authors suggest that cultural differences may contribute to the rates recorded. A systematic review of 21 studies reported a prevalence of UI in older men ranging from 11 to 34%. In the same review, the prevalence of daily UI in men ranged from 2 to 11%. Studies that use a broad definition of urinary incontinence, include older and institutionalised men, and/or use self-reporting methods, tend to report higher prevalence (Thom 1998). For any definition of UI there is an increase in prevalence with age.

Due to differences in pathological anatomy and pathophysiology of urinary incontinence in men and women, there is a different distribution in incontinence subtypes. Hunskaar et al (2005) confirmed previous reports of the predominance of urge incontinence (40–80%) in men, followed by mixed forms of UI (10–30%) and stress incontinence (<10%). The increasing prevalence by age is due to urge incontinence rather than stress.

CAUSES OF LUTS IN MEN

The most likely cause of LUTS is related to the prostate. Symptoms can reflect either storage or voiding problems. Storage problems may be due to reduced capacity, which can be due to a small capacity bladder, incomplete emptying due to bladder outflow obstruction, increased detrusor activity due to idiopathic causes, or irritative problems caused by urinary tract infection, obstruction or bladder cancer. Outflow obstruction may be due to benign prostatic hyperplasia or prostate cancer, urethral or meatal obstruction, penile cancer or detrusor failure due to neuropathy, or may be drug induced with anticholinergics or opioids.

ASSESSING THE PROBLEM

Micturition does not conform to a standard pattern and exhibits wide variation between individuals (see Ch. 2). Few studies have examined voiding patterns of healthy volunteers and further baseline data are needed for both males and females. However, there appears to be little difference, at least in frequency of voiding, between the sexes (Denning 1996).

The urethra and pelvic floor

Males have an 'S'-shaped urethra which is approximately 18–22 cm in length, compared to the shorter, straight urethra in females (3–5 cm). This factor is associated with a lower incidence of urinary tract infections (UTIs) in men compared to women. UTIs are, in turn, frequently cited as causes or risk factors for transient urinary incontinence by increasing sensory input from the bladder and contributing to urgency and detrusor instability. UTI may also exacerbate other types of bladder dysfunction. However, whilst the length and shape of the male urethra may have a protective function with regard to infection, these characteristics can contribute to other problems such as the 'postmicturition dribble' experienced by many men and discussed later in the chapter.

Stress incontinence results primarily from a failure of the external urethral sphincter to accommodate increases in intra-abdominal pressure. The external (voluntary) sphincter is formed by the pelvic floor muscles; any factor contributing to a reduction in the strength of these muscles or in the patency of the seal formed by the urethra is therefore likely to predispose an individual to stress incontinence (see Chs 2 and 3). In fact, genuine stress incontinence is rare in neurologically normal males, although it may result from prostate surgery or chronic retention (RCP 1995).

Postmicturition dribble

Postmicturition dribble (PMD) describes the loss of a small amount of urine after voiding is completed. It is unique to men and is a common and annoying condition in later life and one which can affect quality of life. It can be an important factor in motivating men to consult their doctor. Milliard (1989) suggested that postmicturition dribble that is not associated with obstruction might be caused through the urethra being emptied incompletely by the muscles surrounding it. Denning (1996) suggests that it is caused by pooling of urine in the bulbar urethra which for some reason is abnormally lax and wide. Pelvic floor exercises or bulbar urethral massage are recommended as treatment for this annoying but benign problem. This technique is sometimes referred to as 'milking the urethra' and involves putting the ball of the thumb behind the testicles and pushing up and forward to exert pressure on the urethra, causing the urine to be expelled.

The prostate gland

The healthy prostate is a small gland about the size of a walnut lying just below the bladder. It forms part of the male reproductive system, is attached to the base of the bladder and surrounds the initial 3–4 cm of the urethra; the urethra passes through the centre of the gland to the penis. The main function of the prostate is to make a lubricant as part of the seminal fluid. It is suggested that the prostate acts a bit like a 'junction box' in that it allows the ducts that transport sperm from each testicle and the ducts that drain from the

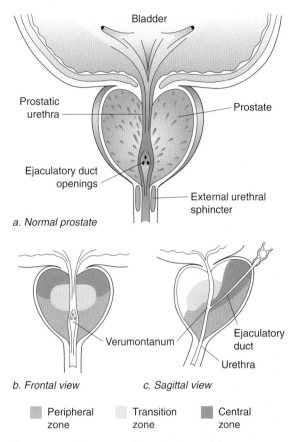

a. Normal prostate

b. Frontal view   c. Sagittal view

Peripheral zone   Transition zone   Central zone

Figure 4.1 Anatomy and morphology of the prostate. Reproduced with permission from Kirby & McConnell (2004).

seminal vesicles to meet and then empty their contents into the urethra during ejaculation.

The prostate gland is divided into two morphologically distinct zones, central and peripheral, that comprise 25% and 70% of the normal prostatic volume respectively. The remaining 5% of the normal gland consists of the transition zone which lies adjacent to the urethra and extends up to the bladder neck (Fig. 4.1). Although the histological characteristics of the transition zone and the peripheral zone are similar, the transition zone is the site of development of benign prostatic hyperplasia, while the adjacent peripheral zone is the more usual site of prostate cancer (Kirby et al 1994).

Three main diseases of the prostate can affect urinary continence:

- benign prostatic hyperplasia
- prostate cancer
- prostatitis.

Benign prostatic hyperplasia

Benign prostatic hyperplasia (BPH) is by far the most common disease of the prostate: 80% of presenting cases, compared with 18% prostate cancer and 2% prostatitis (Kirby et al 1994). BPH increases with age and this may reflect an age-related hormonal imbalance between testosterone and oestrogen. Classic autopsy studies (Ball et al 1981) have shown that histological BPH appears to rise to 50% in men in their 60s and to 90% in men over 80 years of age; however, the proportion of men with palpable prostatic enlargement or symptoms is less, with a prevalence of 21% in men aged 50 and 60 years, rising to 53% in men in their 80s. A population study from Stirling, UK (Garroway & Collins 1991), also reported a prevalence of symptomatic BPH of 43% in men over 60. BPH is one of the most common diseases to affect men beyond middle age and is now so common among older men that its absence could be regarded as abnormal (Webb & Simpson 1997). About half of the men with evidence of BPH (more than 20 g, symptoms of LUTS and a peak flow less than 15 ml/s) reported interference with one or more activities of daily living (Box 4.1).

BPH is rarely a life-threatening condition when appropriately assessed and managed. Deterioration in symptoms and urinary flow is usually slow, and serious outcomes, such as renal insufficiency, are uncommon. The incidence of acute retention increases with prostate size and requires

> **Box 4.1 Adverse effects of symptoms of BPH on activities of daily living**
>
> - Limits fluid intake before travel
> - Restricts fluid intake before bedtime
> - Cannot drive for 2 hours without a break
> - Disruption of sleep
> - Limits going to places without toilets
> - Limits playing outdoor sports
> - Limits participation in social activities, e.g. going to the cinema, theatre or church

urgent treatment. The relatively less serious symptoms of frequency, nocturia and incomplete emptying can nevertheless be very bothersome and may substantially impact on the patient's quality of life. In addition, men with LUTS due to BPH are also prone to erectile dysfunction and disorders of ejaculation (Dorey 2001a). The symptoms of BPH can vary but the typical ones are:

Obstructive symptoms:

- a hesitant, interrupted, weak stream of urine
- straining to void.

Irritative voiding symptoms:

- urgency and urge incontinence
- frequency of urination, especially at night.

As the population ages it seems inevitable that the number of men presenting with BPH will increase. Prostate assessment clinics are a response to this perceived trend. The clinics aim to reduce waiting times, lead to prompt referral of those with severe symptoms and to provide better continuity and quality of care (Webb & Simpson 1997).

Prostate cancer

Prostate cancer is the most commonly diagnosed cancer in men in the UK, accounting for almost one in four of new male cancers diagnosed (Cancer Research UK 2006) and 14% of male deaths from cancer. This represents the second most common cause of male deaths from cancer after lung cancer (Figs 4.2 and 4.3).

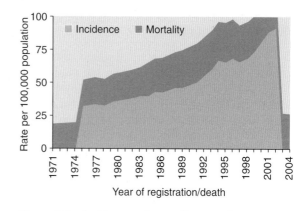

Figure 4.2 Incidence and mortality rates for prostate cancer. Reproduced from Cancer Research UK (2006).

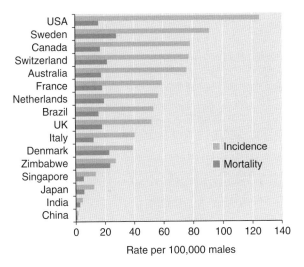

Figure 4.3   Incidence and mortality rates, prostate cancer in selected countries. Reproduced from Cancer Research UK (2006).

Table 4.1   Gleason grading system

Grade	Histological characteristics	Probability of local progression over 10 years (%)
1–4	Well differentiated cancer	25
5–7	Moderately differentiated cancer	50
8–10	Poorly differentiated cancer	75

Ethnic variations appear to exist and death rates are raised in Caribbean and West African men. In terms of prevalence, prostate cancer shows a similar pattern to BPH, in that it is generally a disease of older men and is rare in the under-50 age group. By the age of 80 about half of all men will have a focus of cancer in their prostate, although only 1 in 25 males will actually die from it (DH 2000a).

Treatments for prostate cancer can lead to the unwanted side effect of urinary incontinence. Indeed continence may be the second 'big C' they must confront as they begin to cope with the impact of the cancer treatment. Although bladder disturbance can be temporary, patients view their incontinence as disabling with a negative effect on their quality of life (Butler et al 2001).

The stage and grade of prostate cancer   There are a number of ways to treat prostate cancer depending upon how far the disease has spread. There are four basic stages: by convention the letters 'TNM system' (tumour, node, metastases) is used as a prefix for the stage of the cancer (i.e. T1, T2, T3, T4). Staging is extremely important in the decision-making process; if the cancer has spread beyond the prostate margins surgery will not be curative (Fig. 4.4).

To help decide whether the cancer is likely to progress quickly the tumour grade is scored using a graded scale invented by Dr Donald Gleason. This system assigns a grade ranging from 1 to 5 based on the arrangement of the cancer cells in relation to normal prostate cells. If the cancer cell cluster resembles the small, regular, evenly spaced glands of normal prostate tissue, a Gleason grade of 1 is assigned. If the cancer cells lack these features and seem to spread haphazardly, it is a grade 5. Because prostate cancers often have areas with different grades, primary and secondary grades are given to the two areas that make up the most cancer. The Gleason score is therefore made up of the two grades (e.g. 3 + 2 = 5); the higher the score out of 10, the more likely that the cancer will grow and spread rapidly (Table 4.1).

In view of the non-specific nature of prostatic symptoms, careful diagnosis is important. There are three recognised methods of distinguishing prostate cancer from BPH: prostate-specific antigen (PSA), digital rectal examination and transrectal needle biopsy. The cause of prostate cancer is unknown. However, several risk factors have been identified:

- Having relatives who have had cancer of the prostate
- Belonging to certain ethnic groups (African–Caribbean/African–American)
- Eating a diet high in animal fat and protein (DH 2000a).

The symptoms of BPH and prostate cancer are often similar and the majority of men with these symptoms have benign disease. However, some individuals who have cancer are asymptomatic and, for some, symptoms occur only at the late

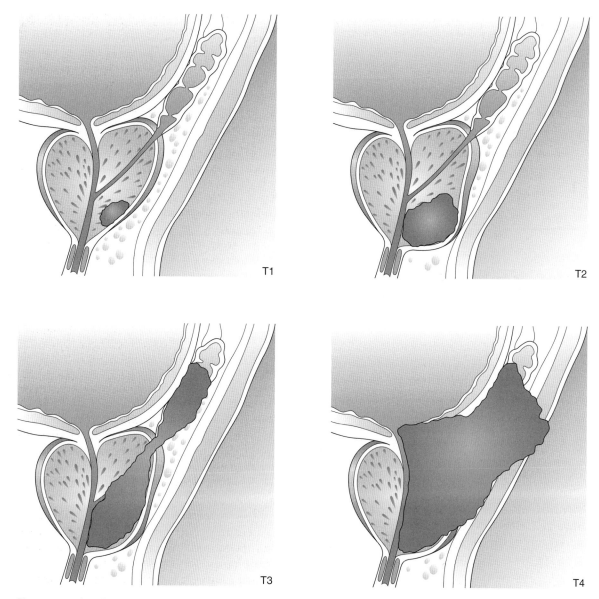

Figure 4.4 Local staging of prostate cancer. The tumour may advance from T1 to T4 with or without the development of metastases. Reproduced with permission from Kirby & McConnell (2004).

stages of the disease. Clearly early diagnosis is important and will be discussed later.

Prostatitis

The prostate is spongy and contains innumerable channels and ducts, which can be prone to infection. If an obstruction such as a urethral stricture occurs distal to the prostate, infected urine maybe forced into the prostatic ducts and cause prostatitis. Acute prostatitis can occur without warning with a systemic illness marked by rigors, fever and muscular pain. Clinically, the patient is very uncomfortable and feels aching in the perineum, which radiates to the thighs and penis. Passing urine is painful and the stream may be thin, with symptoms of frequency and often a high fever (Box 4.2). Palpation reveals a tender, swollen prostate and the urine may or may not grow pathogens on culture. If organisms are identified they should be treated with either a fluoroquinolone or a sulfa-based antibiotic such as trimethoprim that can penetrate the prostatic tissue in adequate quantities. Treatment must be given for 6 weeks for acute flare-ups and 12 weeks for those patients who are chronically symptomatic. Prophylactic or suppressive antibiotics plus prostatic massage may be required in refractory, relapsing or recurrent disease. Surgery, except as definitive therapy for a lower urinary tract problem (e.g. bladder neck stenosis or urethral stricture), should be considered only as a last resort (Kirby R 1997).

ASSESSMENT OF INDIVIDUALS WITH SUSPECTED PROSTATE DISEASE

Urinary incontinence is an embarrassing and unpleasant complaint which many people hide from their families, friends and indeed healthcare professionals. Men seem to be particularly reluctant to seek help, often seeing incontinence as a 'woman's problem' (Hunskaar & Sandvik 1993). Most men with incontinence or evidence of urinary tract outflow symptoms can be managed in primary care. The outcome is likely to be improved if the patient and healthcare professional decide on treatment in partnership, with promotion of self-management (NICE 2000). It is widely accepted that general screening for prostate disease is not practicable but opportunistic questioning can play a vital role in identifying cases of prostatic disease. There are three essential questions:

- Are you bothered by your bladder symptoms?
- Do you get up at night to urinate more than twice?
- Have you recognised a change in your urinary flow?

Further investigation should be offered if the patient answers yes to more than one of these questions (Billington 1999). Completing the International Prostate Symptom Score (I-PSS) (Barry et al 1992), one of several validated tools used to assess the severity of an individual's symptoms (Fig. 4.5), and a full prostatic assessment (Box 4.3) (Billington 1999) provide a qualitative and quantitative assessment of the impact and extent of prostatic symptoms.

Investigations should include the following.

International Prostate Symptom Score (I-PSS)

The I-PSS is used to check the 'bother' factor for the patient. A score of less than 7 indicates mild symptoms, 8–19 moderate symptoms, and more than 18, severe symptoms. Those with a symptom score of more than 19 should be referred for further medical advice. Any assessment should include reference to the impact that the individual's prostate problem is having on their life in general. Although the single question shown in Figure 4.5 will not capture the total impact of symptoms on

Patient Name

Date

		Not at all	Less than one time in five	Less than half the time	About half the time	More than half the time	Almost always	Your score
1.	*Incomplete emptying* Over the past month how often have you had the sensation of not emptying your bladder completely after you finish urinating?	0	1	2	3	4	5	
2.	*Frequency* Over the past month how often have you had to urinate again less than 2 hours after you finished urinating?	0	1	2	3	4	5	
3.	*Intermittency* Over the past month how often have you found you stopped and started again several times when you urinate?	0	1	2	3	4	5	
4.	*Urgency* Over the past month how often have you found it difficult to postpone urination?	0	1	2	3	4	5	
5.	*Weak stream* Over the past month how often have you had a weak urinary stream?	0	1	2	3	4	5	
6.	*Straining* Over the past month, how often have you had to push or strain to begin urination?	0	1	2	3	4	5	
		None	1 time	2 times	3 times	4 times	5 times or more	
7.	*Nocturia* Over the past month, how many times did you most typically get up to urinate from the time you went to bed at night until the time you got up in the morning?	0	1	2	3	4	5	

Total I-PSS score

The total score can range from 0–35 (asymptomatic to very symptomatic). Although there are at present no standard recommendations on grading patients with mild, moderate or severe symptoms, patients can be tentatively classified as follows:

1–7 = mildly symptomatic   8–19 = moderately symptomatic   20–35 = severely symptomatic

	Delighted	Pleased	Mostly satisfied	Mixed – about equally satisfied and dissatisfied	Most dissatisfied unhappy	Terrible
Quality of life due to urinary symptoms If you were to spend the rest of your life with your urinary condition just the way it is now, how would you feel about that?	0	1	2	3	4	5

Figure 4.5 International Prostate Symptom Score (I-PSS). Reproduced with permission from Barry et al (1992).

quality of life, it may serve as a valuable starting point on which to base further conversation between the practitioner and the patient.

Frequency/volume chart

This provides an indication of fluid intake patterns, type of fluid drunk, functional bladder capacity, frequency and the presence and degree of nocturia experienced (see Ch. 2).

Uroflowmetry

Uroflowmetry provides a simple means of quantifying the degree of outflow obstruction. Electronic measurement of urine flow rates is an extremely useful, non-invasive test in most patients with BPH (Fig. 4.6) and is helpful in identifying patients whose peak flow rate is not diminished and thus unlikely to benefit from surgery. Such patients are more likely to be complaining of an overactive bladder rather than BPH. Uroflowmetry measures a number of parameters of obstruction, of which the most important is the peak flow rate. A peak flow rate below 15 ml/s (with voided volume of at least 150 ml) suggests obstruction (Kirby & McConnell 2004) although in older men (70–80 years of age) values of 10 and 15 ml/s may be normal. The presence of a markedly reduced peak flow rate (<10 ml/s) usually indicates some degree of obstruction which is most often caused by BPH. Uroflowmetry is an inadequate test to assess obstruction versus impaired detrusor function as the cause of a low flow rate and is prone to artefact if the bladder volume is less than 150 ml.

Postvoid residual (PVR)

PVR is measured by transabdominal ultrasound and is a useful optional test in the evaluation of BPH, especially in combination with uroflowmetry, as it can help separate patients who are likely to respond to watchful waiting or medical therapy from those who may not. In general, PVR values above 200–300 ml usually indicate a higher likelihood of medical therapy failing, and probably also indicate a higher risk of acute urinary retention (AUR). The test cannot be used to confirm or exclude BPH. It may be useful as a safety measure in monitoring the progress of patients who opt for watchful waiting.

Urinalysis

Urinalysis, either by dipstick or by microscopic examination of sediment, should be performed in all men presenting with LUTS. Urinalysis helps to distinguish BPH from urinary tract infection or bladder cancer, which may produce similar symptoms. If urinalysis is positive, urine microscopy and culture should be carried out and further imaging and evaluation of the renal tract considered. Urine cytology should be requested in those with severely irritative symptoms or haematuria to exclude carcinoma in situ of the bladder. If urine cytology is positive, renal ultrasound and lower tract endoscopy and biopsy are mandatory; CT scan is optional (Kirby & McConnell 2004).

Digital rectal examination

Digital rectal examination (DRE) should be performed on all men with LUTS. Although the prostate is readily palpated by DRE, in its early stages prostate cancer is seldom detectable. DRE is usually performed by the patient's GP, but nurse specialists may also conduct DRE. The test provides vital information regarding size of the prostate, consistency and anatomical limits. A normal prostate feels smooth, about the size of a walnut, with the lateral and cranial borders and medial sulcus of the prostate being identifiable; the seminal vesicles should be impalpable. An enlarged prostate is indicative of BPH, whereas a hardened, nodular prostate, or an immobile prostate, is suggestive of cancer. The examination may feel uncomfortable but tenderness upon examination is an indication of prostatitis (Table 4.2). The examination also allows the nurse to assess rectal muscle strength and skin health in the perianal area. Overall, DRE in isolation is less than 50% accurate in detecting prostate cancer and is usually done in conjunction with PSA (DH 2000a).

Blood tests

Blood tests should be performed for renal function and to measure PSA, a protein produced by the

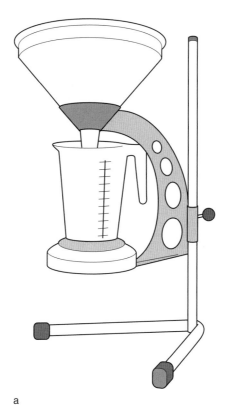

a

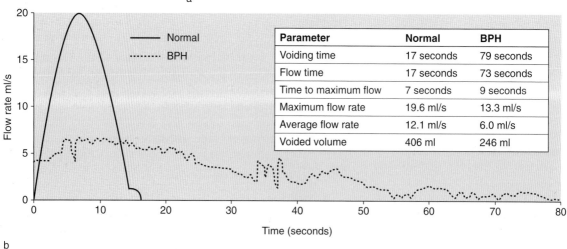

Parameter	Normal	BPH
Voiding time	17 seconds	79 seconds
Flow time	17 seconds	73 seconds
Time to maximum flow	7 seconds	9 seconds
Maximum flow rate	19.6 ml/s	13.3 ml/s
Average flow rate	12.1 ml/s	6.0 ml/s
Voided volume	406 ml	246 ml

b

Figure 4.6 Uroflowmetry using a flowmeter (a) measures a number of parameters of obstruction (b) that are usually altered in patients with BPH. (b) Reproduced with permission from Kirby & McConnell (2004).

prostate. Creatinine and electrolyte levels are measured to check renal function, as some 10% of patients with BPH who have seen a urologist have some renal impairment (Kirby M 1997). Prostate enlargement tends to cause an increase in the level of the PSA, with malignant tumours producing a greater increase than benign enlargement. However, other conditions can also cause PSA to rise, such as a UTI and prostatitis. Although serum PSA testing has fundamentally transformed the

Table 4.2 Assessment through digital rectal examination

Characteristic	Appearance
Size	The normal prostate gland is the size of a walnut; enlargement occurs in both BPH and prostate cancer
Consistency	A normal prostate is smooth or elastic The lateral lobes are symmetric and divided by a palpable sulcus A tender prostate may indicate prostatitis A hard nodular prostate may indicate prostate cancer
Mobility	A malignant prostate gland may be fixed to adjacent structures

diagnosis and treatment of prostate cancer, the ability of PSA to correctly discern cancer from benign disease is imperfect. This has prompted efforts to improve the diagnostic capability of PSA assays. Produced by epithelial cells and secreted into the prostatic ducts, PSA is a serine protease that may enter the systemic blood circulation where it exists in several forms that are classified into two broad categories: unbound or 'free' forms (fPSA) and bound or 'complexed' forms (cPSA).

Three different PSA assays are commercially available and applicable to clinical urology: tPSA, fPSA and cPSA. The oldest, most ubiquitous assay is the tPSA assay, which measures all immunoreactive forms of PSA, free and complexed, present in serum, i.e. total PSA. The tPSA assay is sensitive for prostate cancer detection but suffers from low specificity. Low specificity increases the number of unnecessary biopsies, and it is this diagnostic shortcoming that newer assays have sought to rectify. The fPSA assay provides the percentage of free PSA (%fPSA, the ratio of fPSA to tPSA) which has greater specificity than tPSA for prostate cancer. When applied properly, fPSA may reduce unnecessary biopsies on 20% of men with tPSA in the 4–10 ng/ml range (Catalona et al 1998).

The cPSA assay was also developed to improve specificity. The rationale for cPSA testing is that the proportion of cPSA is greater in men with prostate cancer (Kellogg Parsons & Partin 2004).

cPSA is a versatile assay applicable to population screening and diagnosis, and to prediction of pathological stage and longitudinal serum monitoring in patients with prostate cancer. For detection of cancer, cPSA is significantly more specific than tPSA at all clinically relevant sensitivities, is as specific as %fPSA and is less costly. Kellogg Parsons and Partin recommend that cPSA is used as the initial diagnostic test for prostate cancer with a preliminary recommended threshold of 3.2 ng/ml or greater for biopsy. They also recommend that cPSA could be used in staging nomograms and longitudinal evaluation of patients with prostate cancer. This would have the benefit of reducing the number of unnecessary biopsies, diminish screening costs and potentially minimise the confusion associated with multiple serum assays. Therefore, although a slight elevation in the PSA may indicate prostate cancer, it is by no means definite; approximately two out of three men with a raised PSA will not have prostate cancer. The advantage of PSA testing is that it can find cancer before symptoms develop and may detect cancer at an early stage when treatment could be beneficial. The downside is that it can miss cancer and provide false reassurance; alternately, false positives may cause unnecessary anxiety and medical tests when no cancer is present. It may detect slow-growing cancer that may never cause any symptoms or shorten lifespan. The PSA debate is a complex one.

To screen or not to screen?

Although there is pressure to introduce prostate cancer screening within the UK, the view of the National Screening Committee (2000a,b) is that there is currently no high-quality evidence that screening reduces mortality and that present knowledge about prostate cancer does not conform to the majority of the 10 principles that should govern a national screening programme, proposed by the World Health Organization in 1968. Yet screening is recommended in other countries, particularly the USA. Men or their partners obtain information about PSA from websites and may request or even demand testing. Further ethical issues surround those correctly identified as having prostate cancer as it is often impossible to distinguish between slow-growing tumours that cause no harm and fast-growing tumours that kill (DH 2000a). If screening were to be introduced, some men with low-grade prostate cancer might be subjected to traumatic treatment with the unpleasant side effects of erectile dysfunction and incontinence, who might never have suffered any ill effects from prostate cancer in their lifetime. The National Institute for Health and Clinical Excellence (NICE) is due to report on *Prostate Cancer: Diagnosis and Treatment* in November 2007.

For those men concerned about the possibility of prostate cancer, the PSA test is still available. However, clear information about the benefits and risks of testing should be provided to men to ensure that they are fully informed of the reliability of the test before giving consent. The impetus for improvement in this area of care comes from the Prostate Cancer Risk Management Programme (http://www.cancerscreening.nhs.uk/prostate) which provides information packs for GPs and for patients, with guidance on understanding the PSA test, and through the National Prostate Cancer Programme which funds an extensive programme of research on all aspects of prostate cancer diagnosis and treatment (DH 2000a). At present, prostate screening is not recommended for routine use, based on evidence provided in two systematic reviews of the literature (Chamberlain et al 1997, Selley et al 1997). Further work is being funded in this area, but this does not affect the clinical management of men with symptoms of prostate cancer.

European Randomised Study of Screening for Prostate Cancer (ERSPC)

The ERSPC study is currently the largest randomised controlled trial of prostate cancer screening. It aims to determine whether the effect of early detection and treatment of prostate cancer will reduce deaths from prostate cancer. There are eight participating centres: the Netherlands, Sweden, Finland, Belgium, Italy, Portugal, Spain and Switzerland. Recruitment to the study is still underway and the target is to recruit 180 000 men in total. Each man will be chosen at random to either be screened for prostate cancer (using the PSA test with or without DRE) or join a control group which will not be screened. The first results from the study are expected before 2010.

Transrectal ultrasound and biopsy

When DRE and/or PSA abnormalities are present, transrectal ultrasound (TRUS) provides the most convenient and accurate way of obtaining prostatic biopsies. An automatic biopsy needle is advanced transrectally under ultrasound control and sextant prostate biopsies are taken. With adequate antibiotic cover (typically ciprofloxacin within 24 h of the biopsy), morbidity of TRUS biopsy is minimal and infectious complications occur in approximately 2% (Desmond et al 1993).

Clearly other causes of urinary symptoms (e.g. infection, overactive bladder or stress incontinence) need to be excluded and a comprehensive baseline assessment in keeping with that currently recommended by the Department of Health (2000a) applies equally to those presenting with prostate symptoms. However, when an individual presents with acute urinary retention its immediate relief is an urgent priority if backpressure on the kidneys is to be prevented. Having decided on the diagnosis, treatment options need to be explored.

BPH and prostate cancer: treatment options

The treatment of BPH and prostate cancer do have some similarities, but also marked differences. They are therefore considered separately for ease of discussion. The main treatment options are discussed within this section. For a more comprehensive and detailed account, the reader is referred to more specialist texts.

In males with BPH, if there is no urgent reason to refer, a period of conservative treatment of 3 months is recommended (Abrams 1997, Feneley et al 1999). If the patient has mild to moderate obstructive symptoms, medical management with alpha-blockers and/or 5-alpha reductase inhibitors is generally the first approach. For those with irritative voiding symptoms, bladder training, advice on fluid intake, pelvic floor exercises, plus or minus an anticholinergic drug if the patient is thought to have detrusor instability, may also assist. It is not uncommon for some men to experience a year or more during which their prostate irritates them, only for symptoms to get better without any treatment (Blandy 1998).

Men can be taught how to carry out pelvic floor exercises in the same way as women (see following radical prostatectomy later in the chapter for further details), but have the added advantage that by practising in front of a mirror they can observe muscle contraction at the base of the penis and a scrotal lift. They can also learn to palpate muscle contraction at the perineum 2 cm medially and 2 cm anteriorly to the ischial tuberosity (Dorey 2001b). This is useful when teaching and learning the correct technique but the frequency and intensity of the exercise regime are determined by individual assessment and DRE. Although it is common practice to recommend that men practise pelvic floor muscle training (PFMT) prior to transurethral resection of the prostate (TURP), there are no substantive data to support this practice.

Medical management of BPH has revolutionised the care that men are now receiving and consists primarily of alpha-blockers and/or 5-alpha reductase inhibitors. Surgery has become the secondary rather than the primary treatment for those with mild symptoms. Surgery as the first choice is still indicated for men who are experiencing persistent, moderate or severe symptoms or who have had acute urinary retention. Surgical prostate ablation, by TURP or less frequently open prostatectomy, is still the 'gold standard' and produces the greatest measurable and long-term reduction in both symptoms and bladder outlet obstruction (Feneley et al 1999). Other methods of ablation (e.g. laser techniques) are newer and evidence of their efficacy is currently limited.

Treatment of BPH

As suggested earlier, conservative treatment or 'watchful waiting' is the preferred option for men with mild symptoms as disease progression is uncertain and often slow (Billington 1999). If the patient wishes to try drug therapy an alpha-blocker (e.g. prazosin, indoramin) is usually the treatment of first choice for BPH, since its effects, if any, are immediate (Feneley et al 1999). These drugs improve both filling and voiding symptoms in BPH by relaxing smooth muscle and reducing urethral resistance. Caution is advised in the treatment of older men or those on antihypertensives using this method. However, some drugs are now said to be more urospecific or selective and therefore to have fewer side effects (e.g. alfuzosin). Nonetheless, patients using these drugs should be advised of potential side effects such as postural hypotension and dizziness.

The use of 5-alpha reductase inhibitors to shrink the epithelial part of the gland is another option. The action of drugs such as finasteride is to reduce the size of the prostate by suppressing plasma levels of dihydrotestosterone (DHT), the principal agent causing prostatic enlargement. However, it is suggested that these drugs benefit only a minority of men, with maximum effect taking at least 6 months to be achieved (Feneley et al 1999). Men receiving alpha reductase inhibitors need to be warned of potential side effects such as erectile dysfunction, reduced ejaculate volume and loss of libido (Billington 1999) (Tables 4.3 and 4.4).

Surgical treatment of BPH most commonly involves transurethral resection of the prostate. An instrument is passed along the urethra to the prostate gland and the enlarged prostate is 'pared' away from inside the urethra (Fig. 4.7). The process can easily be visualised if you imagine the coring of an apple. The aim of this technique is to relieve the obstruction at the bladder neck and thereby relieve the retention of urine. The process of TURP may have to be repeated several times as the prostate continues to enlarge and the frequency at which surgery has to be repeated varies between individuals. The procedure is usually performed under general anaesthetic and is a relatively successful option for those who are fit enough to undergo surgery.

Other forms of prostate ablation such as transurethral incision of the prostate and laser therapy are becoming increasingly popular, although TURP is still the more usual procedure. Other alternatives such as the use of radiowaves, microwaves and prostatic stent insertion (a coil-like catheter that is placed in the prostatic urethra) are also used (Downey 2000). However, an open

Table 4.3 Drug dosage and potential side effects

Drug	Dosage	Side effect
5-alpha reductase inhibitor		
Finasteride	5 mg od for 6 months, thereafter continue long term	Impotence 3% or reduced ejaculate
Selective alpha agents		
Doxazosin	1–8 mg od	Postural hypotension or dizziness
Indoramin	20 mg	
Prazosin	0.5–2 mg bd	
Terazosin	5–10 mg, gradually increasing od	
Super selective alpha agents		
Alfuzosin	2.5 mg tds/5 mg bd	
Tamsulosin	0.4 mg od	

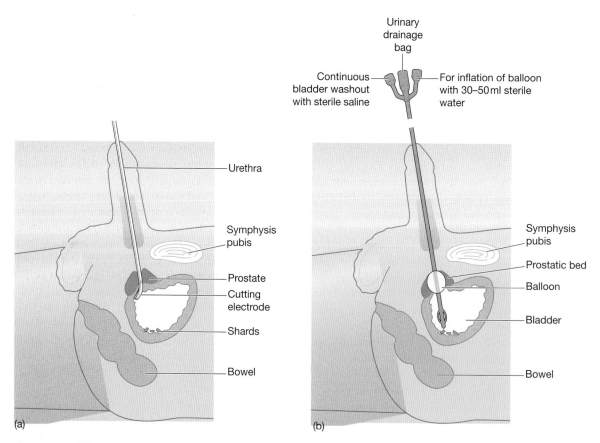

Figure 4.7 (a) Transurethral resection of prostate (TURP). (b) Three-way catheter allowing continuous irrigation of the bladder to remove shards of prostate tissue.

Table 4.4 Side effects of prostate cancer treatments

Treatment	Side effects	Percentage with side effects
Radical prostatectomy	Incontinence	65
	Impotence	80
Radiotherapy	Diarrhoea	10
	Colitis	
	Rectal pain/bleeding	
	Urinary frequency	5–10
	Impotence	40–60
Antiandrogen	Absent libido	90
	Impotence	
	Hot flushes	
	Breast tenderness	
	Cardiovascular problems	
Chemotherapy	Most side effects are temporary and include nausea, vomiting, loss of appetite	100

prostatectomy will be done when men have very enlarged glands as the length of time to remove the tissue endoscopically would be excessive and place the patient at risk of haemorrhage from the resection site and deep venous thrombosis from venous stasis after prolonged leg elevation in stirrups (Game & Farrer 1989).

Complications following TURP

All surgery carries risks. Prostate surgery can result in urinary incontinence and/or retrograde ejaculation, aside from the possibility of immediate postsurgical complications such as haemorrhage and hypovolaemic shock (Morrison et al 1994). Postsurgical urinary incontinence is attributed to the trauma associated with surgery in the area of the bladder neck. Newer treatments such as radiowave (transurethral needle ablation) and laser therapy tend to be associated with less incontinence (Downey 2000).

Nearly all men who have undergone TURP experience retrograde ejaculation. Small numbers of men also suffer from erectile dysfunction for reasons not well understood. Both erectile dysfunction and urinary incontinence are associated with open prostatectomy (Downey 2000). It is therefore particularly important that consent to surgery is informed and that men are aware of the potential urinary and sexual problems that may follow. Sexual problems such as erectile dysfunction can sometimes be the result of anxiety rather than a direct consequence of the surgery. Whatever the underlying cause of the problem, referral to a specialist clinic is the main course of action. The impact that a loss of potency and incontinence can have on an individual in terms of self-image should not be ignored and is considered in more detail later.

A programme to assist the achievement of full continence after prostatectomy should be instigated as soon as possible (see the 'Advice sheet' in Box 4.4). Several options exist to promote postsurgical urinary continence, including pelvic floor re-education and bladder training programmes. Evidence to support the effectiveness of PFMT after TURP is weak and further research is required to elucidate the benefit. A recent Cochrane Review by Hunter et al (2006) of the conservative management of incontinence after TURP concluded that its value remains unclear and that men's symptoms tended to improve over time irrespective of treatment. After radical prostatectomy, there may be modest benefit up to 3 months post surgery of initiating a PFMT routine. Nonetheless, some support for the benefit of pelvic floor re-education and bladder retraining in treating urinary incontinence does exist although more trials are clearly indicated (DH 2000b). Insertion of an artificial urethral sphincter (Fig. 4.8) may be an option for a small proportion of men with intractable postprostatectomy incontinence (Cheater 1996). Venn et al (2000) reviewed long-term outcomes following sphincter implantation and concluded that postprostatectomy incontinence seemed especially amenable to such treatment. Fluid volume or specifically designed bladder training charts such as that reproduced in Figure 2.9 can be useful in helping both the patient and the healthcare professional assess and monitor the improvement of urinary symptoms.

Box 4.4   General postprostatectomy advice sheet

It is anticipated that following the removal of your catheter you will experience a degree of urinary urgency and leakage specifically on movement. To reduce this leakage and help regain bladder control, a programme of pelvic floor exercises and bladder retraining is suggested.

1. Pelvic floor exercises help to retrain the muscles around the bladder neck; try to do the exercises five slow and five fast, 10 times a day (total 100 exercises).
2. After-dribble is also a common problem and can be cured by a simple milking technique (squeeze and lift) or push up behind the scrotum and straighten the penis forward. This dislodges the urine trapped in the bend of the urethra (the tube from the bladder).
3. Bladder retraining will help rectify the frequency and urgency. It is common to have altered bladder sensation following prostate surgery. It is often helpful to keep a diary of how often you pass urine and then try to work on holding on or delaying voiding for a few minutes. As your bladder responds to this training the frequency will reduce.
4. Fluid intake is important. Do not restrict your fluids as concentrated urine will irritate your bladder and make your urgency worse and also increase your risk of urinary infection. Try to consume 8–10 drinks a day and avoid caffeinated fluids as these tend to irritate the bladder and also have a diuretic effect (pass through the body more quickly than water or decaffeinated drinks).
5. Constipation is also a common problem; ask your healthcare professional for advice. A dietary supplement of linseed may help.
6. It is generally advisable to purchase extra protection for a few days. Disposable pads are available in many shapes and sizes. Products are available from most chemists but ask your healthcare professional for advice.

Treatment of prostate cancer

The treatment and care of men diagnosed with prostate cancer depends upon the extent of the disease although the evidence base for these decisions is limited. For early stage cancer the options

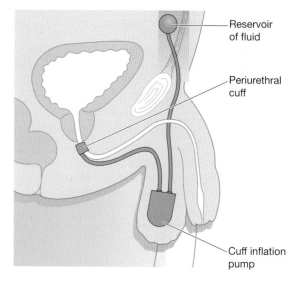

Figure 4.8   An artificial sphincter.

include 'watchful waiting' (to determine whether the cancer is active or slow growing), radical prostatectomy and radiotherapy. For cancer that has spread beyond the prostate, radiotherapy and hormone therapy remain the main treatment options (DH 2000a). Treatment decisions are largely dependent on the stage of the cancer at the time of diagnosis. There are a number of options, each with its advantages and disadvantages, and include surgery, radiotherapy and drug therapy. For early localised disease there are considered two curative options:

1. *Radical radiotherapy* treats cancer by using high-energy rays that destroy cancer cells. For prostate cancer this may be achieved in two ways: using an external beam that produces X-rays that focus on the prostate from outside of the body or using brachytherapy. The latter involves the insertion (under a general anaesthetic) of small radioactive seeds that release radiation slowly over time. Both forms of radiotherapy have side effects, but brachytherapy appears to result in less damage to the bowel and less erectile dysfunction (DH 2000a).
2. *Radical prostatectomy* involves removal of the prostate gland, prostatic capsule, seminal vesicles and prostatic urethra. Intraoperative nerve stimulation techniques have been developed

which theoretically help reduce erectile dysfunction by assisting the surgeon to identify the nerves. Laparoscopic approaches reduce hospital stays but it is unclear whether surgical or oncological outcomes are improved. Cryoablation is rare except in select centres and is accompanied by significant incontinence and erectile dysfunction.

For cancers that have spread beyond the prostate, radiotherapy and hormone therapy are the options of choice. Hormone therapy relies on the fact that most prostate cancers depend on a continuing supply of androgens, mainly testosterone. Reducing the amount of circulating testosterone by removing the testicles (orchidectomy) or by medical castration can help to control prostate cancer and relieve symptoms for months or years. Pharmacological treatment may often be used as an adjunct to surgical intervention when margins are positive and PSA starts to rise after radical prostatectomy (DH 2000a).

There are two main types of pharmacological therapy: luteinising hormone releasing hormone (LHRH) analogues and total androgen ablation or blockade. LHRH analogues act directly on the pituitary gland to inhibit the release of follicle stimulating hormone and luteinising hormone, thus blocking production and release of testosterone. Total androgen blockade is used when a patient no longer responds to other hormonal treatments. Some antiandrogens are given in conjunction with an LHRH analogue or bilateral orchidectomy. This regimen blocks the effect of all circulating testosterone, including that produced by the adrenal glands (Griefzu 2000). These treatments are not without side effects, in particular hot flushes, decreased libido, erectile dysfunction, lethargy, weight gain and mood changes. Moreover, bone loss and osteoporosis are serious consequences of hormone treatment that have, until recently, been overlooked. Men on hormone replacement are at high risk of hip fractures and vertebral compression and must be advised to follow a calcium-rich diet and include a daily calcium supplement.

Cytotoxic chemotherapy using drugs such as methotrexate to prevent growth of the malignant cells may also be employed, but this is a late stage treatment. However, none of the above non-surgical treatments is shown to be superior and none is wholly effective (Marsh 1992, DH 2000a).

At present there is no definitive evidence as to which is the best treatment, especially for early stage tumours, one reason being that some people with early stage disease will often live 10 years or more if no treatment is used. However, it is difficult to predict what course prostate cancer will take in an individual. It is therefore essential that the decision for treatment is shared with the patient and information on outcomes is discussed. The study by Hall et al (2003) shows that factors beyond 'cancer cure' are important to patient treatment decisions (such as risk of incontinence and/or sexual dysfunction) and improved educational approaches are needed to aid decision making.

Radical surgery

Radical prostatectomy (RP) with a nerve-sparing technique is seeing increased popularity in the UK for localised disease. However, considerable morbidity exists following RP, including erectile dysfunction and urinary incontinence, the incidence of which ranges from 2.5 to 87% depending on definitions, method and time of data collection (Krane 2000, Parekh et al 2003). Davidson et al (1996) found that in 188 previously continent men 56% were incontinent following a radical prostatectomy, 21% were incontinent 3 months postoperatively and 14% were still incontinent at 1 year.

Moul et al (1998), using a patient self-reporting incidence, found an 87.4% incidence of incontinence. In a similar study by McCallum et al (2001), of the 180 men questioned, 21 were still incontinent 2 or more years after surgery. Half experienced stress urinary incontinence on urodynamics as well as a component of detrusor dysfunction.

Impaired quality of life and reduced self-esteem following radical prostatectomy have been discussed by many authors (Butler et al 2001, McCallum et al 2001, Alivizatios et al 2003). Quality of life for men with incontinence is negatively affected, with many patients viewing incontinence as the most bothersome symptom. However, Alivizatios et al (2003) suggest that, depending on the individual's opinion, incontinence may be a minor problem which does not have a large impact upon quality of life; their data suggest that erectile dysfunction is the most disturbing complication after radical prostatectomy.

Postprostatectomy incontinence

It is thought that the pathophysiology of postprostatectomy incontinence may be due to sphincteric dysfunction, detrusor dysfunction, or both. MacDiarmid (2001) describes stress urinary incontinence secondary to intrinsic sphincter deficiency but many patients also have bladder dysfunction. In a study by Chao and Mayo (1995), 57% reported sphincter weakness and 39% detrusor dysfunction; 50% presented with a combination of factors. Anastomotic strictures can occur in 5–24% of patients (Chao & Mayo 1995).

It is thought that there are four main factors affecting continence:

1. Pelvic muscle function
2. Trigonal denervation
3. Absence of urethral postvoid milking (Wille et al 2000)
4. Bladder instability following urethral catheterisation.

Electromyography profile

Electromyography (EMG) is the study of bioelectric activity of muscles. The activity is measured in microvolts and is a very useful adjunct when teaching pelvic floor exercises because it enables objective visual and audible measurement of pelvic floor function (see also Ch. 3). EMG units are widely available and are a very useful monitor when assessing pelvic floor contraction. It has been suggested that a low EMG profile is an identifiable risk factor (Rigby 2001); further research is necessary to identify if preoperative low EMG recordings also relate to a postoperative risk of incontinence.

Pelvic floor exercises

A number of uncontrolled, non-randomised studies have suggested benefits of pelvic floor muscle exercise pre- and post radical prostatectomy. Burgio et al (1998) treated 20 men postpros-

tatectomy and showed 70% improvement in symptoms. Van Kampen et al (2000), in a similar study, showed improved outcomes with intervention. However, the most recent Cochrane Review (Hunter et al 2006) notes that studies vary widely in quality, with small varied samples and imprecise outcome measures. Some evidence that PFMT may help is a modest reduction in incontinence up to 3 months post surgery; after that point, however, the benefit is minimal. Sueppel et al (2001) suggested that starting biofeedback and PFMT before surgery improved patient outcomes; their study used biofeedback training.

There remain many unanswered questions about the initiation of exercise both pre- and postoperatively. Of importance, however, is that men value the support they receive from the nurse or the physiotherapist, indicating the importance of regular follow-up and supportive care after major surgery for prostate cancer.

There are many variations on the PFMT protocols. Dorey (2001b) suggests that pelvic floor exercises should be individually taught to make sure the patient is lifting up the pelvic floor and not bearing down. Men can be encouraged to tighten and lift the pelvic floor muscles as in the control of flatus or the prevention of urine flow (Box 4.5). It is important to carefully assess that the exercise are done properly and some units recommend digital rectal examination (Dorey 2001b).

Bladder retraining

Bladder retraining is useful to manage symptoms of urinary urge and frequency (see Ch. 3). Bladder retraining is used to describe the educational and behavioural approach to re-establish bladder control; the purpose is to restore a normal bladder pattern. It is recognised that detrusor dysfunction is a common complication of radical prostatectomy and many patients benefit from combined bladder retraining and anticholinergic treatment.

Fluid intake

Following prostate surgery men are advised to drink enough to keep the urine clear in colour and free from debris. Once the catheter is removed it is important to review fluid intake both in terms

Box 4.5 Pelvic floor exercises for men

STANDING UP

Stand with your feet apart and tighten your pelvic floor muscles as if you are trying to stop the flow of urine. If you look in a mirror, you should be able to see the base of your penis move nearer to your abdomen and your testicles rise.
- Hold the contraction as strongly as you can
- Try to avoid pulling in your abdomen or tensing your buttocks
- Perform three maximal contractions in the morning, holding for the count of . . . seconds
- Perform three maximal contractions in the evening, holding for the count of . . . seconds

SITTING DOWN

Sit on a chair with your knees apart and tighten your pelvic floor muscles as if you were lifting your pelvic floor off a drawing pin.
- Hold the contraction as strongly as you can
- Try to avoid pulling in your abdomen or tensing your buttocks
- Perform three maximal contractions in the morning, holding for the count of . . . seconds
- Perform three maximal contractions in the evening, holding for the count of . . . seconds

LYING DOWN

Lie on your back with your knees bent. With the knees apart, tighten your pelvic floor muscles.
- Hold the contraction as strongly as you can
- Try to avoid pulling in your abdomen or tensing your buttocks
- Perform three maximal contractions in the morning, holding for the count of . . . seconds
- Perform three maximal contractions in the evening, holding for the count of . . . seconds

WHILE WALKING

Try lifting your pelvic floor up 50% when walking.

AFTER URINATING

After you have passed urine, try tightening your pelvic floor muscles strongly to avoid the embarrassing dribble.

THE KNACK

Try tightening just before and during activities which increase your abdominal pressure such as coughing, sneezing, lifting and getting out of a chair.

Reproduced with permission from Dorey (2001b).

of volume and type. There is much confusion over how much we should drink and there is a consensus of opinion that a fluid matrix offers a validated research-based approach (Abrams & Klevmark 1996). As a guide, a matrix suggests intake based on body weight; for example, a 76 kg (12 st) person should aim to consume eight drinks (2.3 litres or 4.2 pints) per day (30 ml/kg).

Bowel care

There are very few data on bowel management postprostatectomy; however, Hall et al (2003), in a study on decision making, found bowel dysfunction to be a common unpleasant surprise after treatment. It is recommended that pre- and postoperative advice be given on avoiding constipation, for which a dietary supplement of linseed can be very beneficial.

Containment advice

Moul et al (1998) reported that 39% of patients needed protection to contain incontinence. Products for men are rarely available in chemists and more frequently they purchase either inappropriate general containment products available in many large retail outlets or resort to female products and even babies' nappies. An overview of containment products and appliances for men is provided below, with more detailed discussion in Chapter 10.

MANAGING INCONTINENCE

Although many people with incontinence can be successfully cured with appropriate management, many others have persistent incontinence that can only be managed symptomatically with appliances such as pads to ensure social continence (see Ch. 10). Alleviating the often unpleasant and undesirable consequences of urinary incontinence may be a short-term measure (during treatment) or a long-term strategy when other options have been exhausted. Management options for males can be grouped into two major categories: containment aids and conduction aids. Examples include small pouches for dribbling incontinence and urinary sheath drainage systems, respectively.

There are some absorbent products for low levels of incontinence specifically designed for males: the 'dribble pouch' is designed to fit over the penis and absorb small amounts of incontinent urine; the 'leaf' fits over both penis and scrotum. These pouches are usually disposable and are held in position by means of a washable jockstrap or tight-fitting underpants.

Conduction aids

Urinary sheaths

The urinary sheath is a method of managing urinary incontinence, which is unique to males, sometimes referred to as condom or external catheters. Sheaths are supplied as one- or two-piece systems, and some of those available come complete with their own applicator. A number of problems have been associated with the use of urinary sheaths such as the sheath becoming detached, irritation of penile skin and difficulty in self-application if manual dexterity is poor. Proper patient assessment, correct fitting and follow-up should ensure best use of the product although not all men can be successful with a sheath system. It is doubtful whether there is one universal best sheath system and it may be advisable to provide the patient with a selection to try.

A number of criteria must be satisfied in order for an individual to be fitted with a urinary sheath, whether it is a two-piece or a one-piece system. The nurse or person fitting the sheath should check that:

- the penis is not retracted
- the skin is not broken or inflamed (although a barrier cream may be used)
- the individual is not confused and at risk of pulling the sheath off or leaving it on indefinitely
- the individual has sufficient manual dexterity if self-caring, or alternatively that the sheath can be applied by a carer or health professional.

Despite the fact that these devices come in a variety of designs and that most manufacturers provide a range of sizes, it is essential that the penis is not too retracted for the successful attachment of a sheath. If the penis is retracted in any way, if the man is obese or if there is herniation around the base of the penis, then it is unlikely that this technique can be applied. It is helpful to try a sheath over a 5-day period to test if this approach is suitable for the individual. If the sheath can be kept in place for more than 12 h then it is probably an appropriate technique. Confused men are very likely to pull off a urinary sheath and this method of management may be unsuitable for such clients (Irvine 1991). This may account for the very low use of urinary sheaths in psychogeriatric units (Stott et al 1990). Sheaths are generally not suitable for men with obstruction, or with symptomatic urinary infection (Button et al 1998). Guidance on fitting a penile sheath is provided in Box 4.6. See also the case study in Box 4.7.

Drainage systems for use with a sheath are similar to those used with an indwelling catheter (see Ch. 10). These include free-standing and smaller body-worn drainage bags. Urine bags are made by several manufacturers and come in a variety of sizes and shapes, with different methods of attachment and a variety of tap fittings. As with other products, patient assessment (including leg length and manual dexterity) and individual patient preference are vital considerations when selecting a product.

Pubic pressure device

A second group of male conduction aids are those generally termed body-worn urinals or pubic pressure devices (see Ch. 10). This form of appliance is most often used in men who are unable to wear either a dribble pouch or a urinary sheath because they have a retracted penis – the penis is effectively too small to hold the appliances in place. Pubic pressure devices work by exerting pressure around the base of the penis and are fitted by an experienced appliance fitter. The device consists of a rubber cone held in place by means of waist and groin straps and attached to a leg drainage bag. Users sometimes complain of discomfort such as sweating and soreness, which is perhaps not surprising given the bulkiness of the device. In suggesting this option, consideration needs to be given to the individual's ability to apply the product and its acceptability.

Box 4.6 Fitting a penile sheath

When a decision has been made to try a penile sheath for managing urinary incontinence, part of the success for the wearer is selecting the right size, type and fitting of the sheath. Most manufacturers offer a one- or two-piece system in a range of sizes from 22 mm to 35 mm.

1. First, the size of the penis can be measured using a specially designed measuring device provided by the manufacturer. The circumference is estimated by placing the device at the base of the penis so that the fit is not too tight or too big. The size of the sheath required is shown on the measuring device at that position.
2. Once the size is chosen, some samples of different makes of sheath should be given for the patient to choose from.
3. Wash and dry the penis but do not apply talc or creams as this may prevent the sheath from forming a secure seal against the skin.
4. Take the sheath from the packet and using the packet, cut a hole in the middle which can go over the penis to keep the pubic hair away from the shaft of the penis. Make sure the foreskin is kept forward.
5. If using the one-piece self-adhesive sheath, place the penis into the sheath leaving a small gap (about 1 cm) at the bulbous end and then gently unroll the sheath the length of the penis and secure firmly by pressing on the penis.
6. If using the two-piece system, carefully stretch the adhesive strip before winding it around the shaft of the penis. This allows for any change in penis size while wearing the sheath. Roll the sheath over the adhesive strip in the same way as described above.
7. Remove the protective 'collar' made from the packet and discard. Attach the drainage bag securely making sure that the tube's connector goes past the 'waist' of the outlet tube and then strap to the leg (straps are provided with bags).
8. Sheaths are durable for 24 h's wear, but sometimes they remain in place for a longer period.
9. To remove a sheath, simply roll it off over the tip of the penis and discard.
10. Wash and dry the genital area thoroughly after removing the sheath and before replacing it with a fresh one.

Indwelling catheterisation

Catheterisation is usually considered a last resort in the management of incontinence, and indwelling catheters are usually only chosen when other strategies have failed. Chapter 10 discusses the issues associated with catheterisation and catheter management. However, catheterisation is the usual choice in cases of AUR to decompress the bladder to prevent ureteric reflux and backpressure to the kidneys.

Acute urinary retention (AUR)

AUR refers to the sudden inability to pass urine and is characterised by painful distension of the bladder. It is a common condition; more than 1 in 10 men in their 70s will experience AUR, while the risk for men in their 80s is nearly 1 in 3 (Jacobsen et al 1997). However, there is some evidence that the incidence is declining, an observation that may partly be explained by a trend towards earlier presentation of men with LUTS (Clifford et al 2000). Our understanding of why men develop AUR is limited, but there are several elements that contribute to its development:

- Events that increase the resistance to the flow of urine (e.g. prostatic obstruction, urethral stricture or increase in muscle tone)
- Interruption of the sensory innervation of the bladder wall (e.g. diabetic cystopathy) or the motor supply to the detrusor muscle or secondary to the influence of drugs
- Events that lead to overdistension of the bladder (e.g. after general anaesthesia, particularly for orthopaedic procedures)
- Prostatic infarction or other causes of inflammation.

The primary management of AUR is catheterisation, which may be undertaken by general practitioners or hospital doctors. A urethral catheter is most commonly used in the UK (Manikandan et al 2004) although some favour a suprapubic approach, particularly if the catheter is going to stay in place for some time.

As a catheter in place at the time of surgery is associated with an increased risk of bleeding and sepsis due to bacterial colonisation, it is preferable

Box 4.7   Case study: Examining the effectiveness of continence care

Henry is a 76-year-old gentleman of previous good health who was admitted to an acute medical ward following a cerebrovascular accident (CVA). He had recovered well from his stroke and was hoping to return home in the near future. However, he was still experiencing problems with his bladder. Although continent during the day, Henry wet the bed most nights. The nurses on the ward had fitted him with a urinary sheath after his attempts to use urine bottles had proved unsuccessful. Henry was unable to fit the sheath himself and even when fitted by the nurses it rarely stayed on all night.

Henry had lived alone prior to admission but planned to live at his daughter's on discharge from hospital. However, there were two practical difficulties: 'Who would apply the sheath?' and 'How would they deal with the washing and the spoiling of bed linen/mattress when the sheath fell off?' The continence nurse specialist was asked to help.

Henry explained his distress, frustration and embarrassment. The care plan in the nursing notes referred to the need to test the patient's urine, assess his constipation risk and do a 3-day continence chart. The evaluation column of the care plan recorded that a urinary sheath had been applied and made reference to a 'wet bed'. The notes indicated that the urine test was 'NAD' and that 'bowels' had been 'well opened' on several occasions. A 3-day fluid volume chart had been partially completed 2 weeks previously and filed in the notes. There was no evidence that the doctor had been informed of the patient's continence problem.

QUESTIONS
- What factors may have influenced the effectiveness of Henry's care?
- What could be done to ensure that his continence care was more effective?

POINTS FOR REFLECTION
It may help to consider the following issues:
- Why was urine bottle use unsuccessful? Had his stroke or another coexisting complaint affected Henry's grip?
- Why wasn't the sheath staying on? There was no reference to the size of the appliance in the care plan. Had the correct sheath size been determined

and communicated to everyone who was involved in assisting Henry to change the appliance?
- Was a sheath appropriate? Henry could not fit it himself and no one was available to help at home. He did not like the sheath. Had he been offered a choice?
- Was Henry's incontinence really intractable? What was really causing it? The fluid volume chart was incomplete. Medical staff were not aware of the continence problem. Would Henry's incontinence problem have benefited from the knowledge of other members of the multidisciplinary team?

WHAT WOULD HAVE CONSTITUTED A DESIRABLE OUTCOME FOR HENRY?
- Option One: Continence.
- Option Two: A management solution, acceptable to Henry and manageable by him with minimal risk of a wet bed with resultant distress.

TREATMENT PLAN
Henry's continence problem was thoroughly assessed and an individual plan of care established. The assessment revealed a high urine output at night, which was also the time Henry was least capable of reaching the toilet/using a bottle because he was tired and had taken sleeping pills whilst in hospital. (He had been unable to sleep through worry.)

Henry was prescribed furosemide (frusemide) at 6 p.m. each evening to eliminate his urine load and reduce the high volume of urine produced at night when he was least able to cope with it. He was provided with a urine bottle with a non-spill adapter, as his grip was weak, especially when tired. He was also weaned off his sleeping pills as these had been started during his hospital stay and had added to his drowsiness when he did need to awaken to pass urine.

OUTCOMES
Henry was continent on discharge (but bought a protective bed sheet and took the continence nurse's contact number just in case!). Effective care had been achieved based upon a comprehensive assessment of the problem, goals that were patient focused and negotiated with Henry and his daughter, and an individualised plan of care which served to ensure that all those involved knew of his requirements.

Box 4.8 Case study: Intermittent self-catheterisation

Mr Williams is a 73-year-old retired gentleman living in his own semi-detached bungalow within walking distance of the shops and his local pub. He worked as a lorry driver for 30 years and considers himself to be pretty healthy. He has been a non-smoker for over 40 years. He was referred by his wife who was nagging him about having to wash underwear smelling of urine. When seen in the continence clinic, Mr Williams complained of: leaking urine with walking, coughing or getting up quickly. He related the problem to the 'pills' the doctor gave him for his prostate. He had gone to see his GP about 3–4 months ago because of increasing difficulty in starting his stream; once started it would stop and start and often dribble at the end. It also took him several minutes to empty his bladder. He had no symptoms of urgency and was only waking up at night once or twice, although he was not sure if he awoke because of a full bladder because he didn't usually feel full even if he went to the toilet. He thought he woke up because recently his penis and anal area had been getting itchy. He was putting cream on a few times a day and at night to help soothe the irritation. His GP had checked his prostate and thought the pills might help. They had improved the volume of the urine stream but made him a bit dizzy when he stood up quickly and seemed to make the 'dribbling' worse.

Mr Williams has type 2 diabetes controlled by diet and hypoglycaemics (Diabinese and Metformin). He rarely goes to his GP and does not remember the results of his most recent blood sugar test or when it was taken. He denies any history of heart disease or hypertension but erectile function is poor. There is no complaint of haematuria, dysuria or UTI; bowels are regular with no straining or flatus or stool incontinence. On examination, his ankles are oedematous extending up to mid-calf and there are signs of venous stasis in both ankles and calves. Abdominal examination reveals an obese abdomen, bladder seems palpable but it is difficult to be certain because of abdominal fat. There is a bilateral, moist, red patchy rash in inguinal creases. Post-void residual ultrasound was 1500 ml after a prolonged void of 300 ml. BP after lying down for 5 min was 163/100. Urinalysis (by dipstick) is positive for protein; glucose; leukocytes.

TREATMENT PLAN

The most probable diagnoses are: incomplete emptying, likely due to diabetic neuropathy; bacteriuria due to chronic urinary retention; hypertension; risk of skin breakdown and infection. Ask Mr Williams what he thinks has contributed to his bladder problems and what his goals for treatment are. Once these are established, explain to Mr Williams that his bladder may not be emptying properly because his diabetes has affected the nerve supply to the bladder muscle so that it doesn't contact well or give him the sensation of having a full bladder. The neuropathy may also be the cause of his poor erections. Explain that poor erections may be a sign of cardiovascular disease and that a visit to his family physician for a check up is warranted. Suggest that he learns how to self-catheterise to drain his bladder effectively and show him how to do this. Ask him to keep a record of how much he drinks and the type of fluid, how much he voids spontaneously and how much he catheterises. Request that initially catheterising should be done 4 times a day (ideally to keep the bladder volume at approximately 500 ml or less); recommend topic antifungal cream for the skin rash on the perianal area and glans penis. Obtain urine for culture and sensitivity and microscopy. Mr Williams should be advised to go to his GP for a full check up, including blood pressure, eyesight changes, blood glucose levels, urinalysis report and review of his medication. He may also benefit from seeing the nurse in the outpatient diabetic clinic for advice on foot and skin care. Request that Mr Williams return to see you in 2 weeks for a follow-up visit, at which time you will review his fluid volume diary and see how he is managing with the catheterisations; you will also check on the status of his skin rash which you explain is common in people with incontinence but is treatable first by the antifungal cream and then by keeping the area dry and protected with a cream. (NB: Mr Williams should not take sulphonamide antibiotics when he is taking Diabinese for his diabetes). Reinforce the importance of having both his blood pressure and blood sugars under good control in order to preserve his eyesight, renal health and cardiovascular status.

that men undergo a trial without catheter (TWOC) after an episode of AUR in the hope that perioperative morbidity will be reduced even if they do not avoid surgery altogether.

A further reason for trying to avoid emergency surgery for this condition is that men who had a prostatectomy following AUR had a worse outcome in terms of symptom reduction and improvements in quality of life than those undergoing planned prostatectomies as demonstrated in the National Prostatectomy Audit (Mebust et al 1989). There is some evidence to suggest that catheter drainage combined with alpha-blockers may be associated with a good chance of successful voiding (McNeill et al 1999, 2004).

Intermittent self-catheterisation

Intermittent self-catheterisation (ISC) is now the option of choice for a wide range of urinary problems involving poor bladder emptying, offering a viable and more convenient alternative to long-term urethral catheterisation (see Ch. 10). ISC is currently regarded as suitable for most patients with bladder symptoms related to incomplete emptying/urinary retention (DH 2000b). The main advantage of ISC is that, after a brief period of training, it can be carried out by the patient in his own home without the need for regular nursing supervision. ISC is suitable for almost any patient, providing they have the necessary cognitive ability, manual dexterity and motivation (see Box 4.8).

Occlusive devices

Apart from artificial sphincters, which are inserted surgically and mentioned above, the only other form of device aimed at preventing outflow of urine is the penile clamp. Penile clamps are an option for a carefully selected group of men who have normal penile sensation, cognitive ability and manual dexterity. They are not recommended for men with neuropathic disorders such as diabetes or multiple sclerosis. Intermittent use (e.g. when swimming) can greatly enhance men's confidence in public places. Good patient teaching about the misuse of the penile clamp is mandatory to prevent skin breakdown, pain or oedema.

Choice of product

Continence appliances are not without their problems and the decision to use/choice of product should be carefully considered (see Ch. 10). Although forming part of a set of consensus guidelines aimed at the primary healthcare team, the following algorithm and five principles are equally helpful in guiding decision making on product use (Button et al 1998):

- The restoration of continence should be the aim for all persons.
- Assessment should precede any issue of aids or appliances.
- Individual patient/client choice should be a key consideration in determining a suitable management strategy.
- Care should include education in the correct use of any aid or appliance issued.
- Product suitability and requirements should be reviewed regularly.

When choosing a product, the National Prescribing Centre (1999) suggests the use of the EASE mnemonic:

- How **E**ffective is the product? (At containing odour and urine?)
- How **A**ppropriate is the product for this patient? (Can they manage it easily, is it comfortable and discreet?)
- How **S**afe is the product? (Is it environmentally friendly, easy to dispose of?)
- Is the prescription cost **E**ffective?

In addition to comprehensive patient assessment and careful choice of product (which includes incorporation of patient views), it is essential that products are used effectively and according to the manufacturer's instructions.

Sexuality and LUTS

The potential impact of urinary incontinence in general and the use of appliances in particular on the individual should not be underestimated. Alterations in body image, relations and sexual activity are issues that it would be all too easy to overlook (Royal College of Nursing 2000). Although these are arguably not subjects to be broached until a sufficiently trusting relationship has been established between the healthcare practitioner and the patient/client, they are important considerations.

The penis is considered by many to be the focus of male sexuality and Lawler (1991) has suggested that compared with female sexuality, male sexuality is more genital, less diffuse and more concerned with power and performance, and is more physical. Physiological changes in an older man such as prostatic disease will affect his genitalia and sexual performance. The argument for healthcare professionals to introduce questions about sexual function into their assessments of men presenting with LUTS is simple. There is now clear evidence that men with urinary symptoms are not only at an increased risk of sexual dysfunction but also that problems with sex significantly reduce the quality of these men's lives. Moreover, knowledge about a man's sexual function can significantly influence the management of his LUTS (Coombe 2003).

The point behind asking questions about a patient's sex life is that the information it reveals can have a significant influence on the choice of management. It is well known that several management options for BPH alone have sexual consequences. Surgery causes ejaculatory dysfunction in around two-thirds of patients, although it may improve erectile dysfunction (Brookes et al 2002). Finasteride can lead to decreased libido, erectile dysfunction and ejaculatory disturbance (Debruyne et al 1998) and the alpha-1A selective blocker tamsulosin may cause a dose-dependent incidence of abnormal ejaculation (Schulman et al 2001). In contrast, the alpha-1 selective blocker alfuzosin has been shown to have no significant link to sexual dysfunction (van Kerrebroeck et al 2000). Choosing the right medication is therefore essential.

With regard to appliances and pads, essentially the message regarding sexuality is that a great deal can be done to maintain sexual image and also to maintain sexual activity. When a man is wearing a urinary sheath or a urinary catheter, provided that the collecting bag has been fitted correctly to the inside of the leg, there is no need for anyone else to know that a device is being worn. On the other hand, the use of pads may be more obvious as many of these are bulky. With improved products, which are smaller and more absorbent, the situation is improving. As with any kind of appliance, good skin hygiene is essential in order to prevent odour and discomfort. These measures will reduce the impact of urinary incontinence on sexuality.

One of the problems arising from the use of devices to manage urinary incontinence is that of altered body image and this is particularly the case where an appliance is being worn (Wheeler 1991). Sexual activity is possible even with an indwelling urinary catheter in situ. The catheter can be taped back along the shaft of the penis, or alternatively it can be removed altogether and replaced after intercourse. Replacement is usually done by the man himself or a partner/carer who has been taught the technique. The outlet to the bladder is blocked during erection of the penis so it is unlikely that urine will leak during intercourse.

Involving a partner in the care of an individual, whether directly in terms of changing catheter bags or continence pads, or indirectly as a source of support, must not be done without careful consideration. Blannin (1987) suggests that where a partner adopts the role of 'nurse' this may produce conflicts in the relationship resulting in a loss of self-esteem and sexual desire. It may also be prudent to emphasise that age is no barrier to experiencing a close sexual relationship (Duffin 1992).

Clearly, consideration of sexuality and sexual function requires a sensitive approach and discussion between partners. It is possible that specialist advice may need to be sought. Any sexual dysfunction as a result of urinary incontinence should be brought to the attention of an appropriate therapist, such as a specially trained counsellor, a continence advisor or general practitioner who may be able to offer help and advice. It may also be appropriate to inform individuals and their carers of the existence of local support groups and services, as well as national organisations such as the Continence Foundation (http://www.continence-foundation.org.uk).

CONCLUSIONS

In the nursing strategy document *Making a Difference* (DH 1999) continence is identified as one of the eight fundamental and essential aspects of care that sometimes fall 'below acceptable standards'. LUTS in men is common and is usually associated with the prostate but it is essential that a thorough assessment of all possible causes is investigated before making a diagnosis. For men, incontinence impacts on every aspect of their life including their sexuality. For any man the diagnosis of prostate cancer is devastating; the treatment can also leave many men with significant incontinence. Through sharing of information and awareness of potential problems, nursing care can improve. As healthcare professionals we are challenged to provide care for a growing cohort of patients with post radical prostatectomy incontinence. There is no doubt that these men need advice and support.

KEY POINTS FOR PRACTICE

- Overactive bladder symptoms are just as common in men as in women, but incontinence is more prevalent in women
- The prostate plays a major role in bladder function in men over the age of 50 years

- Radical surgery for prostate cancer can cause stress incontinence in men. The treatment is the same as for women, i.e. pelvic floor exercises
- Alpha-blockers are recommended as first-line treatment in benign prostatic hyperplasia (BHP); they have a rapid onset of action
- 5-Alpha reductase inhibitors reduce the volume of the prostate and reduce obstruction in BPH

Useful website

http://www.orchid-cancer.org.uk: Orchid Cancer Appeal provides a wealth of information on testicular and prostate cancer ranging from innovative research to patient awareness campaigns. Message boards allow both patients and medics alike to interact on this award-winning site.

ACKNOWLEDGEMENTS

With acknowledgements to Katherine Moore for her contribution to this chapter.

References

Abrams P 1997 Urodynamics, 2nd edn. Springer, London

Abrams P, Klevmark B 1996 Frequency volume charts: an indispensable part of lower urinary tract assessment. Scandinavian Journal of Urology and Nephrology Supplement 179:47–53

Alivizatios G, Skolarikos A, Laguna P 2003 Recent data upon impotence, incontinence and quality of life issues concerning radical prostatectomy. Archivos Españoles de Urología 56(3):321–330

Ball A, Feneley R, Abrams P 1981 The natural history of untreated prostatism. British Journal of Urology 533:613–616

Barry M J, Fowler F J, O'Leary M P et al 1992 The American Urological Association symptom index for benign prostatic hyperplasia. Journal of Urology 148:1549–1557

Billington A 1999 Prostate disease. Nursing Standard 13(25):49–54

Blandy J 1998 Lecture notes on urology. Blackwell Science, Oxford

Blannin J 1987 Incontinence: men's problems. Community Outlook Feb:27–28

Boyle P, Robertson C, Mazzetta C et al 2003 The prevalence of male urinary incontinence in four centres: the UREPIK study. British Journal of Urology 92:243

Brookes S T, Donovan J L, Peters T J et al 2002 Sexual dysfunction in men after treatment for urinary tract symptoms: evidence from randomised controlled trial. British Medical Journal 324:1059–1061

Button P, Roe B, Webb C et al 1998 Consensus guidelines: continence promotion and management by the primary healthcare team. Whurr, London

Burgio K L, Stutzman R E, Engel B T 1998 Behaviour training for post prostatectomy urinary incontinence. Journal of Urology 141(2):303–306

Butler L, Downe-Wamboldt B, Marsh S et al 2001 Behind the scenes: partners' perception of quality of life post radical prostatectomy. Urologic Nursing 20(4):254–258

Catalona W, Partin A, Slawin K et al 1998 Use of the percentage of free prostate specific antigen to enhance differentiation of prostate cancer from benign prostatic disease: a prospective multicenter clinical trial. Journal of the American Medical Association 279:1542–1547

Cancer Research UK 2006 Incidence and mortality rates for prostate cancer. Online. Available: http://info.cancerresearchuk.org/cancerstats/types/prostate/incidence

Chamberlain J, Meilia J, Moss S, Brown J 1997 The diagnosis, management, treatment and costs of prostate cancer in England and Wales. Health Technology Assessment 1:3

Chao R, Mayo M E 1995 Incontinence after a radical prostatectomy. Journal of Urology 154(1):16–18

Cheater F 1996 Promoting urinary continence. Nursing Standard 10(42):47–54

Clifford G M, Logie J, Farmer R D 2000 How do symptoms indicative of BPH progress in real life practice? The UK experience. European Urology 38(1):48–53

Coombe M 2003 Sex and the LUTS consultation. Men's Health 2(2):50–51

Continence Foundation 2000 Making a case for investment in integrated continence services: a source book for continence services. Continence Foundation, London

Davidson P, van den Ouden D, Schroeder F H 1996 Radical prostatectomy: prospective assessment of mortality and morbidity. European Urology 29:168–173

Debruyne F M, Jardin A, Colol D et al 1998 Sustained release alfuzosin, finasteride and combination of both in the treatment of benign prostatic hyperplasia. European Urology 34:169–175

Denning J 1996 Male urinary incontinence. In: Norton C (ed) Nursing for continence. Beaconsfield, London, p 153–169

Department of Health 1999 Making a difference: strengthening the nursing, midwifery and health visiting contribution to health care. DH, London

Department of Health 2000a The NHS prostate cancer programme. DH, London

Department of Health 2000b Good practice in continence services. DH, London

Desmond P V, Thompson I, Zeidman E, Mueller E 1993 Morbidity with contemporary prostate biopsy. Journal of Urology 150:1425–1426

Dorey G 2001a Male patients with lower urinary tract symptoms 2: treatment. In: Pope Cruikshank K, Woodward S (eds) Management of continence and urinary catheter care. BJN Monograph. Mark Allen, London

Dorey G 2001b Conservative treatment of male urinary incontinence and erectile dysfunction. Whurr, London

Downey P (ed) 2000 The prostate. In: Introduction to urological nursing. Whurr, London

Duffin H 1992 Assessment of urinary incontinence. In: Roe B H (ed) Clinical nursing practice: promotion and management of continence. Prentice Hall, New York, Chapter 3

Feneley R C L, Gingell J C, Abrams P et al 1999 Urology guidelines for GPs. Urological Institute, Bristol

Game C, Farrer H 1989 Disorders of the male reproductive tract. In: Game C, Anderson R E, Kidd J R (eds) Medical–surgical nursing: core text. Churchill Livingstone, Melbourne, p 644–653

Garroway W, Collins G R 1991 High prevalence of benign prostatic hypertrophy in the community. Lancet 338:469–471

Griefzu SP 2000 Prostate cancer. Registered Nurse 63(6):26–32

Hall J D, Boyd J C, Lippert M C et al 2003 Why patients choose prostatectomy or brachytherapy for localised prostate cancer: results of a descriptive study. Urology 61(2):402–407

Hunskaar S, Sandvik H 1993 One hundred and fifty men with urinary incontinence. Scandinavian Journal of Primary Health Care 11:193–196

Hunskaar S, Burgio K, Clark A et al 2005 Epidemiology of urinary and faecal incontinence and pelvic organ prolapse. In: Abrams P, Cardozo L, Khoury S, Wein A (eds) Incontinence. Health Publication, Paris

Hunter K F, Moore K N, Cody J, Glazener C M J 2006 Conservative management of post prostatectomy incontinence (Cochrane Review). Cochrane Library Issue 3. Update Software. John Wiley, Chichester

Irvine L M 1991 Continence in later life. In: Garrett G (ed) Healthy ageing: some nursing perspectives. Wolfe, London, p 124–130

Jacobsen S J, Jacobsen D J, Girman C J et al 1997 Natural history of prostatism: risk factors for acute urinary retention. Journal of Urology 158:481–487

Kellogg Parsons J, Partin A 2004 Applying complexed prostate specific antigen to clinical practice. Urology 63:815–818

Kirby M 1997 Making a diagnosis. Benign prostatic hyperplasia. Pulse 4–5

Kirby R 1997 Management of common prostatitis syndromes. Trends in Urology, Gynaecology and Sexual Health Nov/Dec:37–43

Kirby R, McConnell J 2004 Benign prostatic hyperplasia: fast facts, 4th edn. Health Press, Albuquerque, NM, Chapter 2

Kirby R, Fitzpatrick J, Kirby M, Fitzpatrick A 1994 Shared care for prostatic diseases. Isis Medical Media, Oxford, Chapter 2

Krane R J 2000 Urinary incontinence after treatment for localised prostate cancer. Molecular Urology 4(3):279–286

Lawler J 1991 Behind the screens. Churchill Livingstone, Melbourne

McCallum T, Moore K, Griffiths D 2001 Urinary incontinence after radical prostatectomy: implications and urodynamics. Urological Nursing 21(2):113–119

MacDiarmid S A 2001 Incontinence after radical prostatectomy: pathophysiology and management. Current Urology Reports 2(3):209–213

McNeill S A, Daruwala P D, Mitchell I D C et al 1999 Sustained release alfuzosin and trial without catheter after acute urinary retention: a prospective, placebo-controlled trial. BJU International 84:622–627

McNeill S A, Rizvi S, Byrne D J 2004 Prostate size influences outcome following presentation with acute urinary retention. BJU International 94(9):1407–1419

Marsh M 1992 Malignant disease of the prostate gland. Nursing Standard 6(36):28–31

Malmstein U 1997 Urinary incontinence and lower urinary tract symptoms: an epidemiological study of men aged 45–99. Journal of Urology 158:1733–1737

Manikandan R, Srirangam S J, O'Reilly P H, Collins G N 2004 Management of acute urinary retention secondary to benign prostatic hyperplasia in the UK: a national survey. BJU International 93(1):84–88

Mebust W K, Holtgrewe H L, Cockett A T K, Peters C and Writing Committee 1989 Transurethral prostatectomy: immediate and postoperative complications. A comparative study of thirteen participating institutions evaluating 3885 patients. Journal of Urology 141:243–247

Milliard R J 1989 After dribble. In: Bladder control – a simple self-help guide. William & Wilkins, Broadway, NSW, Australia

Morrison M, Shandran T, Smithers F, Fawsett J N 1994 The urinary system. In: Alexander M, Fawsett J N, Runciman P J (eds) Nursing practice: hospital and home. Churchill Livingstone, Edinburgh, p 291–324

Moul J W, Mooneyham R M, Kan T C et al 1998 Preoperative and operative factors to predict incontinence, impotence and stricture after radical prostatectomy. Prostate Cancer and Prostatic Diseases 1(5):242–249

National Prescribing Centre 1999 Prescribing Nurse Resource Pack: urinary incontinence. National Prescribing Centre, Liverpool

National Institute for Clinical Excellence (NICE) 2000 Urinary tract (outflow) symptoms. A guide to appropriate referral from general to specialist services. NICE, London

National Screening Committee 2000a Second report of UK National Screening Committee. DH, Wetherby

National Screening Committee 2000b Information sheet on screening for prostate cancer. DH, Wetherby

Parekh A R, Feng M I, Kirages D, Bremner H, Kaswick J, Aboseif S 2003 The role of pelvic floor exercises on post prostatectomy incontinence. Journal of Urology 170(1):130–133

Rigby D 2001 Urinary incontinence following a radical prostatectomy: is there a need for intervention? British Journal of Nursing 10(supplement 21):8–9

Royal College of Nursing 2000 Sexuality and sexual health in nursing practice: a discussion document. RCN, London

Royal College of Physicians 1995 A report of the Royal College of Physicians. Incontinence: causes, management and provision of services. RCP, London

Selley S, Donovan J, Faulkner A et al 1997 Diagnosis, management and screening of early localised prostate cancer. Health Technology Assessment 1:2

Schulman C C, Lock T M, Buzelin J M et al 2001 Long term use of tamsulosin to treat lower urinary tract symptoms/

benign prostatic hyperplasia. Journal of Urology 166:1358–1363

Stenzelius K, Mattiason A, Hallberg IR, Westergren A 2004 Symptoms of urinary and faecal incontinence among men and women 75+ in relation to health complaints and quality of life. Neurourology and Urodynamics 23(3):211–222

Stott D J, Dutton M, Williams B O et al 1990 Functional capacity and mental status of elderly people in long term care in Glasgow. Health Bulletin 48:17–24

Sueppel C, Kreder K, See W 2001 Improved continence outcomes with preoperative pelvic floor muscle strengthening exercises. Urologic Nursing 21(3):201–210

Thom D 1998 Variations in estimates of urinary incontinence prevalence in the community: effects of differences in definition, population characteristics, and study type. American Geriatric Society 46:473

Van Kampen M, De Weerdt W, Van Poppel H et al 2000 Effect of pelvic-floor re-education on duration and degree of incontinence after radical prostatectomy: a randomised controlled trial. Lancet 355(9198):98-102

van Kerrebroeck P, Jardin A, Laval KU, van Cangh P 2000 Efficacy and safety of new prolonged release formulation of alfuzosin 10 mg once daily versus alfuzosin 2.5 mg thrice daily and placebo in patients with symptomatic benign prostatic hyperplasia. ALFOTI Study Group. European Urology 37:306–313

Venn S N, Greenwell T J, Munday A R 2000 The long-term outcome of artificial urinary sphincters. Journal of Urology 164(3):702–707

Webb V, Simpson R 1997 Older man's burden. Nursing Times 93(5):77–80

Wheeler W 1991 A kind of loving? The effect of continence problems on sexuality. In: Garrett G (ed) Healthy ageing: some nursing perspectives. Whurr, London, p 144–149

Wille S, Mills R D, Studer U E 2000 Absence of post void milking: an additional cause for incontinence after radical prostatectomy. European Urology 37(6):665–669

Wilson, P D, Berghmans B, Hagen S et al 2005 Adult conservative management. In: Abrams P, Cardozo L, Khoury S, Wein A (eds) Incontinence, vol 2. Health Publication, Paris, p 855–964

Chapter 5

Mainly children

June Rogers

CHAPTER CONTENTS

> . . . remember toilet training is a skill acquisition, not a war.
>
> Anon

INTRODUCTION

Achieving continence is a developmental milestone that children reach at varying rates and whilst some children appear to struggle initially the majority of children will be toilet trained by the age of 4 years and be dry at night by 5 years. However, a small number of children may experience ongoing problems and strategies need to be in place to provide for their needs, through the development of integrated paediatric continence promotion services.

> An integrated community-based paediatric continence service, informed by good practice in Paediatric Continence Services, ensures that accessible, high quality assessment and treatment is provided to children and their parents/carers in any setting, including, for example, children looked after and children at boarding schools.
>
> Department of Health (2004)

This chapter will discuss the acquisition of bladder and bowel control and the most common toileting problems, including difficulties with toilet training, daytime wetting, bedwetting, constipation and soiling.

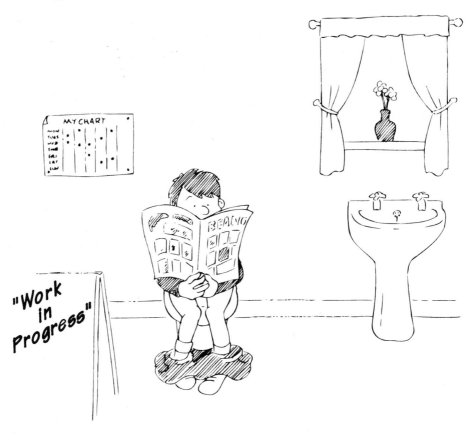

Figure 5.1 Developing toileting skills.

ACQUISITION OF BLADDER AND BOWEL CONTROL

Becoming toilet trained is considered a milestone in childhood development (Fig. 5.1) and there have been a number of longitudinal studies that have identified the age ranges at which children acquire toileting skills. Interestingly, it is increasingly apparent that the average age at which children become toilet trained seems to have shifted from around 2 years of age, 40 or so years ago, to around 3 years of age at the current time. A number of theories have been put forward to explain why this is the case and there is a strong suggestion that the change from washable to disposable nappies may be at least partially to blame. In order to understand why this should be so, it is important to look at the level of physical skills and cognitive development that needs to be in place for the child to gain independent toileting. This knowledge

will also help to inform why some children, particularly those with learning difficulties, appear to struggle with the toilet training process.

The ability to become toilet trained is dependent on the intimate relationship between several factors. First of all there is the need for a level of physiological and physical maturation, whereby the child's bladder capacity has developed such that it can hold on to urine for at least 1–2 h and the child also has the ability to get to and sit on a potty or toilet. Furthermore, the child needs to be able to pull their pants up and down and ultimately wipe their own bottom, flush the toilet and wash and dry their hands. There needs to be a level of understanding, particularly in terms of what 'wees' and 'poos' are all about, and an ability/willingness to cooperate and respond to simple instructions. The child also has to have some awareness of 'self', with a desire to please and imitate and identify with peers, together with a degree of self-determination and independence. Children with autism and other learning difficulties can often struggle with feelings of 'self' and wanting to copy and be like their peers and sometimes this can be interpreted as lack of ability to be toilet trained. In children with normal learning capacity their developing strengths in self-determination are often clearly demonstrated at the 'terrible twos' stage – which is not always considered the best time to start a toilet training programme!

It is easy to appreciate how children who use disposable nappies, and therefore never feel wet, will have difficulties with understanding what 'wees', in particular, are all about. Also the cues that parents previously picked up as a time to start toilet training, such as increasing time intervals between having to change a wet cloth nappy and noticing the child is dry after a nap, are often completely missed with children in superabsorbent disposable nappies. Now the main trigger factor for starting toilet training appears to be starting nursery! If mainstream toddlers appear to have difficulties with understanding about 'wees' and 'poos' due to the absorbency and comfort of disposable nappies, then clearly children with 'special needs' are going to struggle even more (see also Ch. 8).

A study carried out by Bakker and Wyndaele (2000) identified a shift in the age of initiating toilet training from 12 to 18 months by parents born in the 1920s to 1940s to over 18 months with parents born in the 1960s to 1980s. This was felt to be partly due to the labour-saving introduction of disposable nappies, and those of us who can remember soaking buckets of terry towelling nappies, rinsing by hand and then boiling them can vouch for the motivational effect this had on getting the child toilet trained and out of nappies as soon as possible!

MacKeith et al (1973) reported on a toileting 'timetable', suggesting at around 15 months of age the child will start to point to wet clothes or self-made puddles and will use the same word or sound for either urine or faeces. By the time the child is 18 months, separate words will begin to be used and the child will report on soiled or wet nappies. At 2 years of age the child will occasionally announce the need to pass urine and by 3

years will be able to 'hold on' in time to get to a potty or toilet. By the time the child is 4 years the toilet training will be complete, with the child able to use the toilet completely independently with appropriate behaviour such as shutting the toilet door. However, this report was written at a time when the majority of children still wore washable nappies.

A more recent study by Schum et al (2002), which looked at the age of attainment of toileting skills, showed that the average age at which children first reported either during or after passing urine was around 30 months for girls and 34 months for boys. The average age at which they remained dry during the day was 32 months for girls and 35 months for boys. Schum et al also found that the range of normality for attainment of individual skills could vary by as much as a year. Jansson et al (2005) reported the median age for dryness during the day was 3.5 years and the median age for nighttime dryness was 4 years. Nighttime dryness appeared to come around 10 months after the child had become dry in the day. Just under a third of children (31%) developed the ability to recognise bladder signals at 2 years old, 79% at 3 years and 100% at 4 years. However, becoming fully trained involves more than just the ability to recognise bladder and bowel signals. The child has to perceive those signals correctly – leave it too late and there is a risk of having wet pants!

In order for the child to develop full bladder control the normal maturation process affecting micturition needs to have occurred. This involves a compliant bladder which allows filling, an awareness of a desire to void, the ability to postpone voiding until appropriate, the initiation of bladder contraction and sphincter relaxation, and the maintenance of urine flow until the bladder has emptied, after which the cycle starts up again (Berk & Friman 1990). The frequency of voiding varies between individuals, with the normal range varying from four to nine episodes per day in children aged 2–3 years and five to seven episodes per day in a 10 year old (Bloom et al 1993). Boys also have to learn additional skills. They need to learn to stand to urinate if they have been used to sitting on a potty and to understand that a urinal is OK to use but not a bidet! They also have to learn that it is socially acceptable to 'wee' in front of other boys but not in front of girls and that to open your bowels you have to go somewhere private. These social rules are learnt by the majority of children just by watching and copying other children. However, for children with learning difficulties these 'social' rules have to be formally taught.

When in general should the toilet training process start? Blaum et al (2003) carried out a study which looked at the correlation between the age at which toilet training commenced, the length of time it took and the age of the child when it was completed. They found that the initiation of intensive toilet training correlated strongly with the age at completion of toilet training. The earlier the training started the sooner it was complete, except where training commenced prior to around 24 months of age. Early initiation of training was not found to be associated with more toilet training problems, but there appeared to be a 'window' of opportunity to start the training process at around 24–27 months which was associated with both a shorter training time and a younger age of completion. This reflects the author's own specialist experience of children referred with toileting problems.

Many people mistakenly delay starting toilet training children with special needs, saying that the child gives no indication of 'readiness'. However, many children with special needs have the potential to be toilet trained but lack awareness and understanding of social rules and expected behaviours. This can result in them showing no interest in being toilet trained. The key for these children is to identify when they are physically ready and to then commence a training programme, adding in a behavioural and motivational component.

Assessment for toilet training

The difficulties of assessing children with special needs are well documented (Fewell 1991), and the more complex the child's problems the more difficult it becomes to assess the child. The act of communication and the ability to assess a child are inextricably entwined (Wolf-Schein 1998). Consequently, there are distinct risks that judgements may be made which are based on the child's ability to understand what they are being asked to do, rather than on their actual physical or social skills. However, there are children who can communicate but will not cooperate, and vice versa. This presents another source of difficulty since most standard tests assume the practitioner is dealing with a cooperative child who wants to do their best! As a result, children with complex needs are often labelled 'untestable' (Wolf-Schein 1998), with the assumption that they are therefore 'untrainable'.

This is a problem for paediatric continence advisers who may be faced with previous assumptions regarding the ability of some children with learning difficulties to become toilet trained. Such children are frequently 'labelled' as incontinent and automatically issued with nappies, in the belief that they would fail the usual standard toilet training assessment and therefore be unable to be toilet trained. However, relying solely on the standardised, norm-referenced tests may exacerbate, rather than minimise, the developmental delay (Downing & Perino 1992) since the child is likely to be treated according to the level of skill acquisition assigned to them. The most likely intervention is to keep them in nappies rather than recognising their potential for development.

Commencing the assessment early in the child's second year allows for skill development to take place before any 'challenging' or incorrect learned behaviours develop (Taylor & Cipani 1994, Smith et al 2000). This assessment should be a continuous 'dynamic' process as the child's skills develop. Following an initial assessment of physiological maturation and skills, a programme to address any identified skill deficits should be put in place, with further reassessment at appropriate intervals. For example, for the child who will not sit on the potty or toilet, the family should be advised about strategies such as engaging the child in a pleasurable activity that will encourage the child to sit for an increasing length of time. This programme would then continue until the child is able to sit for long enough to complete a void or evacuate their bowels. If the child is unable to sit because of physical difficulties such as lack of balance, a referral to occupational health services should be made so that an assessment for a potty chair or toileting aid can be undertaken. The child should be reassessed approximately every 3 months, with the family given a training programme to follow in the meantime. It is also important to assess the child to exclude any underlying treatable problems, such as constipation, before commencing the formal toilet training programme. The amount of support required for each child will depend upon the individual child's needs and the family dynamics, with some families needing regular review and support and others minimal intervention.

Prior to undertaking the assessment for toilet training readiness, a baseline record needs to be taken of the child's bladder and bowel habits. The main aim of the bladder assessment is to identify a mature bladder that is able to complete a normal micturition cycle. In order for this to be determined, the frequency of voids needs to be recorded but with modern disposable nappies this is difficult for the family to do unless the nappy is left off completely for a number of days, which usually is not practical to do. In this situation the following strategy can be suggested. The family are asked to identify a number of days when they will be at home with the child and to either put cotton pants on the child with the nappy on top, or place a folded kitchen towel that does not disintegrate when wet inside the nappy. The parent/carer then checks the child's nappy at least every hour and records whether the child is wet or dry (see Fig. 5.2 for an example of a record chart).

An infant's bladder holds approximately 30 ml of urine and this increases by 30 ml per year. Thus, by the time the child is around 3 years of age, the bladder capacity is about 120 ml with a frequency of voids of about six to eight per day (Bloom et al 1993). Therefore, when looking for a maturing bladder we would expect a 3 year old to void no less than 2-hourly. A higher frequency (more than eight voids per day) may indicate a urinary tract infection which needs to be investigated, or could be indicative of an overactive bladder. This would warrant further investigation if still occurring at the age of 5 years.

Many children with special needs are prone to developing constipation for a variety of reasons. The bowel assessment should help to identify if this is an underlying problem. The family should

> **Box 5.1   Readiness for toilet training –**
> **assessment checklist**
>
> - Maturing bladder that can hold urine for around $1\frac{1}{2}$–2 h
> - Bowel that is not constipated
> - Ability to sit on toilet/potty for sufficient time
> - Basic level of cooperation

identify the type of stool produced using the Bristol Stool Form Scale (see Fig. 8.8) and record the timing and frequency of bowel action. Normal bowel development follows a pattern of cessation of bowel movements at night at around 1 year of age with awareness of control at around 18 months to $2\frac{1}{2}$ years. Therefore, if a child is still soiling at night at around 2–3 years this may be an indication of an underlying problem such as constipation and a constipation treatment care pathway should be initiated.

A formal toilet training programme can be established once the child is achieving the physical and behavioural skills to enable training to take place (Box 5.1). It must be remembered that this toilet skills assessment checklist will form part of a holistic assessment which should also include, if indicated, urinalysis and a medical check to exclude any underlying pathology.

Summary

Although incontinence was once regarded as an inevitable consequence of learning difficulties (Hyams et al 1992), it has been found that many of these children, even those with profound learning difficulties (Smith et al 2000), respond to behavioural training programmes (Luiselli 1997). This illustrates the importance of early assessment and review of toileting skills and bladder and bowel function, and identification of any skills deficits to help direct individual programme development.

DAYTIME WETTING

Daytime incontinence usually occurs as a result of bladder and/or sphincter dysfunction (Hjalmas

BASE-LINE TOILETING CHART

Child's name: _____   DOB: _____

Date begun: _____

Date	Day 1		Day 2		Day 3		Day 4		Day 5		Day 6		Day 7	
Time	Nappy/ pants	Toilet	Nappy/ pants	Toilet	Nappy/ pants	Toilet	Nappy/ pants	Toilet	Nappy/ pants	Toilet	Nappy/ pants	Toilet	Nappy/ pants	Toilet
7.00														
8.00														
9.00														
10.00														
11.00														
12.00														
1.00														
2.00														
3.00														
4.00														
5.00														
6.00														
7.00														

Pants:
W = wet
D = dry
P = poo/soiled

Toilet:
W = wee
P = poo

Figure 5.2   Base-line toileting chart.

1992a), with the exception of those children who are incontinent as a result of an organic cause, such as spina bifida or sacral agenesis.

Terminology

Whilst some symptoms of daytime wetting, such as bedwetting and daytime wetting accidents, are considered normal in toddlers, they can be pathological in the school child. A variety of terms have been used in the past to describe daytime wetting problems and symptoms, including diurnal enuresis, diurnal incontinence, detrusor instability, detrusor overactivity and overactive bladder (OAB). In order to clarify terminology and definitions, the Standardisation Committee of the International Children's Continence Society has produced a set of guidelines (Neveus et al 2006). Some of the most common terms are presented below and it should be noted that some of the recommended definitions can only be quantified following investigations such as urodynamics.

Urgency

Urgency is the sudden and unexpected need to void caused by detrusor instability which produces unstable bladder contractions. Urodynamic studies have shown that more than half of these children have unstable contractions during the filling phase. It is also reported that up to 40% of children with urgency also have associated vesicoureteral reflux and up to 60% have a history of urinary tract infection (Meadows 1990, Hannson 1992, Hjalmas 1992a, van Wijk & van Gool 1995).

Detrusor overactivity

Detrusor overactivity (also termed overactive bladder or OAB) is characterised by involuntary detrusor contractions during the filling stage and is usually associated with a history of urgency and frequency with small amounts of wetting interspersed with dry periods (Hjalmas 1992b, van Gool et al 1992). Diagnosis can only be confirmed by urodynamic studies. When associated with children with a neurological condition the term used is 'neurogenic detrusor overactivity' which replaces the older term 'detrusor hyperreflexia'.

Detrusor underactivity

Detrusor underactivity is defined as a contraction of reduced strength and/or duration, resulting in prolonged and incomplete bladder emptying. It was previously termed 'lazy bladder syndrome' and was felt to be the end result of long-standing interrupted and incomplete voiding (van Gool et al 1992). These children often void by abdominal pressure alone with significant residual volumes of urine, which can be detected clinically. Current thinking is that persistent residual volumes of 20 ml or more or 10% of the child's maximum voided volume are significant and worthy of further investigation.

Dysfunctional voiding

Dysfunctional voiding is characterised by involuntary intermittent contractions of the periurethral striated muscle of the external urethral sphincter during voiding. The term cannot be truly applied unless confirmed by repeated uroflow measurements showing curves with repeated staccato pattern. This condition relates to children who are neurologically intact.

Detrusor sphincter dyssynergia

Detrusor sphincter dyssynergia applies to children with neurogenic bladder disturbance and is identified urodynamically by concurrent detrusor voiding contractions with an involuntary contraction of the urethral and/or periurethral striated muscle.

'Giggle' micturition

This is an uncommon form of wetting characterised by a normally dry child experiencing complete bladder emptying on giggling or laughing. These children have normal bladder and sphincter control and no evidence of 'stress incontinence'. In children with this condition it is thought that detrusor contractions are induced by centrally mediated electrical discharges from the hypothalamus that occur with laughter (Cisternino & Passerini-Glazel 1995).

Structural problems

For children who are always wet (usually girls) with no period of dryness, the possibility of an ectopic ureter needs to be considered. In this instance the ectopic orifice can open into the urethra, the vestibulum or the vagina (Jaureguizar & Pereira 1992). These children will require surgical referral.

Urodynamic stress incontinence

Urodynamic stress incontinence can be identified during filling cystometry and is defined as the involuntary leakage of urine during increased abdominal pressure, in the absence of a detrusor contraction. Children, notably girls, who report wetness following exercise or abdominal straining could have stress incontinence due to a wide bladder neck anomaly (Hjalmas 1992b, Jaureguizar & Pereira 1992). Although it tends to improve with age there may be a predisposition to stress incontinence in later adult life (Meadows 1990). It must be remembered, however, that genuine stress incontinence in childhood is extremely rare.

ASSESSMENT OF DAYTIME WETTING

A standardised, structured approach to history taking is important (Norgaard et al 1998), together with discussions with parents and child aimed at demystifying the problem. The symptoms of wetting need to be explained and put in perspective in relationship to the child's overall development, and should be discussed with the parents. A baseline frequency/volume chart will give an indication of the degree of wetting and frequency of voiding. Previous studies have identified that 3 days of recording are required to reflect a true picture of bladder function (Mattsson 1994, Mattsson & Lindstrom 1995). However, in practice this can be difficult because of schooling. The baseline assessment also includes fluid intake and the families are asked to record the amount, type and times the drinks are taken. It is generally recommended that children consume at least six to eight drinks spread out evenly during the day, but Almond (1993) identified that during the school day some children may take very little or no fluids for 7 h or more.

> **Box 5.2   Key aspects of physical assessment**
>
> - Assessment of perineal sensation
> - A check of lumbosacral reflexes
> - Inspection of external genitalia
> - Exclude asymmetry of buttocks, legs or feet
> - Check spine for subcutaneous lipoma, skin discolouration or hair growth
>
> Based on Norgaard et al (1998).

Any underlying constipation should be excluded and a note made of any previous urinary tract infections and relevant surgery as well as a general medical history. The child's functional bladder capacity can be estimated by asking the child to pass urine into a jug, when they feel the urge to go, and measuring and recording the contents. The bladder capacity can be estimated by multiplying the child's age by 30 and adding 30 (Rogers 1996a).

Physical examination

The general physical assessment should include the areas indicated in Box 5.2, based on Norgaard et al (1998). The child should be referred on for further investigation if the assessment identifies a history of more than one confirmed urinary tract infection, always being wet (usually girls), and an association with long-term bowel problems and/or previous failed management programmes (where non-compliance was not an issue).

If the child is still wetting during the day at age 5 years (or earlier if any of the above indications are present), they should be seen by a specialist for a full physical examination and a pre/postmicturition ultrasound scan of the renal tract. The scan is a non-invasive test and can identify such abnormalities as hydronephrosis, duplex system anomalies, any residual urine or thickening of the bladder wall (Olbing 1992, Rickwood 1992, Rogers 1996b).

Investigations

Possible investigations are listed in Box 5.3.

Box 5.3 Investigations

Investigation	Indication
Urinalysis	Screen for urinary tract abnormalities/urinary tract infection
Ultrasound of renal tract	Screen for urinary tract anomalies
Bladder scan	Assess bladder emptying/check for residual urine
Urine flow meter	Evaluate voiding in a child with postvoid residuals or suspected voiding dysfunction
Urine concentrating capacity	When polyuria/polydypsia are present
Urodynamics	When previous conventional therapy has failed or non-invasive investigations indicate possible problem
Serum creatinine	Polyuria or documented urinary tract disease
Plain X-ray	Screen for spinal anomalies and renal calculi

Treatment options for daytime wetting

Treatment options may involve one or more of the following:

- Frequency/volume chart for baseline and monitoring outcomes
- Encourage regular fluid intake
- Regular/timed voiding
- Correct posture for micturition
- Cognitive bladder retraining
  - education
  - motivation
  - biofeedback
- Pelvic floor awareness
- Anticholinergic medication
- Antibiotic prophylaxis.

Advice for families

Clear advice, in the form of oral and written information, should be given regarding drinks and regular toileting (Olbing 1992, Rogers 1996a). Star/incentive charts (Fig. 5.3) may be appropriate to aid motivation and compliance in some instances, but it is important to remember that the rewards should be given for achievable processes which are readily understood by the child, such as increasing drinks, rather than the outcome of a 'dry day'.

Cognitive bladder training in the community

The basis of treatment for children with daytime wetting is bladder re/training in the form of modified cognitive bladder training. Cognitive bladder training teaches these children how to void, when to void and also the correct number of voidings, by means of education, motivation and biofeedback (Rogers 1996a).

The cognitive bladder training programme was originally developed for children aged 7 years and older as hospital inpatients; however, it can be adapted and simplified for the younger child. The family are made aware that the programme may have to be followed for several weeks before any improvement is noted, and it will then need to be continued until the child is completely symptom free. The core components of the programme are education, motivation and biofeedback.

Basic information is given to the child about their bladder and kidneys as appropriate for their age. There are several *My Body* type of books available with helpful illustrations and children are often fascinated about how their body works. A soft-bodied doll, which has been adapted by sewing a felt bladder and kidneys on its tummy, is also useful with a younger child.

The child is taught about the correct way to sit on the toilet with their feet flat on the floor or a stool, to relax, not strain, and to use their detrusor muscles not their abdominal muscles to pass urine. The child is also told to try and pass urine in one go and not to stop and start. An instruction sheet is provided and the child encouraged to empty their bladder regularly. For those children who may not empty their bladder completely, 'double micturition' can be taught. This involves the child going to the toilet to pass urine, then going to their bedroom, sitting down, counting to 30 (or waiting for 1–2 min depending on their age) then returning to the toilet to try and pass urine again. The children are also advised to drink regularly

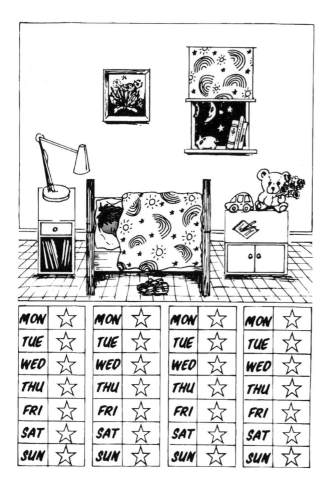

Figure 5.3   Example of a star chart. The child receives a star for each dry night.

MON	☆	MON	☆	MON	☆	MON	☆
TUE	☆	TUE	☆	TUE	☆	TUE	☆
WED	☆	WED	☆	WED	☆	WED	☆
THU	☆	THU	☆	THU	☆	THU	☆
FRI	☆	FRI	☆	FRI	☆	FRI	☆
SAT	☆	SAT	☆	SAT	☆	SAT	☆
SUN	☆	SUN	☆	SUN	☆	SUN	☆

throughout the day, taking extra drinks into school if necessary. Many children restrict fluid intake in the mistaken belief that it will reduce the wetting episodes and they need to understand that this can make the problem worse rather than better.

The advantages of being dry are discussed with the child and positive reinforcement is emphasised with the parents. The child is also encouraged to follow the programme by using 'incentive' charts and coloured stickers. Ongoing support is important and frequent contact needs to be made, either by telephone or home visits, to ensure continued motivation and compliance with the programme.

Although initially the child is encouraged to go to the toilet as soon as they feel an urge, for some children the number of times per day they pass urine is important. For example, some children do not go to the toilet often enough, either because

they don't like the toilet facilities available or for other reasons. Instead they will 'hold on' and put off going for as long as possible until they finally wet themselves. The aim is for the child to eventually learn to pass urine at an average of around seven times per day.

A form of 'biofeedback' can be adapted for the community setting using the following approaches. For those children who continue to pass urine an inappropriate number of times, either too frequently or not often enough, numbered stickers (from 1–7) can be given to stick on a chart. The child is aware, for example, that they have to have used sticker number 3 by lunchtime. Counting the number of times they pass urine acts as a feedback for the child.

The child is told to listen to the sound as they pass urine – does it come in one go, or does it spurt? The child is made aware that the urine should come out in one go. The child also measures the amount of urine they pass. By knowing their expected bladder volume the child can identify whether they are passing a full bladder or just a partial amount. For those children who 'deny' being wet, a wetting alarm can be used. This is worn in the pants and signals when the child starts to wet, and the parent then sends the child to the toilet straight away. (The alarm would only be used at home for obvious reasons!)

Pelvic floor therapy

Most children with daytime wetting learn to suppress the urge to void by contracting their pelvic floor instead of using central control. Left unchecked this could go on to develop into dysfunctional voiding with failure of the pelvic floor to relax during micturition. Teaching the child to relax the pelvic floor is therefore important. A training programme of pelvic floor relaxation and biofeedback was shown to be effective in treating recurrent urinary tract infections (UTIs) in 83% of girls with dysfunctional voiding causing incomplete bladder emptying (De Paepe et al 1998).

Medication

For those children with detrusor overactivity (OAB) who fail to respond to bladder retraining alone, a trial of oxybutynin can be tried. Oxybutynin is an anticholinergic and antispasmodic agent (see Ch. 9), and although some side effects (e.g. dry mouth, constipation and drowsiness) have been reported, it has been found to significantly reduce daytime wetting (Hjalmas 1992a). Oxybutynin is rapidly absorbed from the gastrointestinal tract and maximum effect is seen within 3–4 h. The usual starting dose for children over 5 years is 2.5 mg two to three times per day, with the last dose before bed. It must be stressed that medication is not a substitute for bladder retraining and correct relaxed regular voiding.

For those children with recurrent symptomatic UTIs, prophylactic antibiotic therapy can be beneficial. However, there is no confirmed benefit for children with asymptomatic infection whose wetting persists following eradication of symptoms of infection.

NOCTURNAL ENURESIS

Nocturnal enuresis has been defined as the involuntary passage of urine, during sleep, in a child aged 5 years and above, in the absence of any congenital or acquired defects of the nervous or renal system. However, most children with nocturnal enuresis are not offered advice or treatment until they are at least 7 years old. This can result in several years of anxiety and frustration for the child and family as they struggle to cope with the bedwetting alone.

Although there is a reported spontaneous cure rate of 15% per year (Stenberg & Lackgren 1995) without any active intervention, a study by Houts et al (1994) showed that children who are treated for nocturnal enuresis are more likely to stop wetting than those who are not. It is also known that approximately 1–2% of children will continue wetting into adulthood (Blainey 1995) and all children with nocturnal enuresis should be offered appropriate advice and treatment. Nocturnal enuresis is a multifactorial condition with no single main consistent cause. Each child is a unique individual, living within a particular setting of family dynamics and therefore a child-centred 'holistic' approach must be taken to ensure treatment strategies are appropriate.

Assessment

All children with nocturnal enuresis should have a documented assessment to help identify any underlying problems (e.g. constipation) and also to facilitate effective decision making regarding the most appropriate treatment. The assessment should identify the child's level of motivation to become dry and any environmental or social factors that may contribute to the problem.

Family setting

It is known that between 74 and 98% of children with nocturnal enuresis have a family history of bedwetting (Hogg 1996). Such families are normally more sympathetic towards the child, with an increased understanding of the problem. It is useful to know whether the child has their own room or shares a bedroom or bed and the location of the nearest toilet (e.g. upstairs or downstairs). Is there a burglar alarm switched on when everyone goes to bed? Such issues could influence the child's willingness to get out of bed at night to pass urine. A potty in the bedroom next to a night light could be a solution. If an enuresis alarm is to be considered it will be important to take into account how other members of the family may be disturbed.

Child's details

Nocturnal enuresis can be primary where the child has never been dry or secondary where the child recommences wetting after being dry for 6 months or more. A 1–2-week baseline assessment identifying the number of wet beds, the degree of wetness and the approximate time of voiding (estimated by the parents checking the child's bed at their own bedtime) is helpful when monitoring progress. The baseline can also aid identification of those children who may benefit from synthetic antidiuretic hormone medication (desmopressin) which can reduce urine production at night.

The baseline record should also include fluid intake during the day and the number of times the child passes urine. This should be done a few days prior to the first appointment with a continence specialist, including school days and weekend, if possible. This will help to establish if there are any problems with access to drinks or toilets during the school day. The child's general health should also be checked and urine tested for any abnormalities (by dipstick). Although there may be no reported history of daytime wetting the child should be questioned carefully about any frequency and urgency which may be present. Any daytime problems should always be addressed first. The child's functional bladder capacity (maximum voided volume in millilitres) can be estimated, as indicated earlier, by multiplying their age by 30 and adding 30. Constipation needs to be excluded as a loaded rectum may affect bladder capacity and is thought to contribute to unstable bladder contractions (Eller et al 1997).

If any previous advice or interventions have been tried these need to be identified and the degree of success or lack of it discussed. It will be helpful to know how long the treatment was tried

Box 5.4   Key points for implementing treatment

- Engage both parents and child
- Ensure that improvement is seen as a possibility
- Ensure that parent and/or child take an active part and responsibility for the treatment
- Set in place some practical help
- Ensure that there is regular monitoring by the professional, reducing in frequency as improvement occurs
- Focus on the gains, however minimal these are initially

and the family's perceptions about why the child failed to respond on those occasions. Both the child and family's understanding of the problem and their attitude towards it is important as this may influence the treatment offered (Butler et al 1990). Careful explanations are needed in order to ensure the child and family understand the problem of nocturnal enuresis and have an informed choice regarding treatment options (Boxes 5.4 and 5.5).

Treatment methods

There are two main treatment methods: the enuresis alarm and the antidiuretic hormone desmopressin. However, treatments should not be used in isolation and the child's motivation, individual personality and family dynamics should always be taken into account. The professional should also consider practical issues and daytime toileting and fluid intake. Incentive charts can help the child's motivation, and regular contact and review will help support the family and ensure any problems are identified early.

The enuresis alarm

The enuresis alarm has been cited as the most successful method of treating nocturnal enuresis with an appropriately selected group, with a success rate of around 70% (Forsythe & Butler 1989, Houts et al 1994). There are two main types of alarm available – the bed or pad and buzzer alarm, and

Box 5.5 Enuresis information sheet

You have asked for advice because your child is not yet dry at night. It may be that you have just begun to think that it is time that the wetting stopped. It may be that you are fairly desperate as the wetting has been a problem for years, because trips away from home are difficult and because you have tried everything. You may be somewhere between these stages.

The reasons why your child is not yet dry at night may be straightforward or more complex.

It may be one of the following or a combination of these:

- Age
- Developmental level
- Physical ability or maturation
- Emotional state
- Events relating to school or family
- Practical difficulties.

In order to implement a plan of action tailored to your child's individual needs and to the family, it is important to consider all possible factors and to form a clear picture of the pattern of wetting. Treatment plans may include star charts and enuresis alarms. All involve record-keeping.

REMEMBER

- Wetting is not usually deliberate.
- Irregular patterns of wet and dry nights can be quite normal.
- As with any developing skill, children vary in the age and stage when they become dry.
- Restricted drinking will not help develop control and may impede the process.
- Research studies do not confirm the view of many parents that deep sleep is the cause.
- Lifting helps to keep beds dry but the child needs to be awake when urinating.
- Most children grow out of it eventually.

It is important to start keeping a record of the pattern of night wetting even before your referral to someone who can help. The person giving you this sheet can advise you.

Name .... Profession ....

Can be contacted at ....

the body or mini alarm (Rogers 1998). The bed alarm consists of a sensor mat which goes on the bed under a sheet on which the child sleeps. The sensor mat is connected to a sound box which is usually placed at the side of the bed. The body alarm consists of a smaller sensor which fits inside the child's underwear and is connected to a mini sound box which is attached to the child's pyjamas.

The principle of this approach is that when the child wets, the sensors trigger the alarm which will wake up the child. The child then needs to get out of bed and try to complete the voiding episode in the toilet before coming back to change the bed and reset the alarm if necessary. The child obviously needs to have a level of understanding and motivation to comply with the alarm treatment and most children will need help and support from family members initially. Since there is an inevitable degree of disruption to other family members, the level of cooperation required from the whole family makes it important that alarms are only issued after careful counselling of the child and family.

An alarm should *not* be issued in the following circumstances (without very careful counselling of the family) due to risk of failure and increased intolerance/stress within the family:

- obvious parental intolerance
- an unstructured household
- child's sleeping arrangements not conducive, e.g. sleeps with sibling
- child shows reluctance to use alarm
- parents/carers unable to or not motivated to manage alarm
- child not able to cope with alarm due to physical problems
- child immature or known to be frightened of loud noises.

Prior to issuing an alarm the various aspects of the treatment should be discussed with the family. The child and family should be made aware of the types of alarm available, with the child being allowed to choose the type if possible. There should be a practical demonstration of the alarm with written instructions. The family needs to understand that it is like having a 'new baby' in the house and to expect to be woken up by the sound of the alarm at any time during the night. The enuresis alarm is not a 'magic box' that will get the child dry overnight and on average it may take 4–6 months. Therefore, it is usual to suggest an initial trial period of around 6 weeks. If the child has made no response to the alarm during this time it should be discontinued. It can be reintroduced at a later date when the child may be more responsive. However, the family needs to be aware that there may be a series of signs which are indicative of progress. The first stage may be simply that the child wakes to the alarm by themselves. Then, over a period of time, they wake more quickly to the alarm and the wet patch gets smaller with more urine passed in the toilet.

The healthcare professional involved needs to check if the family has enough spare sheets to cope with the frequent bed changes. Any spares should be kept in the child's bedroom so that there is less disruption when changing the bed during the night. The child also needs to know what to do with any wet bedding.

Following the issue of an alarm the family should be contacted during the next week to ensure there are no immediate problems, and thereafter every 2–4 weeks. For practical purposes these reviews may be a combination of home/clinic/school drop-in clinics or telephone.

Alarm troubleshooting

If the alarm stops working, then the batteries should first be checked. In the case of a continuing problem there should be a clearly defined system whereby a faulty alarm can be returned for repair. Families are encouraged to purchase spares and change the batteries if the sound becomes low to avoid disruption in the treatment. If the families complain of frequent false alarms then the professional needs to check that the sheets are always changed, even if only slightly damp, as this could set off the alarm. The alarm can also be triggered by the child sweating excessively and so the type of bedding and bedding protection needs to be checked, especially if plastic covers are used. Body alarms are more sensitive than bed alarms so the family needs to ensure that the sensor is adequately covered and not in direct contact with the child's

skin. It may be necessary to change to a different alarm if the false alarms persist.

Many families complain that the child does not wake to the alarm so one strategy is to try altering the sound of the alarm by changing the position of the sound box or placing it in a biscuit tin, for example. If a parent needs to get up to wake the child in the early stages of trialling the alarm, they may find using a baby alarm in their room helps them to hear when the enuresis alarm sounds. Another strategy is to use the alarm as a wake-up call in the morning so that the child gets used to associating the sound with waking up. If the child still fails to wake up to the alarm despite these various strategies, then changing from a body alarm to a bed alarm, which has a louder sound, or to a body alarm which incorporates vibration, may help. In the author's continence service it has been found that combining alarm use with desmopressin treatment has helped those children who fail to respond to an alarm alone. Another concern voiced by parents is that the alarm wakes and disrupts siblings. In this case, if using a bed alarm, try switching to a body alarm which has a quieter sound or discuss with the family the possibility of changing bedrooms for the period of alarm treatment.

Unfortunately, many areas have waiting lists for alarms so if the child has to wait they could practise waking during the night with an alarm clock and then going to the toilet from lying in bed. Commencing a short course of desmopressin while on the waiting list may also help to give everyone a respite from the bedwetting.

Desmopressin

Desmopressin (Desmotabs/DesmoMelt) is the synthetic analogue of the antidiuretic hormone vasopressin. Normally there is an increased secretion of vasopressin overnight, resulting in production of more concentrated urine (increased urine osmolality), with reduced urinary output. However, not all children with nocturnal enuresis secrete larger amounts of vasopressin at night and consequently they continue to produce large volumes of dilute urine which can often result in a wet bed (Norgaard et al 1998).

Desmopressin can be taken in the form of DesmoMelt (0.120 µg). This preparation has been designed to build on the efficacy and safety profile of Desmotabs. The Melt does not require water to aid swallowing and when it is put in the mouth it dissolves immediately into the saliva which is then swallowed in the normal way. DesmoMelt is absorbed from the mouth, pharynx and oesophagus as the saliva passes through to the stomach. This enhanced bioavailability facilitates effective outcomes at lower doses than the tablet form and the melt formulation also makes it particularly easy for children to take.

The use of desmopressin and its mode of action should be discussed in detail with the child and the family before any treatment begins. Written information should be provided which includes the different formulations available (i.e. tablet, nasal spray, melt), the dose and the timing of administration. The family needs to be aware of the importance of restricting fluid intake following administration of desmopressin since less urine will be produced. The medication should also be used with caution if the child has been swimming in the evening since large amounts of water may have been ingested! For a child with cystic fibrosis it is particularly important to obtain medical advice prior to any treatment with desmopressin.

Around 70% of children have been shown to respond to desmopressin (Hjalmas 1995), with predictors of good response including a family history of bedwetting, a normal bladder capacity, a wet bed before midnight and being a multiple wetter (Stenberg & Lackgren 1995). In those children who also have some daytime symptoms, combined therapy which includes an anticholinergic such as oxybutynin with desmopressin has been found to enhance the response rate (Caione et al 1995). Desmopressin can be administered from the age of 5 years and can be used until the child is mature enough to cope with an alarm.

Other indications for treatment with desmopressin include:

- when there is stress in the family and/or intolerance
- if the child is experiencing low self-esteem

- an alarm non-responder
- when the alarm is not appropriate
  - younger child
  - older immature child not able to cope with alarm
  - children with behavioural difficulties who may 'sabotage' alarm
  - for holidays/nights away from home
  - during stressful periods, e.g. examinations
- if more than one bed wetter in the family
- no adequate washing/drying facilities
- children with learning disabilities
- to aid management and removal of 'nighttime' nappy
  - combined therapy with alarm.

The long-term effects of untreated nocturnal enuresis are well documented (Rogers 1998). These include low self-esteem and social isolation as children with bedwetting will not take part in sleepovers or school trips away from home. Therefore no child should be denied appropriate treatment, including pharmacological methods where needed, because of their age, family circumstances or the perceived cost (Box 5.6). Unfortunately, 'this understanding has been a long and tragic time in coming' (Arnold 1997).

FUNCTIONAL CONSTIPATION

Constipation has been cited as one of the commonest conditions of childhood (DH 2004) and is said to account for 3% of all hospital outpatient visits and up to 25% of referrals to a paediatric gastroenterologist (Agnarsson & Clayden 1990). Constipation has a reported prevalence of around 34% in 4–11 year olds, with 5% experiencing chronic constipation lasting more than 6 months (Yong & Beattie 1998).

Terminology

The term 'constipation' describes a symptom rather than a diagnosis and comes from the Latin word 'constipare' which means 'to crowd together'. Constipation has been defined as the difficulty, delay or pain on defecation (Drugs and Therapeutics Bulletin 2000) without necessarily implying

> **Box 5.6   Case study 1**
>
> Ben, aged 5, was taken to the school nurse by his mother because of his problem with bedwetting. She was finding it difficult to cope with all the washing and was complaining about the smell in his bedroom. Ben was also reluctant to have friends round to play because he was worried that the smell might reveal his 'secret'.
>
> An initial assessment including dipstick urine test did not reveal anything abnormal and the family were reassured that there did not appear to be any underlying pathology as the cause of the bedwetting. However, it was noted that Ben appeared to be very wet at night, often wetting the bed within a few hours of going to sleep. This suggested that nocturnal polyuria could be the cause of the wetting.
>
> The family was given practical advice regarding management of the wetting and treatment options were discussed. Ben's parents were also advised to ensure that Ben had 6–8 drinks during the day, went to the toilet regularly throughout the day and had a last 'wee' before sleep.
>
> Since the wetting was causing some degree of stress and upset within the family, a follow-up appointment was made for the next week. At this appointment it was decided to start Ben on a trial of desmopressin and he commenced DesmoMelt (0.120 µg) with one Melt at bedtime. Ben was reviewed a week later when a delighted mum reported that Ben had had four dry nights with reduced wetting on the other nights. The DesmoMelt was therefore continued with regular reviews including a Melt-free week every 3 months to check response. Six months later he was completely dry and the medication was discontinued.

that the stools are hard (Buchanan 1992). The number of 'normal' bowel movements varies per individual but generally ranges from three times per day to three times per week (Weaver & Steiner 1984, Leung et al 1996). Therefore, any fewer than three bowel movements per week would be considered a risk factor for constipation (Leung et al 1996).

Overflow soiling – functional retentive soiling

Soiling is the involuntary passage of stool into the child's underwear as a direct result of chronic con-

stipation (Clayden 1992, Rogers 2000). Importantly, it may be the first symptom that the child presents with (Benninga et al 1993) although the constipation may have existed undetected for many months previously. In fact, chronic constipation is thought to be the cause of soiling in 95% of affected children (Loening-Baucke 1997). A variety of factors may influence the occurrence of soiling, including possible oversecretion of mucus due to rectal irritation, some straightening of the anorectal angle (Read & Abouzekry 1986) and decreased rectal sensation (Loening-Baucke 1997). This is combined with reflex relaxation of the anal sphincter, all of which are provoked by the retained stool in the lower bowel (Buchanan 1992).

Encopresis – functional non-retentive soiling

Encopresis is a term used to describe the passage of normally formed stools in a socially unacceptable place, in a child over the age of 4 years, and is thought to be behavioural in origin (Clayden 1992). These children form only a very small percentage of children who soil and do not normally have any underlying constipation.

Normal defecation

In most cases the cause of paediatric constipation is functional and occurs as a result of a combination of closely linked factors (Clayden 1992). An understanding of the normal defecation process will help in the detection of those factors and direct appropriate treatment (see also Ch. 8). When stool descends from the sigmoid colon into the rectum, pressure is put on the rectal wall which activates the stretch receptors. Impulses are then sent to the defecation centre in the sacral spinal cord (S2–S4). These actions result in the simultaneous awareness of an urge to defecate with resultant reflex relaxation of the internal anal sphincter (rectosphincteric reflex) and contraction of the external anal sphincter (anus). If sufficient stool is present, the initial contraction of the external sphincter is followed by total relaxation of the external and internal sphincters leading to defecation (Donatelle 1990).

If it is inconvenient to defecate, the stool can be retained by voluntary contraction of the external anal sphincter and the puborectalis muscle, which helps constrict the anal canal. When the call to defecate is voluntarily suppressed, the rectum accommodates the retained stool by adaptive compliance and eliminates the reflex relaxation of the internal sphincter and the urge to defecate. Some of the stool in the rectum is returned to the descending colon by retroperistalsis.

When it becomes convenient to defecate, the external sphincter is consciously relaxed and intra-abdominal pressure can be increased voluntarily by performing the Valsalva manoeuvre which helps force the stool along. During this process the pelvic floor is elevated which lifts the sphincter up over the faecal mass and allows the stool to be expelled (Leung et al 1996).

Causes of constipation

There is a general consensus of opinion that functional constipation often develops in childhood as a result of a number of contributory factors, all of which need to be identified and addressed to ensure good treatment outcomes and prevent relapse (Clayden 1992, Leung et al 1996). The constipation often develops when the child begins to associate pain with defecation and once pain is associated with bowel movements the child begins to withhold stools in an attempt to avoid discomfort. The rectum gradually enlarges to accommodate the increasing retained stool, and the normal urge to defecate slowly disappears. The passage of infrequent, very large, hard stools reinforces the child's association of pain with defecation, resulting in worsening stool retention and the cycle continues.

Diet/fluid intake

Lack of fibre in the diet can result in low faecal bulk with resultant decrease in mass peristaltic movements of the colon. A survey of children with constipation identified that 48% were 'faddy eaters' and 47% were reported to have a poor appetite. Appetite improved in half of these children following passage of the retained stool

(Clayden 1992). Drinking large quantities of milk to the detriment of solid food may predispose a child to passing hard stools and some children develop constipation as a result of intolerance to cow's milk (Lacano et al 1998). Inadequate fluid intake or excessive fluid loss (from diarrhoea/vomiting or febrile illness) may cause hardening of the stool and can be an important cause of constipation, especially in infants (Clayden 1992, Leung et al 1996).

'Withholding'

If the urge to defecate is continually ignored then the brain may become less responsive to further defecation urges. If the parent fails to notice that the child has not 'been' for a number of days the child will eventually become constipated. Conflicts around potty training have been cited by some authors as a contributory factor in younger children (Clayden 1992, Borowitz et al 2003). Older children may voluntary inhibit defecation if they are busy playing or deterred from using school and public toilets because they are unclean, lack privacy or are perceived by the child as cold, dark or scary (Pilapil 1990). However, the commonest reason children 'hold on' is because of pain or discomfort (Borowitz et al 2003) (Fig. 5.4). An anal fissure is one of the many causes of painful defecation, particularly when associated with the passage of large hard stools. Other causes are Group A streptococcal perianal infection and skin diseases such as epidermolysis bullosa and severe eczema (Clayden 1992). Sexual abuse is fortunately a very rare occurrence but something which may need to be considered.

If left untreated, constipation can result in a variety of other problems including anorexia, abdominal pain and overflow soiling (Doig 1992) with the development of a megarectum (Clayden 1992). Constipation has also been reported to account for 27% of cases of daytime wetting, 32% of nocturnal enuresis and 3% of UTIs in boys and 42% of UTIs in girls (Loening-Baucke 1997). Vesicoureteral reflux and upper urinary tract dilatation have also been linked to constipation (O'Regan et al 1986, Dohil et al 1994). In the absence of soiling, these other problems may be the first indication that chronic constipation is present.

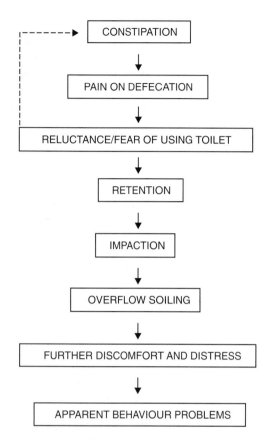

Figure 5.4 Sequence leading to retentive soiling.

Assessment

A carefully documented assessment should encompass a history of bowel habits including a check on passage of meconium, stool frequency and type using the Bristol Stool Scale (see Ch. 8), any soiling and associated problems such as abdominal pain and withholding behaviour. Diet and fluid intake need to be assessed, as well as a check on any medication and general health. Family history should be noted and any social issues discussed. Any previous interventions, including results of any investigations, need to be evaluated and recorded.

A clinical examination should be carried out to check the child's general health and to exclude any underlying pathology such as sacral agenesis. The abdomen should be palpated and examined for evidence of distension and faecal loading. Rectal examination is not necessary just to detect constipation since it can be distressing for the child and

may be perceived as physical abuse if force or coercion is used (Clayden 1992). A routine abdominal X-ray may be helpful to confirm overflow soiling as a result of faecal impaction in a child who initially presents with loose stools, particularly if the retained stools are soft and difficult to palpate. Combining the X-ray with a bowel transit time study may provide useful information and the resultant X-ray is also valuable as an educational tool to reinforce the message to the child and parents regarding the extent of the faecal loading and demystifying the cause of the soiling problem (Clayden 1992).

Treatment

The diverse needs of children with constipation and soiling are best met through a multidisciplinary team approach including nursing and medical staff as well as the support of a dietitian and psychologist. The general principles in managing functional constipation in children are to soften and clear any faecal impaction, establish a regular, pain-free pattern of defecation and prevent relapse by supportive management, including demystification and education for the child and family (Clayden 1992, Baker et al 1999).

Diet/fluid advice

The child should be encouraged to drink regularly throughout the day, aiming to have six to eight water-based drinks per day. In hot weather, extra drinks should be given, with such things as ice lollies and jellies providing extra fluid for the reluctant drinker. The average daily recommended fibre intake for adults is 18 g but there is currently no specific daily recommended intake for children. However, the general consensus of opinion appears to recommend, as a rough guide:

Child's age + 5 = daily amount (g) of fibre intake.

Any increase in fibre should be done on a gradual basis in conjunction with the increased fluid intake.

Lifestyle/behavioural advice

The child should be encouraged to sit on the toilet at regular intervals throughout the day. In our continence service we have found it more beneficial to encourage the child to actively 'push' a set number of times, then get off the toilet to come back and try again later if nothing happens, rather than asking the child to sit for an extended period of time with no result.

For effective straining the child needs to sit comfortably on the toilet with the feet supported on a step if necessary so that the knees are slightly higher than the hips (Loening-Baucke 1997), preferably after a meal as this makes use of the gastro-colic reflex. The toilet area should be warm and inviting with positive reinforcers used to encourage compliance if necessary.

Laxatives

If dietary and lifestyle changes are not sufficient to overcome the constipation, and certainly if the child is impacted, then the introduction of laxative therapy would be the next step. Clearance of impaction is necessary prior to initiation of bowel maintenance therapy (Baker et al 1999). Clinical experience with an iso-osmotic laxative comprising polyethylene glycol (PEG) 3350 with electrolytes (Movicol) has been found to be very effective in treating faecal impaction in children (Vincent & Candy 2001). This treatment was found to be well tolerated by the children and eliminated the need for invasive procedures such as enemas. In a comparative study with lactulose, Movicol was also found to be more cost-effective (Christie et al 2002). It is licensed for all children with constipation from aged 2 years and above and for clearance of impaction from aged 5 years.

Box 5.7   Case study 2

Adam, aged 4 years, was referred to the paediatric constipation clinic by the GP because of ongoing problems with constipation and soiling. Adam had been constipated on and off for as long as his mother could remember and when he started potty training he would happily wee on the potty but refused point blank to do a 'poo' except in a nappy. Once Adam started nursery, his mother felt he was now too old to use a nappy and insisted he used the potty/toilet. However, this seemed to make the constipation worse as he then refused to do a poo at all and began soiling as well.

This caused great problems in nursery as well as at home and Adam's mother also felt that his behaviour deteriorated at this point, as he would become very aggressive and disruptive at times. Adam had been on senna and lactulose on and off in the past but they were no longer effective and sometimes his mother felt that Adam was soiling on purpose just to annoy her! Adam had always been a lively child and not easy to manage. He was the oldest of three boys: James (2.5 years) and Nicholas (8 months) and, indeed was expected to be the 'big boy'. The younger boys had been more placid and easier to establish with a routine.

Adam was seen by the paediatric continence advisor who spent a long time with Adam and his mother and father to explain how constipation develops and how overflow soiling then occurs. She explained that this overflow soiling occurred outside Adam's control and that in order to resolve the problem they would need to clear out Adam's bowel with laxatives and then keep him on a maintenance dose for at least 6 months. Adam commenced on Movicol Paediatric Plain and the nurse explained how to increase the dose until his bowel was cleared and check with the Bristol Stool form chart for when his poo had become the right consistency. Charts were kept to record progress and the nurse kept in touch by phone until the evacuation was complete and Adam was on the maintenance dose.

Adam's mother encouraged him to sit on the toilet regularly after meals and provided lots of support and encouragement. (She had previously discussed feeling very guilty about blaming Adam for the soiling but was reassured by the nurse that it was a common response and to move on from that and to now provide lots of support and positive reinforcement.) At the follow-up appointment, his mother reported that although Adam was now passing soft stools he was reluctant to open his bowels on the toilet. As he was still asking for a nappy, it was decided to allow Adam to have a nappy on to do a poo provided he did it sitting on the toilet! This allowed Adam to be more relaxed about the process and alleviated any 'holding on' behaviour.

A few weeks later, Adam's mother reported that Adam had now overcome his fear completely and was now proudly doing all his poos on the toilet with no nappy on. Over the next 6 months, contact was maintained with the family and although there were a couple of relapses, one when his mother forgot to renew the prescription, overall progress was maintained and Adam was finally discharged with no further problems. However, his mother was advised to continue to monitor the frequency and consistency of his stools over the following months and to contact the service at any time for any further advice and support if necessary.

An alternative to single line treatment is a step approach to evacuation of the rectum. The retained mass should be softened first by the administration of a softener such as docusate sodium which has a detergent-like property that helps break up the stool and also acts as a rectal stimulant. The usual dose is 2.5 mg/kg three times per day. The second phase involves evacuation of the now softened stool using a stimulant such as senna (5–10 ml) at night and adding weekend doses of sodium picosulfate (5 ml) if necessary. Senna is a natural laxative which stimulates defecation through its effects on intestinal motility and fluid and electrolyte transport.

The maintenance phase involves establishing regular bowel movements. A combination of a softener and stimulant may be necessary in some cases if the child is 'withholding'. Lactulose is a synthetic disaccharide which is hydrolysed to acids by the colonic flora. Due to the osmotic effects of lactulose and its metabolites the water content of the bowel increases with resultant softening of the stool (Loening-Baucke 1997); however, flatulence and abdominal cramps are frequently reported side effects (Baker et al 1999). Continuing the laxative therapy for several months will be necessary (Leung et al 1996, Baker et al 1999) and there is a general level of agreement that children with chronic constipation will have to continue with laxatives for at least a year (Clayden 1992). It is important to eliminate any pain associated with the passage of stools and to aim for the passage of at least three soft stools per week which are easily evacuated without straining.

Summary

Functional constipation is a common childhood condition and in the majority of cases the constipation develops as a result of a complex accumulation of factors including specific triggers such as reduced fluid intake following a viral infection or periods of restricted access to the toilet. The passage of large painful stools perpetuates the problem when the child begins to associate pain with defecation.

The management of constipation can often be a challenge in children who initially may be reluctant to sit on the toilet. The key to successful treatment includes taking a child-focused approach with effective initial evacuation and appropriate maintenance therapy.

KEY POINTS FOR PRACTICE

- Presumptions should not be made regarding the cause of wetting and soiling in children, particularly those with 'special needs'
- Children should not be issued with continence products without first undergoing a full assessment to exclude any underlying pathology
- An 'holistic' child-centred approach, including taking into account the level of the child's ability to undertake treatment programmes and the family dynamics, should always be employed

Useful addresses/resources

ERIC
34 Old School House
Britannia Road
Kingswood
Bristol BS15 2DB
Tel: 0117 960 3060
Fax: 0117 960 0401
Email: enuresis@compuserve.com, info@eric.org.uk
Websites: http://www.eric.org.uk, http://www.trusteric.org (young people's website)
ERIC is a national registered charity that provides information and support to children and young people, parents and professionals on childhood bedwetting, daytime wetting, constipation and soiling, and incontinence in children with special needs. It also provides resources such as books, bedding protection and enuresis alarms.

ERIC runs conferences and seminars for professionals and can provide cost-effective bespoke seminars tailored to suit in-house needs. For further details contact training@eric.org.uk.

ERIC School Campaign websites:
1. http://www.wateriscoolinschool.org.uk. This is a national campaign to improve water facilities and access to fresh drinking water for children in schools.

2. http://www.bog-standard.org.   Bog Standard is a national campaign to improve the standard of school toilets and pupils' access to better quality facilities.

PromoCon
Disabled Living
Redbank House
St Chad's Street
Manchester M8 8QA
Tel: 0161 834 2001
Email: promocon@disabledliving.co.uk
Website: http://www.promocon.co.uk

PromoCon, working as part of Disabled Living Manchester, provides impartial advice and information regarding products and services for children and adults with bowel and/or bladder problems.

PromoCon has produced a series of *Talk about...* booklets which are aimed specifically at children to help them understand the problems they are having. Topics in the series include constipation, daytime wetting, bedwetting, going to the toilet. Contact Promo-Con for further information.

http://www.childhoodconstipation.com: website providing downloadable information for families.

IMPACT Paediatric Bowel Care Pathway, Norgine 2005. Resource pack for the treatment of constipation.

Care pathways – daytime wetting/nocturnal enuresis. PromoCon 2005

References

Agnarsson V, Clayden G S 1990 Constipation in childhood. Maternal and Child Health 15(8):252–256

Almond P 1993 Constipation: a family centered approach. Health Visitor 66(11):404–405

Arnold S J 1997 No more bedwetting. John Wiley, New York

Baker S S, Liptak G S, Colletti R B et al 1999 Constipation in infants and children: evaluation and treatment. A medical position statement of the North American Society for Pediatric Gastroenterology and Nutrition. Journal of Pediatric Gastroenterology and Nutrition 29:612–626

Bakker E, Wyndaele J J 2000 Changes in the toilet training of children during the last 60 years: the cause of an increase in lower urinary tract dysfunction? BJU International 86:248–252

Benninga M A, Buller H A, Taminiau J A 1993 Biofeedback training in chronic constipation. Archives of Disease in Childhood 68:126–129

Berk L B, Friman P C 1990 Epidemiological aspects of toilet training. Clinical Pediatrics 29(5):278–282

Blainey J L 1995 Practical considerations in large scale treatment programmes for nocturnal enuresis in children. Proceedings of the 3rd International Children's Continence Symposium 16–17 October 1995. International Children's Continence Society Monograph Series No. 1. Wells Medical, Kent, p 45–46

Blaum N J, Taubman B, Nemtheth N 2003 Relationship between age at of toilet training and duration of training: a prospective study. Pediatrics 111(4):810–814

Bloom D A, Seeley W W, Ritchey M L, McGuire E J 1993 Toilet habits and continence in children: an opportunity sampling in search of normal parameters. Journal of Urology 149:1087–1090

Borowitz S M, Cox D J, Tam A et al 2003 Precipitants of constipation during early childhood. Journal of the American Board of Family Practitioners 16(3):213–218

Buchanan A 1992 Children who soil. Assessment and treatment. Wiley, London

Butler R J, Redfern E J, Forsythe W I 1990 The child's construing of nocturnal enuresis: a method of inquiry and prediction of outcome. Journal of Child Psychology and Psychiatry 31:447–454

Caione P, Giorgi P L, Passerini-Glazel G et al 1995 Desmopressin (DDVAP) and oxybutynin in nocturnal enuresis: results of a multicentre trial. Proceedings of the 3rd International Children's Continence Symposium 16–17 October 1995. International Children's Continence Society Monograph Series No. 1. Wells Medical, Kent, p 77–81

Christie A H, Culbert P, Guest J F 2002 Economic impact of low dose polyethylene glycol 3350 plus electrolytes compared with lactulose in the management of idiopathic constipation in the UK. Pharmacoeconomics 20:49–60

Cisternino A. Passerini-Glazel G 1995 Bladder dysfunction in children. Scandinavian Journal of Urology and Nephrology 173:25–29

Clayden G S 1992 Management of chronic constipation. Archives of Disease in Childhood 67:340–344

De Paepe P, Hoebeke C, Renson E et al 1998 Pelvic-floor therapy in girls with recurrent urinary tract infections and dysfunctional voiding. British Journal of Urology 81(supplement 3):109–113

Department of Health 2004 National Service Framework for children, young people and maternity services. TSO, London

Dohil R, Roberts E, Jones K V et al 1994 Constipation and reversible urinary tract abnormalities. Archives of Diseases of Childhood 70:56–57

Doig C M 1992 Paediatric problems – 1. British Medical Journal 305:462–464

Donatelle E P 1990 Constipation: pathophysiology and treatment. American Family Physician 42:1335–1342

Downing J, Perino D M 1992 Functional versus standardised assessment procedures: implications for educational programming. Mental Retardation 30(5):289–295

Drugs and Therapeutics Bulletin 2000 Managing constipation in children 38(8):57–60

Eller D A, Homsy Y L, Austin P F et al 1997 Spot urine osmolality, age and bladder capacity as predictors of response to desmopressin in nocturnal enuresis. Scandinavian Journal of Nephrology Supplement 183:41–45

Fewell R R 1991 Trends in the assessment of infants and toddlers with disabilities. Exceptional Children 58:166–173

Forsythe W I, Butler R J 1989 Fifty years of enuresis alarms. Archives of Diseases of Childhood 64:879–885

Hannson S 1992 Urinary incontinence in children and associated problems. Scandinavian Journal of Urology and Nephrology 141:47–57

Hjalmas K 1992a Functional daytime incontinence: definitions and epidemiology. Scandinavian Journal of Urology and Nephrology 141:39–44

Hjalmas K 1992b Urinary incontinence in children: suggestions for definitions and terminology. Scandinavian Journal of Urology and Nephrology 141:1–6

Hjalmas K 1995 SWEET, the Swedish Enuresis Trial. Scandinavian Journal of Urology and Nephrology Supplement 173:89–92

Hogg R J 1996 Genetic factors as predictors for desmopressin treatment success. Scandinavian Journal of Urology and Nephrology 183(supplement 31):37–39

Houts A C, Berman J S, Abramson H 1994 Effectiveness of psychological and pharmacological treatments for nocturnal enuresis. Journal of Consulting and Clinical Psychology 62:737–745

Hyams G, McCoull K, Smith P S et al 1992 Behavioural continence training in mental handicap: a 10 year follow up study. Journal Intellectual Disabilities and Research 36:551–558

Jansson U B, Hanson M, Hellstrom A L et al 2005 Voiding pattern in healthy children 0–3 years old: a longitudinal study. Journal of Urology 164(6):2050–2054

Jaureguizar E, Pereira L 1992 Structural incontinence. Scandinavian Journal of Urology and Nephrology 141:20–25

Lacano G, Cavataio F, Montalto G 1998 Intolerance of cow's milk and chronic constipation in children. New England Journal of Medicine 339:1100–1104

Leung A K C, Chan P Y H, Cho H Y H 1996 Constipation in children. American Family Physician 54(2):611–618

Loening-Baucke V 1997 Fecal incontinence in children. American Family Physician 55(6):2229–2236

Luiselli J K 1997 Teaching toilet skills in a public school setting to a child with pervasive developmental disorder. Journal of Behavioural Therapy and Experimental Psychiatry 28:153–168

MacKeith R C, Meadow S R, Turner R K 1973 How children become dry. In: Kolvin I, MacKeith R C, Meadow S R (eds) Bladder control and enuresis. Clinical and Developmental Medicine 48(49):3–32

Mattsson S 1994 Voiding frequency, volumes and intervals in healthy school children. Scandinavian Journal of Urology and Nephrology 28:1–11

Mattsson S, Lindstrom S 1995 How representative are single frequency-volume charts? In: Norgaard J P, Djurhuus J C, Hjalmas K et al (eds) Proceedings of the Third International Children's Continence Symposium. Wells Medical, Kent, p 97–99

Meadows S R 1990 Day wetting. Pediatric Nephrology 4:178–184

Neveus T , von Gontard A, Hoebeke P et al 2006 The standardization of terminology of lower urinary tract function in children and adolescents: report from the Standardisation Committee of the International Children's Continence Society (ICCS). Journal of Urology 176(1):314–324

Norgaard J P, van Gool J D, Hjalmas K et al 1998 Standardization and definitions in lower urinary tract dysfunction in children. British Journal of Urology 81(supplement 3):1–6

Olbing H 1992 Management of the incontinent child in general practice. The paediatrician's viewpoint. Scandinavian Journal of Urology and Nephrology 141:126–134

O'Regan S, Schick E, Hamburger B 1986 Constipation associated with vesicoureteral reflux. Urology 28:394–396

Pipapil V R 1990 A horrifying television commercial which led to constipation. Pediatrics 85(4):592–593

Read N W, Abouzekry L 1986 Why do patients with faecal impaction have faecal incontinence? Gut 27:283–287

Rickwood A M K 1992 Management of the incontinent child in general practice. The paediatric urologist's viewpoint. Scandinavian Journal of Urology and Nephrology 141:117–125

Rogers J M 1996a Cognitive bladder training in the community. Paediatric Nursing 8(8):18–20

Rogers J M 1996b Single-minded action. Nursing Times 92(4):78–80

Rogers J M 1998 Nocturnal enuresis should not be ignored. Nursing Standard 13(9):35–38

Rogers J M 2000 The causes and management of constipation in children. Community Nurse 6(3):39–40

Schum T R, Kolb T M, McAuliffe T L et al 2002 Sequential acquisition of toilet-training skills: a descriptive study of gender and age differences in normal children. Pediatrics 109(3):E48

Smith L, Smith P, Lee S K 2000 Behavioural treatment of urinary incontinence and encopresis with learning disabilities: transfer of stimulus control. Developmental Medicine and Child Neurology 42:276–279

Stenberg A, Lackgren G 1995 Desmopressin tablet treatment in nocturnal enuresis. Scandinavian Journal of Urology and Nephrology Supplement 173:95–99

Taylor S, Cipani E 1994 A stimulus control technique for improving the efficacy of an established toilet training programme. Journal of Behavioural Therapy and Experimental Psychiatry 25(2):155–160

Van Gool J, Vijverberg M A, de Jong T P 1992 Functional day time incontinence: clinical and urodynamic assessment. Scandinavian Journal of Urology and Nephrology 141:58–69

van Wijk J A E, van Gool J D 1995 Urodynamic follow-up in girls with recurrent uncomplicated urinary tract infections. In: Norgaard J P, Djurhuus J C, Hjalmas K et al (eds)

Proceedings of the Third International Children's Continence Symposium. Wells Medical, Kent, p 127–129

Vincent R, Candy D 2001 Movicol for the treatment of faecal impaction in children. Gastroenterology Today 11(2):50–52

Weaver L T, Steiner H 1984 The bowel habit of young children. Archives of Diseases in Childhood 59:649–652

Wolf-Schein E G 1998 Considerations in assessment of children with severe disabilities including deaf-blindness and autism. International Journal of Disability, Development and Education 45(1):35–54

Yong D, Beattie R M 1998 Normal bowel habit and prevalence of constipation in primary school children. Ambulatory Child Health 4:27

Chapter **6**

Vulnerable groups

Frail elderly *Sharon Eustice*
Mental health needs *Mary Kennedy*
Neurological disability *Collette Haslam*

The fact than an opinion has been widely held is no evidence whatsoever that it is not utterly absurd. Indeed, in view of the silliness of the majority of mankind, a widespread belief is more likely to be foolish than sensible.

Bertrand Russell (1929)

INTRODUCTION

The principles of promoting continence and management of incontinence form the central theme of this book, and are largely applicable to all patient/client groups. However, there are a number of discrete groups for whom continence problems and access to services may pose a particular problem (DH 2000). This chapter examines some of the specific issues for three groups: frail elderly, people with mental health needs and people with long-term physical disabilities through neurological dysfunction. Chapter 7 focuses on continence care for people with intellectual disability.

FRAIL ELDERLY

This section focuses on the frail elder with urinary and faecal incontinence. Although the volume and quality of the research-based evidence to support continence care for this group is generally limited, it is important to recognise that current population trends are moving towards increasing numbers of older people and therefore greater understanding of their needs is crucial. Modernisation and redesign within healthcare services requires motivation of commissioners to deliver quality services for those who are frail that are based close to home and avoids hospital admission where possible (DH 2006).

Prevalence of incontinence in the frail elder person

Older people are often afflicted by urinary and faecal incontinence, not because it is inevitable, but due to many factors within and outside the lower urinary tract and bowel. Most prevalence rates reported for older people target all those >65 years (Peet et al 1995, RCP 1995, Hunskaar et al 2003) (see Ch. 1). However, prevalence figures for

the frail elderly are less available. Brandeis et al (1997), in their study on 2014 frail nursing home residents using a minimum data set, identified that 49% had urinary incontinence. It is not clear, however, how the researchers have defined the frail older person and the study suggests that all residents within the nursing home setting were classified as frail.

Developing services designed for frail elders poses several challenges for healthcare delivery. The first relates to clear identification of the population in question and the second to providing services which facilitate dealing with the potential multiplicity of problems experienced by individuals. Since most healthcare services are traditionally focused around a specific component of the human system, dealing with more than one at a time requires a shift in ethos towards greater patient centeredness in dealing with frailty (Rockwood & Hubbard 2004).

Defining the frail elderly

Although there does not appear to be a clear definition on what factors would constitute frailty, the literature does provide some consistency in the descriptions. Fonda et al (1998) defined frail older people as those over 65 and homebound or institutionalised. More recently, Gammack (2004) suggested that frailty is characterised by a loss of physiological reserve, resulting in a greater risk of injury and illness due to less ability to compensate for the environment and maintain functional status. This can range from mild to severe stages, leading to disability (Ferrucci et al 2004). Ferrucci et al go on to say that cognitive impairment may be a result of frailty, but that if it precedes it, then this is classified separately. Perhaps the greatest clarity on what factors make a person frail is offered by Fried et al (2001). They propose that frailty is a clinical syndrome and can be measured by markers such as weight loss, exhaustion, weakness in grip strength, slow gait speed and reduced physical activity.

The literature does not specify clearly if urinary incontinence is most likely to occur as a result of frailty, although Miles et al (2001) suggest that it may be an early indicator for the onset of frailty. In their population-based survey of 2660 people

Figure 6.1   A paradigm for continence. Reproduced with permission from Fonda et al (2005).

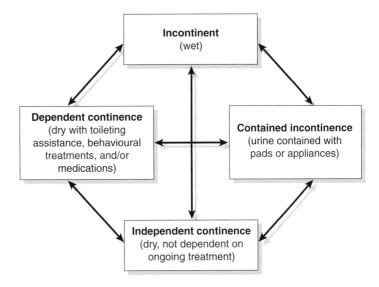

over 65 years, they found that incidence of incontinence was associated with a greater risk of impairment than prevalence of incontinence at base-line (Miles et al 2001). However, Holroyd-Leduc et al (2004), in their study on 6506 people aged 70 and over, found that those with urinary incontinence at baseline were more severely ill. Therefore, they concluded that urinary incontinence is a marker for frailty. Baztan et al (2005) concurred with this on the basis of their own work. In their investigation of 205 patients admitted to a geriatric rehabilitation unit, they found that urinary incontinence was associated with increased mortality or institutionalisation at 6 months following admission. Premorbid incontinence was considered a risk factor for this association.

A key consideration is whether or not incontinence can be cured in this group. Fonda et al (2005) suggest that while it may depend on types of treatment and aim of that treatment, cure is doubtful for particularly frail patients. They emphasise that quality of life is a fundamental issue and that incontinence which cannot be cured may still be open to improvement. Schnelle and Smith (2001) have developed quality indicators to guide healthcare professionals in systematic assessment. Their stance is that frail elders should have the same access to therapeutic care as other patient groups with incontinence.

Developing a care plan for a frail patient requires an attitude and approach that recognises the particular characteristics and uniqueness of this group. In terms of outcome, a shift from dependent urinary or faecal incontinence to independent continence may be unrealistic (Fig. 6.1) and often this means that incontinence problems are not adequately addressed where there is a prevailing belief that independent continence cannot be attained. However, by implementing treatment or management strategies which focus on achievable targets this should help to reduce avoidance of dealing with the additional complexity of incontinence in a frail patient. It has been suggested that admission to a nursing home facility is twice as likely for women with incontinence and three times as likely for men, compared with those who are not incontinent (Thom et al 1997). However, by setting appropriate and realistic goals it may be possible to reduce caregiver stress and burden to facilitate the cared-for person to remain in their own home.

AGEING AND THE AETIOLOGY OF URINARY AND FAECAL INCONTINENCE

Understanding the effects of ageing on the lower urinary tract and bowel in the frail elderly as opposed to natural ageing processes (see Ch. 2) is hampered by the paucity of published literature. What the literature does consistently emphasise is the multifactorial nature of urinary and faecal incontinence in the frail elder (Fonda et al 2005).

In a study on 249 frail elders living at home, Shimanouchi et al (2000) identified that stroke was the most common diagnosis. They also found that women (average age 83.3 years) had a higher tendency towards severe urinary incontinence than men (average age 79.5 years). However, other groups have reported comparable occurrence of symptoms between elderly men and women (Madersbacher et al (1998). Resnick et al (1995) challenged the concept of 'normality' and the ageing lower urinary tract when they found that normal urodynamic function was actually an exception in their study population of 56 volunteers between the ages of 65 and 101 years. Asymptomatic detrusor overactivity was identified in a third of the volunteers and contractility of the detrusor muscle was shown to decline with age. Fonda et al (2005) make reference to a particular age-related change that results in decreased vaginal blood flow leading to vault shortening and narrowing, which can render examination in the frail female difficult. Alteration of vaginal shape with consequential pelvic organ prolapse can also be a factor that contributes to the development of incontinence in frail elderly women.

In summary, it seems likely that increased risk of incontinence in the frail elderly group is more about a failure to compensate for additional stressors than an increased risk due to specific physiological changes in the lower urinary tract.

Detrusor hyperactivity with impaired contractility

Detrusor hyperactivity with impaired contractility (DHIC) is a condition commonly present in the frail elder (Resnick & Yalla 1987). This is where the bladder is overactive on filling, but has poor contractility on voiding. The condition presents with urgency, frequency, nocturia and urge incontinence. However, because the bladder muscle is weak, it fails to empty completely and therefore a residual volume of urine develops. Distinguishing these symptoms from other lower urinary tract conditions can be challenging and requires rigorous assessment. Treating DHIC may require both antimuscarinic medication and intermittent catheterisation (Nordling 2002).

Urinary tract infection

The treatment of asymptomatic bacteriuria, especially in the frail elder where aetiology of urinary incontinence is not fully understood, is often a controversial issue. Urinary tract infection (UTI) accounts for 25% of community-acquired bacterial infections in the frail elderly and 25–30% in those living in care homes (Richards 2004). While recurrent symptomatic UTIs might be a result of age-related changes in immune function, they may also be related to urinary incontinence and be treatable (Fonda et al 2005). However, treating asymptomatic bacteriuria is not generally recommended and McMurdo and Gillespie (2000) caution overdiagnosis and overtreatment of UTI in the frail elder. It is not uncommon in clinical practice to send a urine sample for microbiological analysis on the basis of a routine urine screen. This can lead to prescription of antibiotics for cases where symptoms are vague and non-specific, so misdiagnosis occurs. Exposing frail elderly people to antibiotics may result in unwanted side effects, overuse of medication, antimicrobial resistance and increased cost of therapy (Nicolle 2001). Further research is needed in the diagnosis of UTI, particularly in this patient group, to assist clinicians to make sound clinical judgements. In the meantime, the clinical condition of the patient should be fully assessed, including a search for other diagnoses and new symptoms localised to the lower urinary tract (McMurdo & Gillespie 2000). A minimum set of criteria for antibiotic therapy has been proposed by Loeb et al (2001). They recommend initiating antibiotics only for those patients who present with acute dysuria alone or fever (>37.9°C) and at least one of the following:

- new or worsening urgency
- frequency
- suprapubic pain
- macroscopic haematuria
- costovertebral angle tenderness
- urinary incontinence.

Nocturia

Nocturia can have a significant impact on frail elderly people and it is suggested that over 50%

of both men and women (>60 years) may be affected by this condition (Lundgren 2004). A study on 6517 people (predominantly working men) found that almost a third (28.5%) woke at least twice to void overnight. This increased to 60% for those over 69 years (Yoshimura et al 2004). There was no direct association with age alone, although risk factors for nocturia were prostatic hyperplasia in men, hypertension, cerebro- and cardiovascular disease, type 1 diabetes and poor renal function.

Nocturia is defined by van Kerrebroeck et al (2002) as waking one or more times during sleep to void, which is preceded and followed by sleep. Generally, nocturia is a commonly misunderstood condition and may be a contributing factor for the risk of falls in the frail elderly person (Brown et al 2000, Kron et al 2003). Weiss and Blaivas (2000) have reviewed the multifactorial nature of nocturia and, more recently, Marinkovic et al (2004) classified the major contributing factors/conditions as polyuria/nocturnal polyuria (urine over-production), overactive bladder and bladder outlet obstruction, each of which would require specific treatment approaches (Fig. 6.2). It is important that reporting of this condition is encouraged and treatment directed at the cause. A key consideration will be the level of bothersomeness caused by the nocturia and this should guide the degree of therapeutic input.

Faecal incontinence

Faecal incontinence is a very distressing condition and in the frail elder is usually a result of constipation (Fonda et al 2005). This may be explained partly by neurological diseases, reduced mobility, constipating medications and a reduced ability to increase abdominal effort (Muller-Lissner 2002). Very little has been written on this subject specifically in the frail elder population, although there is an extensive literature on constipation in older people in general (see Ch. 8); however, it is important that the underlying causes are identified and treated.

Other factors influencing incontinence in the frail elderly

The major precipitating factors that impact on the lower urinary tract can be classified as comorbid medical illnesses (e.g. type 1 diabetes, congestive cardiac failure), neurological and psychiatric conditions (e.g. stroke, Parkinson's disease, dementia), medications, functional impairments (e.g. mobility, impaired cognition) and/or environmental factors (e.g. inaccessible or unsafe toilets) (Fonda et al 2005). Since frailty diminishes an individual's ability to compensate for age-related changes in the lower urinary tract/bowel that an age-matched contemporary who is fit and well might achieve, it is imperative that reversible causes of incontinence are recognised and treated. Failure to treat the transient causes of incontinence can lead on to chronic incontinence. Work by Resnick and Yalla (1987) and Resnick (1996) is commonly quoted in the literature. Their mnemonic DIAPPERS (Box 6.1) provides a useful tool in summarising the causes that can initiate a new episode of incontinence or worsen established incontinence. However, one criticism of the use of this mnemonic is that it may reinforce an association between incontinence in older age and management of incontinence by containment alone (Keilman 2005).

Tannenbaum et al (2001), from their review of literature spanning 30 years or more, speculate that behavioural and pharmacological approaches to the management of incontinence can be implemented successfully in the frail elderly, even in cases of 'established incontinence', a term used to describe persistent incontinence despite the transient causes being addressed (Lekan-Rutledge 2004).

COMPREHENSIVE ASSESSMENT

When should incontinence be considered intractable? Certainly, it should not be identified as such until non-invasive therapies have been tried. Improving quality of life and reducing morbidity is just as valuable in the frail elder population as any other group. Ouslander (2000) has emphasised the need for comprehensive initial assessment and suggested that labelling incontinence as

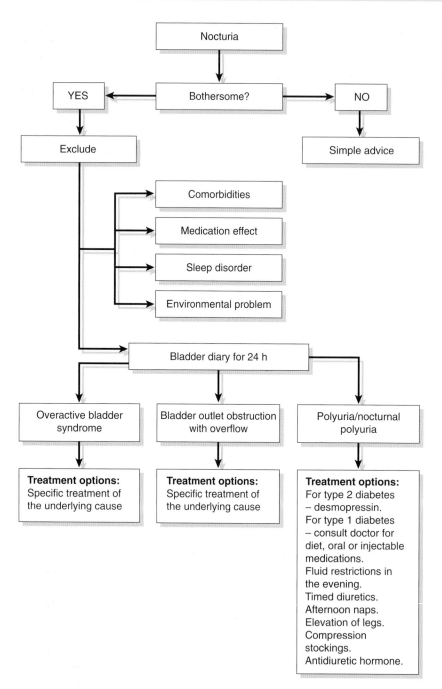

Figure 6.2 Nocturia algorithm. Adapted from Eustice & Wagg (2005) with permission from *Nursing Times.*

intractable is a 'self-fulfilling prophecy'. These views were supported by Landi et al (2003), who studied 5372 frail elder patients (mean age 77 years) in need of home care interventions. They found urinary incontinence in 51% of their sample and concluded that failure to treat reversible causes, which were strongly associated with the onset of urinary incontinence, was an indicator of inadequate quality care. Earlier work by Brandeis et al (1997) suggested similar results, but also raised an interesting point about a lack of guidelines to support clinical management. Chapter 2

Box 6.1 Causes of transient incontinence –
DIAPPERS (after Resnick 1996)

Delirium	May result from drugs, surgery or an acute illness
Infection	Symptomatic urinary tract infections can cause urinary incontinence
Atrophic urethritis/ vaginitis	Thinning, friable, irritated tissues that may cause or contribute to incontinence
Pharmaceuticals	Drugs include sedatives, narcotics, antimuscarinics, calcium channel blockers, loop diuretics, angiotensin-converting enzyme inhibitors, non-steroidal anti-inflammatory drugs and alpha-receptor agonists/antagonists
Psychiatric	Can cause incontinence if severe depression
Excess urine output	Can result from large fluid intake, caffeinated drinks and endocrine problems
Restricted mobility	Arthritis, pain, postprandial hypotension, poor use of assistive devices or fear of falling
Stool impaction	Can cause both urinary and faecal incontinence that can be corrected with disimpaction

details the components of general assessment strategies.

Other important factors contribute to and influence the management of frail elder men and women, such as the role of healthcare professionals, other caregivers and the goals of continence care. Thus a positive approach is needed, while taking into account reduced energy levels of the frail elder and being able to skilfully communicate with other professionals and non-professionals in delivering care to this group (Lekan-Rutledge 2004). Gitlin et al (1999) demonstrated in their evaluation of environmental modifications for frail elders ($n = 75$) that bathrooms and toileting were the most challenging aspects of self-care. Following supportive interventions from the occupational therapy department, 85% of frail elders were able to use their new equipment.

Improved quality of care is not simply dependent on the implementation of effective assessment skills but is also affected by infrastructure issues, such as enough staff, common guidelines, education and audit, as well as other incentives needed to make a real difference (Ouslander & Johnson 2004). Although their reference point is care homes, there is a sensible debate for transferring this concept to primary care. Reuben et al (2003) demonstrated that primary care physicians could improve care to older people using a multimethod approach, which includes condition-specific information, medical record prompts, educational material for patients and decision support. Even though this appears encouraging, effective translation into practice, from a healthy older population presenting with urinary incontinence to the frail elderly population, remains challenging. It has emerged from the findings of a recent audit of continence care for older people within parts of the UK that assessment for older people remains relatively poor, despite government drivers to improve care (RCP 2005).

ACHIEVING CONTINENCE

Addressing the reversible causes of incontinence may resolve or improve the continence status of the frail elder person. However, achieving continence may also be influenced by the health beliefs held not only by the individual sufferer but also by health professionals. Mitteness (1990) suggested there are significant characteristics that need to be considered. These are principally a lack of knowledge by the layperson of the causes of incontinence and a belief that the incontinence is inevitable and a non-reversible part of the ageing process. Through action and non-action, healthcare professionals contribute to lay knowledge and can either promote better understanding of incontinence or continued belief in its inevitability as part of the ageing process. Mitteness and Barker (1995) have commented on the management strategies employed by older people to maintain the secrecy about their incontinence. If the sufferer becomes frail, then self-imposed strategies such as scheduling activities to be near toilets, 'just in case' voiding to prevent leakage, dealing with increased laundry, etc. are vulnerable to failure and the individual's loss of control exposes the incontinence. Robinson (2000), in her qualitative investigation into nursing home residents living with incontinence, identified a range of coping strategies employed by older people, including:

- 'limiting' own activities or behaviours
- 'improvising' to reduce accidents
- 'learning' new skills to deal with incontinence
- 'monitoring' themselves against others
- 'speaking up' about their incontinence
- 'letting it go', which can be accidental, deliberate or negotiated voiding.

How people feel about themselves can have a notable impact on their ability to manage difficult situations such as coping with incontinence. 'Feeling old' may involve fears of helplessness, loss of control over one's life, feeling different and 'being able to identify when beginning to feel old' (Nilsson et al 2000). Baltes and Smith (2003) raise poignant issues about the 'fourth age' (the very old), which brings dysfunction and decreased likelihood for development/improvement in function. If incontinence is an additional feature in the older person's experience, how does this impact on their overall perceptions of their health? According to Johnson et al (1998), urinary incontinence is associated with poor self-rated health. However, the strongest association was for people with urinary incontinence who did not have other impairments to activities of daily living. For those with impairments, an association between urinary incontinence and poor self-rated health was less apparent. The experience of incontinence is unique to each individual, but health professionals' commitment to effective communication and therapeutic care may help to reduce misconceptions and maximise health outcome (Robinson 2000).

Conservative treatments

Although there is limited research-based evidence to guide practice for conservative treatments in the frail elder population (Engberg et al 2004), this does not necessarily mean they should be precluded from options that would be suitable for a fitter, older population (Gnanadesigan et al 2004). An algorithm to assist healthcare professionals

with systematic assessment and treatment has been developed by Fonda et al (2005). The recommendations include the need for sufficient fluid intake, reduced caffeine and management of constipation, and although the algorithm is mainly based on expert opinion, successful implementation should go some way to reducing poor care.

Lifestyle interventions

Lifestyle interventions to improve continence status are advocated by many healthcare professionals and may include advice on good fluid intake, smoking cessation and weight loss regimes. In a postal survey of 7046 women, of whom 435 (6.2%) were over 80 years, carbonated drinks were associated with both overactive bladder and stress urinary incontinence (Dallosso et al 2003). Dowd and Jones (1996) studied the effects of increased fluid intake on urinary incontinent episodes in 32 older women who were randomly assigned to one of three groups. Women were asked to increase their fluid intake, maintain their fluid intake or decrease it. The results showed no significant differences in incontinence episodes between the groups/regimes. However, the women commented that their awareness was raised about their need to increase fluid intake. In a study that targeted frail older people in nursing homes, fluid consumption during mealtimes was not found to increase despite improved activity in exercise and a scheduled toileting regime (Simmons & Schnelle 2004). In this study, exercise intervention also did not increase stool frequency. In a summary of the evidence for diet and fluid management to aid continence, Fonda et al (2005) drew attention to the limited scientific basis to inform practice.

Behavioural therapies

Behavioural therapies have been developed for the frail elder suffering from urinary incontinence as a method to restore or improve symptomology. Specific interventions include prompted voiding (Eustice et al 2006), habit training (Ostaszkiewicz et al 2004a), timed voiding (Ostaszkiewicz et al 2004b) and combined exercise and toileting schedules (Simmons & Schnelle 2004). Other interventions such as bladder retraining, biofeedback and pelvic floor muscle exercises have been less well studied in the frail elder population.

A systematic review on prompted voiding found that for people over 65 years of age, who were mobile but cognitively impaired, this technique produced short-term benefits (Eustice et al 2006). These conclusions were derived from a meta-analysis of the findings from nine randomised controlled trials, which had small sample sizes but well-defined inclusion criteria. The technique is underpinned by operant conditioning theory and involves prompting the person to use the toilet, with the aim of increasing self-initiated toileting (Palmer 2005). Although the long-term benefits are yet to be studied, the resources needed to work with a prompted voiding protocol are predominately labour intensive.

Habit training involves implementation of a toileting schedule that is generated from an individual's bladder diary and therefore the schedule is personalised to avoid wet episodes. Ostaszkiewicz et al (2004a) systematically reviewed the literature and found only three trials on which to assess its efficacy. No conclusions could be made about this intervention due to the limited data. In a study on 78 frail elder people living at home, 75% of the experimental group (n = 31) improved their continence status through a modified version of habit training, called pattern urge-response toileting (Colling et al 2003). Notable findings from this work were the reduction of skin problems and reduced carer burden. The latter may have resulted from increased information and education of the caregiver, enabling them to manage better, but the overall evidence was inconclusive.

Ostaszkiewicz et al (2004b) also looked at the most long-standing of toileting interventions, timed toileting. This technique relies not on individual bladder diaries or any prompting, but is based on trying to establish fixed time intervals to void (e.g. every 2 h). A review of the literature identified only two trials worthy of further investigation. However, the data were too few to make any decisions or recommendations about the impact of timed toileting.

Some studies have used combined exercise and toileting schedules to investigate outcome measures such as improved skin health. Bates-Jensen et al (2003) found that where toileting schedules were effective in reducing wet episodes, then skin health improved. Therefore, focusing on those patients who can respond to intervention is likely to produce the most benefit. For those who are unable to respond to such interventions, then alternative devices for managing incontinence to prevent skin exposure to moisture and destructive digestive enzymes are needed. However, apart from health professionals' own experience and marketing information, there is little in the way of robust evidence to inform which products or devices work best (Newman et al 2004). For further detail on management and containment options, see Chapter 10.

The majority of studies or reviews that investigate behavioural interventions tend to exclude the frail elderly (Burgio et al 1998, Berghmans et al 1999, Teunissen et al 2004). From the findings available it would seem that individuals with appropriate mobility, with or without cognitive impairment, can respond well to behavioural interventions but there is a need for a high level of staff or carer involvement and associated high costs, usually due to the increased dependence of the frail elder needing assistance to toilet. Unless assistance from caregivers is available, then behavioural interventions are likely to be less successful (Bear et al 1997). In advancing frailty, urinary incontinence has been identified as one measure that implies functional dependence prior to death (Covinsky et al 2003). Recognising when or when not to pursue implementation of interventions to promote continence requires sensitivity and skill on behalf of the healthcare professional so that a sense of balance is achieved between what the patient can realistically attain and their functional dependence (Box 6.2).

Medications

Special consideration is necessary for frail elders when prescribing medication (see Ch. 9). Pharmacokinetics (the absorption, distribution and elimination of a drug) and pharmacodynamics (the response of the drug on the body) can be altered in the older patient compared to younger adults (Bressler & Bahl 2003); for the frail elder, the changes can be profound (Shah 2004). For those frail elders where the reversible conditions have

Box 6.2   Case study 1

Mrs E is an 89-year-old lady who lives at home with her daughter, who is her principal carer. Mrs E has a medical history of hypertension, a stroke leaving a left-sided hemiparesis, diabetes, arthritis and reduced vision. She is occasionally incontinent of urine at night and also needs to go frequently. Her daughter needs to help her mother get to the bedside commode several times a night. Her mother rings a small hand bell. Mental status implies mild cognitive impairment.

By day, Mrs E is continent, but is dependent on her daughter to get her to the toilet on time. She does need to go quickly and can be on and off the commode several times a day. Mrs E is getting increasingly tired during the day, with low mood, as is her daughter, who has called Social Services for extra help and is asking for nighttime cover to help her have a good night's sleep.

Mrs E also complains of chronic constipation. Physical examination by the GP was negative. The district nurse team carried out an assessment of the situation. Bladder diaries confirmed urgency and frequency of voiding by day and night, with low bladder capacity. Urine test was clear, but postvoid residual urine was present. This was verified on three occasions by a portable bladder scan, which indicated residual volumes ranging between 200 and 400 ml.

Following discussion of the findings with Mrs E and her daughter, a treatment plan was agreed that would focus on the chronic constipation initially, with the use of regular toileting after meals to establish a pattern. A bulking agent was prescribed and fluid intake increased which resulted in bulkier stools and better stool evacuation. Combination treatment of antimuscarinic medication (one that did not impair cognition) and daily intermittent catheterisation, performed by the daughter, enabled reduced nocturia and incontinence. Both Mrs E and her daughter were able to sleep better, leading to an improved quality of life.

been addressed and behavioural intervention trialled if appropriate, drug therapy may have a place in treating urinary and faecal incontinence. Siegler and Reidenberg (2004) present a case study where combined use of anticholinergic drugs for urinary incontinence and cholinesterase inhibitors for dementia in the same patient was clinically effective. However, Ancelin et al (2006) suggest caution in that cognitive functioning is altered in elderly people who are long-term users of anticholinergic drugs. They found that users of these drugs might be identified as having mildly impaired cognition, compared with non-users. Healthcare professionals therefore need to assess carefully, be vigilant for drug interactions and avoid situations where the risk of adverse events is high. Fonda et al (2005) reviewed 28 studies and concluded that some drugs, such as immediate-release oxybutynin and tolterodine, were associated with impaired cognition.

Adverse events can affect up to 35% of older people living in their own homes and need to be detected (Hanlon et al 1997). Urinary incontinence associated with the use of medications can occur in those frail elders taking benzodiazepines (Landi et al 2002). To reduce adverse events, Rochon et al (1999) suggest an initial low-dose drug therapy approach where potential for lack of tolerance is high. Antimuscarinic medications are well known for their unpleasant side effects, such as dry mouth, constipation and increase in postvoid residual urine. The frail elderly are already at risk of these conditions and therefore selecting drug therapy warrants careful monitoring. For instance, postvoid residual urine should be measured by bladder scanning prior to commencing any antimuscarinic medication (Fonda et al 2005).

SUMMARY

Frailty challenges a person's ability to remain continent due to loss of compensatory skills. Therefore, recognising the causes of transient incontinence and reversing these can improve quality of life. A fundamental challenge for health care is to demonstrate a positive, interprofessional approach that is patient centred in order to tackle the complex, multifactorial issues raised by frailty. There is evidence to suggest that behavioural interventions and some pharmacotherapy can be successful for carefully selected patients and, indeed, they should have access to therapeutic care where comprehensively assessed. Service redesign programmes need to demonstrate that they can grasp and deal with frail elderly care in the climate of increasing longevity.

KEY POINTS FOR PRACTICE

- Becoming frail may be a clinical syndrome compounded by comorbid medical illnesses, neurological and psychiatric conditions, functional impairment and environmental issues
- Inability to compensate for these factors can lead to urinary and faecal incontinence
- Common conditions affecting the lower urinary tract and bowel in the frail elder are detrusor hyperactivity with impaired contractility (DHIC), nocturia and constipation
- Frail elders should be offered comprehensive assessment and not excluded from treatment or management strategies
- Always investigate and treat the reversible causes of incontinence first
- Behavioural interventions can be successful if there is availability of caregiver assistance and pharmacotherapy is useful in carefully selected frail elders
- Treatment of symptomatic bacteriuria is appropriate whereas asymptomatic bacteriuria is not
- Healthcare professionals need to be watchful for adverse events and drug interactions when prescribing medication
- Interprofessional working is fundamental in achieving better outcomes in managing the complexity and multifactorial nature of frail elder care

MENTAL HEALTH NEEDS AND INCONTINENCE

This section explores the relationship between urinary incontinence and mental illness, and the vulnerability of people who experience both conditions. People with mental health problems are acknowledged to be more vulnerable to poorer physical health than the general population, including an increased risk of diabetes and of mortality from cardiovascular disease and respiratory infection (Phelan et al 2001, Mentality 2003, Nash 2005). People with schizophrenia are recognised as being at increased risk of type 2 diabetes because of the side effects of medication, poorer health care, poorer physical health and less healthy lifestyles (Ohlsen et al 2005). Although those with a mental illness experience the same range of physical health needs as the general population, they may encounter various issues associated with their illness or its management that can make addressing the problem or accessing services more difficult.

ATTITUDES, STIGMA AND VULNERABILITIES

Loss of urinary control can lead to stigmatisation, social isolation, shame, hopelessness and depression (see Ch. 1), but individuals with mental health problems may also experience prejudice and discrimination as a consequence of stigma associated with mental illness, negative attitudes and stereotyping (Faulkner & Layzell 2000, Nash 2002). Both urinary incontinence and mental illness are surrounded by taboos and misconceptions, and share similar negative characteristics. The stigma associated with either condition can lead to discrimination and social exclusion, reducing the likelihood that those affected will actively seek professional help (Faulkner & Layzell 2000, Roe & Doll 2000). In a report by the Mental Health Foundation (2000) it was identified that people with mental health problems felt ostracised and frequently discriminated against. The consequence of this was lowered self-esteem, social isolation and exclusion, depression and anxiety. Similarly, urinary incontinence is considered socially unacceptable and as it can attract ridicule and blame it remains a 'hidden' problem for many people. Failure to conceal the problem may lead to social exclusion and isolation, and feelings of guilt, shame and embarrassment can make seeking help difficult (Ashworth & Hagan 1993, Saltmarche & Gartley 2001).

The fear and stigma associated with being incontinent in public comes early in life and loss of bladder control may be viewed as a violation of social norms, with severe psychological and social consequences for the individual concerned (Palmer 1994, Mitteness & Barker 1995). People who suffer discrimination or social exclusion because of illness may experience feelings of vulnerability, such as hopelessness and helplessness, through a perceived loss of control over their life (Rogers 1997, Mowforth 1999). Incontinence is often equated with a lack of self-control which can reflect in a derogatory way on the individual's self-perception, making them feel that they have regressed to a childlike state. Since continence control is an ability normally learned during childhood it is understandable that many adults who develop problems in later life feel this symbolises a threat to their maturity.

Coping with a stigma such as incontinence may involve the individual making a decision about whether to disclose their condition, risking further stigma, or attempt to conceal it and pass for normal (Goffman 1963, Joachim 2000). As discussed by Smart and Wegner (1999), individuals who have a 'concealable stigma' may be very motivated to engage in deliberate efforts to keep it concealed, even though this may require a great deal of mental control. For the individual with incontinence this can result in a complex set of coping strategies that can take up a considerable amount of time and energy (Shaw 2001). In an effort to conceal their condition individuals may face an internal struggle (Smart & Wegner 1999) which for clients with mental health problems may have serious psychological consequences.

It has been suggested that health professionals may reinforce incorrect and negative beliefs about incontinence, such as those related to age or stigma (either consciously or unconsciously) (Mitteness 1990). This not only affects the way in which health professionals interact with patients but can also influence the quality of care provided (Smith 1998, Henderson & Kashka 1999, Vinsnes et al 2001). The Department of Health's guidance on *Good Practice in Continence Services* (DH 2000a) draws attention to the personal costs of incontinence, identifying social embarrassment and social exclusion together with limitations on employment, education and leisure opportunities. These issues have a known damaging effect on mental and physical health and are major contributors to health inequalities (Acheson 1998, DH 2002). Those people with mental illness are among the most excluded groups when it comes to issues of employment, standards of living, housing and social support (Mentality 2003).

Prevalence of mental illness

Within the UK, approximately six million people consult their GP each year about a problem with

a mental health element (Nolan & Badger 2002). A high percentage of problems presented are psychosocial, with around 30% of all consultations and 50% of consecutive visits concerning some form of mental health problem, predominantly depression or anxiety (Kessler et al 1999, Mentality 2003). Depression is also reported as being much more common in people with physical health problems (Peveler et al 2002), with an estimated lifetime prevalence of 26% for women and 12% for men (Sobieraj 1998). Although estimates suggest that an average GP practice of 2500 individuals will identify 300 patients with a nonpsychotic mental illness a year, a significant number of patients with depression remain unrecognised (Lloyd & Jenkins 1995). This may include people with incontinence since several studies have reported an association between urinary incontinence and higher levels of anxiety and depression (Berglund et al 1994, Valvanne 1996).

Urinary incontinence and depression

The relationship between common mental health disorders and urinary incontinence is highly complex and as yet is not well understood (Melville et al 2002). It has been suggested that the symptoms and disability associated with a chronic illness such as urinary incontinence may be a contributing factor in the development of depression (Zorn et al 1999, Dugan et al 2000, Melville et al 2002). Depressive symptoms and urinary incontinence have been reported as two of the most common disabling illnesses that can affect women (Melville et al 2002). Hunskaar et al (2004) reported a 35% prevalence of urinary incontinence in women, and Singleton et al (2000) reported that approximately 20% of women suffered from depression.

In a study by Dugan et al (2000) it was reported that people who were incontinent often experienced shame, disgust, embarrassment and reduced social contact that may lead to depression. About 35% of those with urinary incontinence reported some depressive symptoms, which is slightly higher than the national average, and approximately 30% indicated that urinary incontinence interfered with their daily activities. The authors were of the opinion that depression associated with incontinence may make it more difficult for

Box 6.3   Case study 2

A 72-year-old gentleman was admitted to hospital with depression. During his admission he became incontinent of urine and was referred by the nursing staff for a continence assessment. Staff reported that he appeared unaware when he was incontinent and required encouragement and assistance to wash and change. Some of his behaviour was thought to be related to his depression but communication was also a problem as he was partially deaf. Although he normally wore a hearing aid he was not inclined to use this when first admitted. He had one previous admission to hospital with depression and at this time had responded well to treatment with antidepressants.

Following assessment he was found to be in retention with overflow and with his consent an indwelling urethral catheter was inserted. His wife reported that this had also happened on his last admission and at the time it was thought to be a side effect of his antidepressant medication. He had not experienced any problems prior to his admission. Following discussion with the ward team it was agreed to monitor the situation until his mood had stabilised and his medication could be reviewed.

As his mood did not improve with antidepressants, and his mental state continued to deteriorate, he was started on a course of electroconvulsive treatment. During this time he became distressed about having a catheter in situ and a trial without catheter (TWOC) was agreed. This was unsuccessful and another catheter was inserted. Following review with the urologist an alpha-blocker was recommended to try to relieve possible outflow obstruction, and an abdominal ultrasound scan was arranged which was found to be normal. After a period on alpha-blockers he had another unsuccessful TWOC and it was arranged for him to be seen in the urology outpatient clinic.

By the time he received his appointment his depression had improved significantly and he was due to be discharged home. He was still not happy about having a catheter and was hoping this could be removed if the urologist was able to recommend treatment. Although he was accompanied to his appointment by a nurse he had also written down a number of questions he wanted to ask. As it was important to him that he was able to express his worries and concerns, every attempt was made to create an environment where he felt he was listened to and his opinion was acknowledged. To ensure the urologist understood some of his problems, information was provided beforehand regarding his recent mental health problems, his urinary symptoms and his hearing impairment.

Unfortunately, even with such intervention, the gentleman found the consultation a traumatic experience. For the purpose of prostate assessment he had to undergo a digital rectal examination (DRE), which was handled in an insensitive manner with little regard for the invasive nature of the procedure. Although he had some understanding of what this may involve he was given little explanation and was subjected to a lot of hand waving as a way of communicating with him. During the consultation the conversation was mainly directed towards the nurse, who was informed following the DRE that further investigations would be required. When the gentleman was asked by the nurse if he understood what was being said the urologist's response was to raise his voice and to start shouting at him. On handing him the questions he had written down the urologist glanced at them briefly and said he would know more once the investigations had been completed. The urologist's final comment was that a letter would be sent to his GP and his psychiatrist detailing his recommendations.

---

those individuals to engage in treatments such as pelvic floor exercises and bladder training, which may help reduce episodes of incontinence.

At times, having a history of mental illness such as depression may act as a barrier to effective treatment and can result in both physical and psychological needs not being met (Box 6.3).

Older people and mental health problems

Continence problems in older people have been discussed earlier in this chapter but it is important to recognise the needs of older people with mental health problems, as their physical needs can sometimes be overlooked because of their mental illness. Older people often have a number of physical disabilities, such as sensory impairments or limited mobility, which can make maintaining continence difficult. Even though depression, apathy, loss of interest and social withdrawal can all contribute to incontinence, it is important not to exclude a physical cause for the incontinence, such as bladder infections, prolapsed uterus in women or prostate problems in men. Unfortunately, incontinence in older people is still too often seen as an inevitable part of ageing, and management strategies, such as the inappropriate use of pads, are often implemented without proper assessment.

Urinary incontinence and dementia

Older people living with dementia have multiple cognitive problems which can have a profound effect on their daily life. The loss of intellectual, personality and planning skills can all have an impact on the person's ability to remain continent. A number of cognitive skills are required for successful toileting (Box 6.4) and for the person with dementia these can break down at any point. They may have difficulty finding the toilet or identifying what it is for; decreased attention span can mean they are easily distracted and may get up from using the toilet before they have finished; and the ability to plan and carry out daily activities independently, such as using the toilet, can be lost.

The way in which people with dementia behave and communicate may be interpreted wrongly and can result in their physical, psychological and social needs being unmet. If the person has lost the skills necessary to communicate, and is not able to understand what is happening, then feelings of fear and frustration are likely to build up. As identified by Kitwood and Benson (1995) this can result in the person attempting to communicate behaviourally and what is commonly referred to as 'challenging behaviour' (e.g. restlessness, shouting or physical aggression) can be the end result.

Box 6.4 Skills required for successful toileting

- Recognise the need to use the toilet
- Be motivated to use the toilet
- Identify an appropriate place
- Locate an appropriate place
- Have the physical ability to get there
- Hold on until an appropriate place is reached
- Maintain goal-oriented behaviour
- Able to adjust clothing and use toilet once reached

Although getting information from the person about their incontinence may be difficult, this should not be a barrier to thorough assessment and in such circumstances information can be provided by the family or carers involved. The person's incontinence could simply be due to them having difficulty getting to the toilet and with some help and supervision the problem could be resolved. Observing the person's behaviour may also be a good indicator of when they need to use the toilet. Characteristic signs may include restlessness, agitation or pulling at clothing. Strategies to promote continence and/or manage incontinence include habit training or prompted voiding (see Frail elderly section above and Ch. 3).

Sexual abuse

People with dementia are particularly vulnerable to risk of physical or psychological abuse, as discussed in the *No Secrets* guidance published by the Department of Health (2000b). Healthcare professionals who care for older people need to be alert to possible actions which may be considered as abuse. For example, catheterising a person suffering with dementia would not be appropriate, as apart from difficulty in obtaining their consent, they are unlikely to remember what the catheter is for and why it is there. The likelihood is they will try to remove the catheter by pulling on it, leading to unnecessary self-injury and urethral trauma.

Another area of concern is associated with female survivors of sexual abuse who may have experienced problems at various times throughout their lives when gynaecological procedures involving examination of the pelvic area have been performed. In a paper exploring sexual abuse, Kitzinger (1990) provides an enlightening example of an elderly blind woman being held down by four nurses to be catheterised and who during the procedure repeatedly cried out 'please don't do it daddy, please don't do it daddy'. Although the woman's past history was not known, from Kitzinger's own work with survivors of childhood sexual abuse she was aware that medical procedures can often bring back overwhelming memories of sexual violence. This can

Box 6.5   Case study 3

A 35-year-old man was referred for assessment via the urology clinic following a problem with teaching him to do intermittent self-catheterisation (ISC). He had a history of depression and anxiety and was under the care of the mental health services. At his first appointment he was extremely anxious and expressed concern about how this problem could be managed if he was unable to do ISC. He complained of urinary frequency, urgency, occasional urge incontinence and nocturia five or six times a night. He also had a feeling of incomplete bladder emptying and on previous investigations was found to have high residual urine volumes.

He was concerned about the impact his symptoms were having on his relationship and he was now avoiding going to places without easy access to a toilet. He was anxious to improve the management of his symptoms and asked if he could be shown again how to catheterise. It was agreed that should he experience any pain or discomfort during the procedure it could be stopped, or alternatively, as he was in the best position to decide how much pain he could tolerate, he could take over the catheterisation. The catheter was passed without any difficulty and he decided he could now try doing this himself. Having been provided with instructions and catheters, another follow-up appointment was arranged.

At the beginning of his next appointment he immediately disclosed that he had been sexually abused as a child and wondered if this was related to him having problems with emptying his bladder. He also reported that although he had no problems passing the catheter, and had noticed an improvement in his symptoms, he did find it unpleasant touching his genitals as this provoked memories of the sexual abuse. He hoped that eventually he would be able to overcome this as he did want to continue with the ISC. Time was spent exploring his concerns and issues he had with regards to this. It was acknowledged that to continue he would need ongoing help and support from the service.

create strong feelings of vulnerability and is not only restricted to women. An example of a management problem with intermittent self-catheterisation in a male survivor of sexual abuse is provided in Box 6.5.

Physical health care

A relative lack of adequate training and skills in physical health care has been identified as an important issue in the provision of care to mental health clients (Phelan et al 2001, DH 2005). One of the most frequently expressed forms of discrimination cited by people experiencing mental health problems is their physical illness not being taken seriously or being attributed to mental distress or psychosomatic sources (Mental Health Foundation 2000). As a result, people with mental illness often have significant health issues resulting from neglect of their physical health or from the effects of long-term medication. These issues were noted in a study by Kennedy (2006) in which mental health clients were interviewed about their experience of living with urinary incontinence.

The relationship between medication and UI

Many of the drugs used in the management of mental health problems can have a potent effect on bladder function (Kelleher 1997, Iqbal et al 2003). For example, lithium carbonate can cause excessive thirst, with polydipsia and increased diuresis, and the anticholinergic effects of antidepressants can cause voiding difficulties leading to urinary retention with overflow and the risk of urinary tract infections (British National Formulary 2004). An association with psychotic illness and increased urinary incontinence has previously been identified (Warner et al 1994). In some cases this is thought to be due to high doses of antipsychotic drugs, and in particular to clozapine, which appears to have a higher incidence of urinary incontinence compared with other antipsychotic drugs such as olanzapine and risperidone (Fuller et al 1996). There has also been an identified link between antipsychotic drugs and nocturnal incontinence, as the drugs can reduce alertness and impair bladder sensation, increasing the risk of nocturnal incontinence (Koch et al 2002).

ASSESSMENT AND INVESTIGATIONS

Incontinence is unlikely to improve on its own and it is essential that a comprehensive assessment includes physical, psychological and social aspects to ensure effective treatment and management. The assessor needs to recognise there may be particular problems for people with mental illness which contribute to heightened feelings of humiliation, alienation and vulnerability, and can have a damaging effect on the person's self-esteem and self-confidence, increasing the risk of social exclusion.

Antipsychotic medication not only places the mentally ill at risk from a number of physical conditions, but can also cause a problem related to antipsychotic-induced weight gain (Ohlsen et al 2005). The psychological effects of being overweight, with added threats to self-esteem and self-image, can be particularly damaging and can result in non-adherence to treatment and subsequent relapse (Ohlsen et al 2005). This can mean that priority is not always given to physical health needs and they may be overlooked as interventions are focused on the mental illness and stabilising psychotic symptoms (Nash 2005). In such circumstances it would not be uncommon for continence problems to be neglected or seen as part of the person's mental illness.

Where the person is acutely unwell or experiencing high levels of distress it may be difficult or inappropriate to attempt assessment of continence until their mental health has stabilised. For those people with severe and enduring mental health problems it may be difficult to obtain accurate information or consent for investigations. There may be a lack of motivation and compliance with treatment may be a problem. As a result of underlying psychosis the person's mental state may fluctuate and they may experience apathy and disorganised thinking which may contribute to episodes of incontinence. Typically, they may lack motivation with poor self-care skills which can impact on the treatment and management of their incontinence.

TREATMENT AND MANAGEMENT STRATEGIES

The strategies for treating incontinence presented in other chapters are equally applicable to those people with mental health problems if they are able to comply with them. However, there are some particular issues to consider which are discussed below.

Self-management

It may be difficult to motivate or engage clients who are depressed, anxious or psychotic in treatment programmes, especially any which involve long-term treatment such as bladder training. Also, suggesting pelvic floor exercises to someone who is depressed is unlikely to have any impact when they lack the motivation or concentration to follow the advice given. The first solution may be to offer pads for protection and to introduce exercises once the depression has improved. Because of the symptoms of their illness, clients may be socially isolated, and where they experience delusional ideas or paranoia, they may be unwilling to accept help or adhere to treatment (Wood & O'Neill 2005). How this is approached, and the treatment offered, will depend on their ability and motivation to deal with the problem (Sells & McDonagh 1999). A significant amount of time may be needed to establish a trusting relationship before any progress can be achieved, but providing ongoing psychological support is essential if the person is to develop effective ways of coping with their incontinence and not remain socially isolated or excluded.

Lifestyle changes

There are a number of lifestyle factors that make people with mental health problems more vulnerable to poor physical health, including a tendency to poorer diets, obesity, cigarette smoking, substance misuse and physical inactivity (Ohlsen et al 2005). The *National Service Framework for Mental Health* (DH 1999), the National Institute for Clinical Excellence (2002) and the *Review of Mental Health Nursing* (DH 2005) have all recognised the need to explore ways of helping people with mental health problems to engage in making healthy living choices and identified improved physical care as a priority within mental health services, including dietary changes to tackle obesity and manage weight loss.

Many people who experience urinary incontinence will restrict their fluid intake in an attempt to prevent incontinence. However, they need to be made aware that this is not advisable as a low fluid intake can irritate the bladder, increasing urinary frequency and urgency, and leading to the risk of bladder infections (see Ch. 3). Increased fluid consumption can be a particular problem for people with schizophrenia who experience poly-dipsia, and as a result may increase their intake of caffeine (McNeill 2001). This is often made worse by medication as many of the psychiatric drugs can cause a dry mouth, which again can promote increased fluid intake. Smoking is also signifi-cantly higher among people with mental illness, with the prevalence highest among those with a psychotic disorder (McNeill 2001). As smoking can increase the elimination of caffeine, some may be inclined to take more caffeine to make up for the elimination caused by heavy smoking. The likelihood is that this will either cause or aggra-vate urinary symptoms and ideally a combined approach would be needed to look at moderating the intake of caffeine and to offer support with stopping smoking. However, in reality, this may be difficult to achieve and the individual would need to demonstrate an appropriate level of moti-vation before a programme of treatment could be agreed.

CONCLUSIONS

The mentally ill are a vulnerable group with poorer health care, poor physical health and less healthy lifestyles. They do not always have easy access to resources and in many instances are reliant on support from mental health profession-als to assert their rights to appropriate treatment (Gardner & Smith 2004). Urinary incontinence is a multifaceted problem and people can experience a range of physical, psychological and social needs related to this. For the mentally ill to be able to access services and treatment on equal terms to the general population, there is a need to develop a shared care approach that supports multiprofes-sional working and ensures the delivery of holistic care that takes into account the entire well-being of the person (Gardner & Smith 2004, Kennedy 2006).

Mental illness and urinary incontinence are sig-nificant public health problems that affect a wide range of the population (DH 2000a). In order to combat the taboo, stigma and social exclusion associated with both conditions there is a need to increase public and professional awareness (DH 2004, 2005). Health promotion and education are important aspects of health care and all health professionals have a responsibility to actively engage in initiatives that promote health-ier lifestyles.

KEY POINTS FOR PRACTICE

- It is not unusual for urinary incontinence and mental illness to coexist
- There are a number of studies dedicated to the psychological aspects of urinary problems amongst 'normal' populations, but there are very few concerning those with established mental illness
- People who suffer with urinary incontinence are significantly more depressed, have higher levels of anxiety and feel more stigmatised than those without the problem
- Having a mental health problem often carries considerable stigma and it is not uncommon for people with mental illness to be ostracised and discriminated against. Combined with the nega-tive impact of incontinence, this can result in loss of self-esteem, feelings of helplessness, self-disgust, self-hatred and somatisation, leading to depression, anxiety and social isolation
- People that suffer discrimination or social exclu-sion because of illness may experience feelings of vulnerability through a perceived loss of control over their life
- People who are mentally ill are more vulnerable to poorer physical health than the general popu-lation, with higher levels of morbidity and mor-tality than the general population

CONTINENCE PROBLEMS IN NEUROLOGICAL DISABILITY

CONSEQUENCES OF NEUROLOGICAL DAMAGE ON THE BLADDER

Continence problems are common in people with neurological disability. The precise type of bladder disorder which occurs due to neurological damage

Box 6.6   Neurological bladder problems

Functional problem	Cause
Failure to store	Neurogenic detrusor overactivity
Failure to empty	Detrusor areflexia
	Detrusor–sphincter dyssynergia
	Poorly sustained detrusor contractions
Combined storage and emptying failure	A combination of the above

Box 6.7   Pathophysiological consequences of neurological lesions

- Suprapontine lesions
  - Neurogenic detrusor overactivity
- Suprasacral lesions
  - Neurogenic detrusor overactivity
  - Detrusor–sphincter dyssynergia
  - Unsustained detrusor contractions
- Sacral, cauda equina and pelvic nerve lesions
  - Detrusor areflexia or hyporeflexia (acontractile or hypocontractile detrusor)
- Pudendal nerve lesions
  - Incompetent urethral sphincter

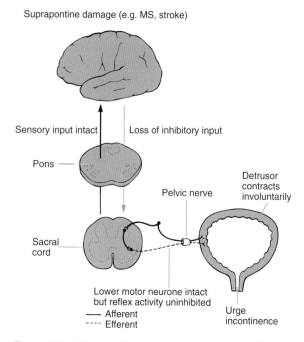

Figure 6.3   Neurogenic detrusor overactivity: mediation of the micturition reflex in the sacral cord. MS, multiple sclerosis. Adapted with permission from Popovich & Stewart-Amidei (1991).

depends on which area of the central nervous system (brain and spinal) is affected. Neural control of the lower urinary tract is complex, but the main functions are limited to storage and voiding, with the reciprocal association of the higher centres and spinal pathways (see Ch. 2 for normal bladder function). The key pathophysiological consequences of neurological lesions are outlined in Boxes 6.6 and 6.7.

Suprapontine damage

Damage above the pons leaves the spinal–bulbar–spinal reflex intact. Coordinated sphincter relaxation and detrusor contraction for voiding are therefore preserved but the inhibitory input to delay micturition may be lost or impaired. The result is an excess of reflex bladder activity, hence *detrusor overactivity* (DO); the person is aware of the need to pass urine but is unable to hold on (Fig. 6.3). This results in urinary frequency, urgency and urge incontinence. If the bladder dysfunction is part of a recognised neurological condition the term *neurological detrusor overactivity* (NDO) is used (Abrams et al 2002).

Suprasacral damage

Lesions that occur above the sacral area and below the pons (i.e. spinal lesions) cause disruption to the spinal–bulbar–spinal reflex pathways. This results in the loss of the normally coordinated activity of the bladder and sphincter and results in *detrusor–sphincter dyssynergia* (DSD). The urethral sphincter does not relax as the bladder contracts and voiding is obstructed. The bladder may then generate high pressures, which can result in ureteric reflux and renal damage, particularly in patients with traumatic or congenital spinal cord

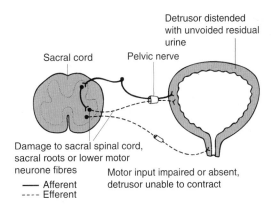

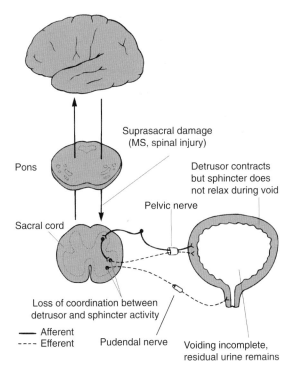

Figure 6.5   Detrusor areflexia. Adapted with permission from Popovich & Stewart-Amidei (1991).

Figure 6.4   Detrusor–sphincter dyssynergia. MS, multiple sclerosis. Adapted with permission from Popovich & Stewart-Amidei (1991).

injury. Some urine may be passed if the detrusor contraction persists and the sphincter finally relaxes, but the bladder will often not empty completely (Fig. 6.4). Additionally, the detrusor may not be able to sustain contractions during voiding, contributing to incomplete emptying of the bladder.

Pelvic nerve, pudendal nerve and infrasacral damage

Damage at and below the sacral spinal cord (i.e. to the axons of the parasympathetic neurones or to the pelvic nerves) causes loss of motor supply to the bladder. The bladder becomes hypocontractile or acontractile – *detrusor areflexia*. When an attempt is made to pass urine the bladder does not empty properly and residual urine remains (Fig. 6.5).

A summary of the pathophysiology of bladder and bowel function associated with neurological

disease at different neuroanatomical sites is provided in Table 6.1.

CONSEQUENCES OF NEUROLOGICAL DAMAGE ON THE BOWEL

As with urinary continence, faecal continence is dependent on the integration of the autonomic and somatic divisions of the nervous system. Peristaltic movements propel food from the stomach, through the small intestine and into the colon. These movements are controlled by the enteric nervous system of the gastrointestinal wall. Parasympathetic stimulation generally increases the rate of peristalsis whilst sympathetic stimulation has an inhibitory effect (see Fig. 8.1 for the innervation of the lower bowel).

Diseases of the central nervous system are unlikely to have any direct effect on bowel function, except when the sacral spinal cord (levels S2–S4) is involved; provided the spinal reflexes remain intact, defecation can occur. Constipation is the most common complaint in neurological conditions and this may be a result of the effect on gut transit time, secondary to autonomic dysfunction. If the neurological disease affects the somatic sacral nerves there may be external anal sphincter weakness, resulting in faecal incontinence. The general effect of reduced mobility, swallowing function and conscious control of some neurological conditions may cause bowel constipation as can the medication prescribed to ease symptoms

Table 6.1 Pathophysiology of bladder and bowel function associated with neurological disease at different neuroanatomic sites

Level of lesion	Neurological disease	Bladder dysfunction	Bowel dysfunction

Suprapontine	Dementia
	Parkinson's disease
	Cerebral vascular accident
	Cerebral tumour
	Cerebral palsy
	Multiple system atrophy
		Inappropriate toilet behaviour
		Neurogenic detrusor overactivity
		Hyperreflex with coordinated
		  external sphincter and bladder
		  neck activity
		Incontinence
			Inappropriate toilet behaviour
			Incontinence
			Faecal impaction following
			  immobility

Suprasacral	Multiple sclerosis
	Traumatic injury
	Compression (e.g. tumours,
	  cervical spondolysis)
	Myelitis
	Spina bifida
		Hyperreflexic with uncoordinated
		  external sphincter and uncoord-
		  inated bladder neck if above T6
		Sensory impairment
		Incontinence
			High cord lesions – colonic
			  mobility reduced and
			  delayed colonic transit
			Low cord lesions – colonic
			  mobility increased,
			  reduced compliance,
			  instability in rectum
			Loss of voluntary control over
			  sphincters, pelvic floor and
			  abdominal muscles
			Rectal prolapse
			Mixed incontinence

Infrasacral or conus	Sacral agenesis
	Cauda equina disease
	Pelvic surgery
	Childbirth injury
	Diabetes mellitus
		Areflexic/underactive with
		  denervated/underactive
		  external sphincter but
		  coordinated bladder neck
		Sensory impairment
		Incontinence
			Weakness or loss of pelvic
			  floor and sphincter muscle,
			  voluntary control and spinal
			  reflexes
			Rectal prolapse
			Impaired pelvic sensation
			Areflexic rectum
			Mixed incontinence

(Craggs & Vaizey 1999, Wing et al 2003) (see Ch. 8 for normal bowel function).

NEUROLOGICAL DISORDERS AND BLADDER AND BOWEL DYSFUNCTION

The following section considers the effects of four common neurological disorders on continence and the management of the symptoms.

Multiple sclerosis

Urinary problems

Multiple sclerosis (MS) is characterised by demy-elinated areas (plaques) that can occur anywhere in the central nervous system; pathways to and from the bladder may therefore be disrupted at any level. Urinary problems are a common feature of multiple sclerosis, occurring in up to 75% of people (NICE 2003). For some people urinary symptoms may occur early on in the disease as part of a spinal cord syndrome. In general, bladder dysfunction has been found to correlate with lower limb deficits (Betts et al 1993). Therefore, as the patient's general condition deteriorates and lower limb function worsens, symptoms of bladder dys-function will be more troublesome and treatment options may become more involved (Box 6.8).

NDO has been found to be the most common problem: studies reporting urodynamic findings

Box 6.8 Summary of measures* which may be effective in bladder dysfunction in MS at each stage (see algorithm in Fig. 6.6)

- ADH (antidiuretic hormone)
- BoNT/A (botulinum neurotoxin type A)
- Buzzer, suprapubic vibrating stimulus
- CBME (cannabis-based medical extract)
- CISC (clean intermittent self-catheterisation)
- IDC (indwelling catheter)

* As monotherapy or in combination.

have found a frequency of 52–97% (Litwiller et al 1999). DSD may also occur and this combined with poorly sustained contractions causes bladder emptying problems. Gallien et al (1998) examined 149 patients with MS and urinary symptoms and confirmed that NDO and DSD were the main dysfunctions. Hyporeflexia or areflexia seems to occur much less frequently in this group of patients.

Bowel problems

Bowel problems in MS are common, including constipation and/or difficulty with defecation. These symptoms may be caused by loss of the coordinated activity of the pelvic floor (Chia et al 1995), but may also result from the use of constipating drugs such as anticholinergic medication. Loss of mobility is also very likely to contribute to or cause constipation in this group of patients and alterations in diet and fluid intake due to dysphagia and bladder dysfunction may also play a part.

Faecal incontinence in MS patients may be caused by a variety of factors. There may be impairment of the external anal sphincter (Waldron et al 1993) or of the normal cortical inhibition of colonic motor activity resulting in high intracolonic pressures. It can also be due to faecal overload. Constipation and faecal incontinence can occur independently or coexist and this is reported in 39–73% of MS patients (Bakke et al 1996, Hennessey et al 1999).

Stroke

Urinary problems

Of the many people who experience a stroke each year, a proportion become incontinent as a result. Incontinence has been reported to occur in 32–79% of people admitted to hospital after stroke (Brittain et al 1998, Patel et al 2001). Studies have shown that incontinence is a strong predictor of poor outcome regarding general functional status, mobility, cognition and discharge destination (home or residential care) (Di Carlo et al 1999, Thomas et al 2005). Brocklehurst and colleagues (1985) found that about 40% of people regain continence during the first 2 weeks following the stroke; however, at 1 year post stroke, incontinence is still a problem for about 15% of people. Brocklehurst et al consider this could be a consequence of altered consciousness, immobility and dependence, although this prevalence rate is similar to that in the general elderly population. Barer (1989) suggests that one of the reasons that the association between continence and good recovery is so strong is that continence is important for morale and self-esteem.

NDO is the most frequent urodynamic finding in people who have had a stroke, with patients complaining of urinary frequency, urgency and incontinence (Khan et al 1990); incomplete bladder emptying problems are also frequent. Whilst urinary incontinence is frequently caused by stroke, this symptom may have been a problem beforehand. Borrie et al (1986) reported that 17% of their patients already had incontinence before their stroke, and Jawad and Ward (1999) found that premorbid incontinence was the most significant variable predicting poor functional outcome.

Bowel problems

Bowel function is recognised as a considerable problem following a stroke, with constipation affecting 60% of those in rehabilitation wards (Robain et al 2002), and faecal incontinence affecting more than 56% acutely, 21% at 3 months and ≤22% at 1 year (Baztan et al 2003, Harari et al 2003). Faecal incontinence may be due to impaction and overflow and/or may be associated more with disability-related factors such as ability to self-toilet and medication, rather than the actual cause of the stoke (Harari et al 2004). Other impairments which are common following a stroke may also indirectly affect bowel function. These include functional problems, in particular immobility, aphasia, dysphagia and cognitive problems or mood changes.

Parkinsonism

Urinary problems

Bladder problems are not inevitable with Parkinson's disease (PD), although many patients do have some form of bladder dysfunction as the disease advances (Sakakibara et al 2001). Neuronal degeneration in the areas of the brain that control micturition is responsible for a variety of bladder symptoms in this group of patients. It seems likely that, in health, basal ganglia have an inhibitory effect on the micturition reflex and, with the cell loss in the substantia nigra that occurs in PD, bladder overactivity occurs. Whilst it is generally accepted that NDO is the commonest cause of urinary symptoms in patients with PD, it has also been suggested that symptoms may be compounded by bradykinesia of the bladder sphincter, i.e. a failure of the sphincter to relax when voiding (Araki & Kuno 2000). This disorder is particularly difficult to distinguish from symptoms due to benign prostatic hyperplasia and careful pressure voiding studies are mandatory if prostatic surgery is being considered (Chandiramani & Fowler 1999). The symptoms can include frequency, urgency, urge incontinence and those of incomplete emptying. Urinary symptoms in PD are often noticeably worse in the 'off' state when the condition is failing to respond to medication (Raudino 2001).

Estimates of the prevalence of urinary symptoms associated with PD in the past may have been complicated by the inclusion of patients with multiple system atrophy (MSA). MSA is characterised by degeneration of several areas in the nervous system which are involved in bladder control, including the motor nucleus of the urethral and anal striated sphincter (Onuf's nucleus).

> **Box 6.9 Sphincter electromyography**
>
> Sphincter electromyography (EMG) is a method of examining the innervation of the striated muscles of the pelvic floor. A concentric needle electrode is inserted into the urethral or anal sphincter and motor unit potentials (electrical activity) are recorded. The duration of each motor unit is measured. The average motor unit duration in normal subjects is about 6 ms. Motor units of prolonged duration are indicative of denervation (and reinnervation).
>
> EMG may also be used as part of a urodynamic investigation to record sphincter activity during filling and voiding. It is particularly useful for the detection of detrusor–sphincter dyssynergia.

People with MSA often present with severe incontinence, and in men this is almost always associated with erectile dysfunction (Beck et al 1994a, Chandiramani et al 1997, Sakakibara et al 2000). There may be a combination of DO, incomplete emptying and sphincter weakness. Denervation of the urethral sphincter can lead to stress incontinence in women. Men, in whom the correct neurological diagnosis has not been recognised, may be guided towards prostatic surgery. This, however, is to be avoided since it may exacerbate incontinence (Beck et al 1994b). Sphincter electromyography (Box 6.9) has been found to be valuable in the differential diagnosis of parkinsonism, although the results have been found to depend on the method used to capture and analyse the motor units (Podnar & Fowler 2004).

Bowel problems

Constipation is an early and troublesome feature of PD and MSA, and gut transit times may be slower in this group of patients (Sakakibara et al 2003, Lui et al 2005). Constipation is likely to be exacerbated by immobility and swallowing problems. Haboubi et al (1988) found prolonged orocaecal transit times in elderly patients with PD compared with elderly patients without the disease. Faecal incontinence can also occur, caused by reduced anal tone during resting and voluntary contractions (Stocchi 1999).

Anorectal function studies using manometry in patients with MSA and idiopathic PD by Stocchi et al (2000) showed an abnormal pattern during straining. However, manometric patterns did not differentiate patients with MSA from those with idiopathic PD.

Spinal cord injury

Urinary problems

Bladder management after a spinal cord injury (SCI) is critical from the outset. In the past there was a high incidence of morbidity and mortality from upper renal tract disease; nowadays, however, better awareness and more astute management have reduced the risks (Horton et al 2003). Immediately following spinal injury there is a period of 'spinal shock' – which can last days or weeks – and refers to the cessation of spinal reflex activity in areas below the level of injury as well as sometimes in segments immediately above it (Arnold 1999). During this time there is an absence of the usual bladder emptying mechanisms and the bladder must be drained to prevent overdistension, usually by means of a urethral or suprapubic catheter.

The type of continence problem experienced will depend on the site of injury, with sacral and cauda equina lesions giving rise to detrusor areflexia with a flaccid bladder and weak sphincters. Suprasacral lesions cause DSD and NDO, resulting in a small capacity, overactive bladder with incomplete emptying due to failure of the external sphincter to relax and poorly sustained detrusor contractions. Once reflex activity has resumed, intermittent catheterisation should be instigated to ensure complete bladder emptying; if detrusor overactivity is present, anticholinergic medication is likely to be necessary. If able, the patient should be instructed in the technique as soon as possible for self-management. Some patients may benefit from other forms of long-term management as will be discussed in treatment strategies.

Autonomic dysreflexia is a potentially life-threatening condition and is reported in 50–70% of SCIs. It is the result of an uncontrolled sympathetic response that is precipitated by such activities as catheterisation or manual evacuation of the bowel, and may lead to mass sympathetic overactivity below the level of the injury, usually T6 and above, although it has been reported in patients with lower level lesions. Autonomic dysreflexia is due to disruption to the control normally exerted from the higher centres when input is lost, and spinal reflexes are activated. This causes symptoms such as sudden hypertension, sweating and headaches, and flushing/blotching of the skin above the level of injury. It is essential that note is taken as to whether the patient has a history of any autonomic dysreflexia before undertaking investigations and procedures that may precipitate such an event and expert advice sought if necessary (Bycroft et al 2005).

The management of continence problems for patients with SCI differs greatly from those with progressive neurological disease. Patients with spinal injury are usually younger and do not face the problem of increasing disability; however, they are at higher risk of upper urinary tract damage. These patients will usually require life-long follow-up to monitor renal function and to ensure that continence is managed optimally (Arnold 1999).

Bowel problems

Suprasacral lesions will leave the lower motor neurones to the lower colon and anal sphincters intact but there is a degree of loss of voluntary control. SCI usually results in substantial bowel problems, with 11% reporting faecal incontinence weekly or more, and slightly over a third (39%) declaring reliable continence of bowels (Glickman & Kamm 1996). A survey by Krogh et al in 1997 of people with paraplegia showed that less than a quarter had a normal desire to defecate and more than half used digital stimulation to trigger defecation. Injury to the sacral region and damage to the cauda equina may affect the lower motor neurones supplying the internal and external anal sphincters and the lower colon. Loss of lower colonic movement causes severe constipation, and faecal incontinence may occur due to lack of sphincteric muscle tone. In many published studies SCI subjects ranked bowel dysfunction as one of their main problems due to the associated time and effort required for bowel management.

There are various bowel programmes used to manage this problem but most are not research based. Bowel evacuation consists mainly of conservative, assistive and pharmacological methods; however, for a few patients, surgical intervention may have to be considered (Weisel & Bell 2004).

ASSESSMENT AND INVESTIGATIONS OF URINARY DYSFUNCTION

Despite the variety of bladder disorders that are caused by neurological problems, the treatment options available can be limited (although improving) and therefore assessment needs primarily to answer two main questions:

- Is there a failure of bladder emptying?
- Is there a failure of bladder storage?

It has been suggested that once this information is obtained the results of further urodynamic or other investigations are unlikely to influence management (Fowler 1996).

Investigations

Measurement of residual volume

The simplest method of identifying if there is a failure of bladder emptying is to measure the post-micturition residual urine volume. This can be done by asking the patient to void and then carrying out a residual scan by ultrasonography or, if a scanner is not available, inserting a size 10 Ch intermittent catheter. More than 100 ml on repeated measurements is considered to be clinically significant and interventions to improve bladder emptying are usually required. Decisions about the management of bladder symptoms based on measurement of postmicturition residual volume have been presented as an algorithm that can be applied to all groups of neurological patients (Fig. 6.6).

Further urodynamic studies

Neurological disabilities can make performing urodynamic studies difficult (Andrews 1994). It is reasonable to limit the use of investigations such as cystometry to those with complex problems in whom preliminary treatment is unsuccessful.

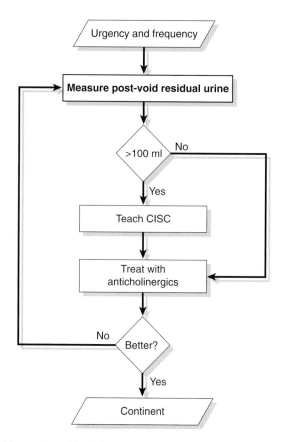

Figure 6.6 Algorithm for the treatment of neurogenic incontinence. CISC, clean intermittent self-catheterisation; PVR, postvoid residual. Reproduced with permission from Fowler (1996).

However, if any invasive treatment such as surgery is contemplated it is particularly important to determine the nature of the bladder dysfunction and probably best accomplished using a video-cystometrogram (see Ch. 2).

History

As with all groups of patients, a detailed history is important and it is worth remembering that people with a neurological condition may have a non-neurological cause for their bladder and bowel symptoms.

Charting

The use of a continence chart or diary is invaluable to identify the frequency of passing urine and episodes of incontinence. This information also provides a baseline from which to measure improvement once interventions have been initiated. Where possible, patients should be responsible for keeping their own chart, but cognitively impaired people and those with upper limb involvement may be unable to do so. In this case carers may be able to check pads hourly to record this information.

Observations

Disabilities due to neurological disorders often have a severe effect on toileting, which may be a crucial factor in losing or gaining continence. Ouslander et al (1987) found a strong association between functional disability and incontinence in nursing home settings, and suggested a functional assessment of toileting skills is important. The extent and nature of disabilities are also likely to affect the implementation and success of management strategies.

MANAGEMENT OPTIONS

Finding the most acceptable and effective form of continence management for a person with neurological disorders is usually a question of compromise and balance. For people with static conditions (e.g. cerebral palsy, spinal injury, spina bifida), preservation of renal function should be a top priority and emphasis needs to be placed on achieving effective bladder emptying; for those with progressive disease (e.g. MS, PD), the emphasis must be on reducing symptoms of detrusor overactivity. The importance of achieving continence needs to be balanced against the impact that the strategies used will have on the individual's independence and lifestyle.

Treatment strategies for neurogenic detrusor overactivity

Bladder retraining

Bladder retraining is a method for improving control over frequency, urgency and urge incontinence, although its value in patients with neurogenic detrusor overactivity, rather than idiopathic

detrusor instability, has yet to be demonstrated. Following completion of an initial baseline chart, the patient is asked to increase the interval between voiding (usually by 15–30 min). Progress is monitored and intervals are then increased gradually until frequency is reduced to 3–4-hourly and incontinence is improved or absent.

Behavioural methods

Cognitive impairment in neurological disease may mean that the person does not recognise the need to pass urine and/or is not aware of the appropriate places where urine (or faeces) should be passed. Behaviour modification techniques (see above) have been used extensively with other groups of people, such as those who have congenital neurological disabilities (e.g. cerebral palsy), but to a lesser extent with people who have acquired neurological disorders in later life. However, with similar perseverance by the neurological patient and their carer, improvement in bladder (and bowel) habit may be obtained.

Pelvic floor exercises (PFE)/electrical stimulation

Although the benefit from PFE/stimulation is not well documented in neurological patients with bladder dysfunction, a study by Vahtera et al (1997) showed that patients with MS in a rehabilitation setting could benefit symptomatically after a number of sessions. The guidelines from the National Institute for Clinical Excellence have suggested that MS patients should be 'considered for a course of pelvic floor exercises preceded by a course of electrical stimulation of the pelvic floor muscles' (NICE 2003). Patient selection is important as the patient's general neurological condition will have a bearing on the outcome if it is to be successful.

Pharmacological treatment

Chapter 9 provides a detailed discussion of various types of medication but some of those used most commonly to treat continence problems in neurological disability are also considered here.

Oral medication

Anticholinergic medications are the mainstay for the treatment of symptoms of neurogenic bladder overactivity. The rationale for this treatment is that the parasympathetic innervation of the detrusor muscle will be blocked, but because their effect is to increase capacity and reduce urgency it may be that they have a more complex mode of action (Anderson 2001). There are a number of anticholinergic medications available, all with essentially similar profiles and common side effects (e.g. dry mouth). Prior to prescribing this type of medication a bladder scan should be carried out to ensure a postvoid residual of ≤100 ml (see intermittent self-catheterisation below).

Intravesical medication Intravesical medication has been used as an alternative to oral medication with the aim of minimising side effects. Oxybutynin chloride delivered directly into the bladder at frequent intervals (one to four times per day) was found to be effective (Pannek et al 2000, Lose & Norgaard 2001). Atropine given intravesically is a potent anticholinergic which has been demonstrated to increase bladder volumes and decrease frequency in patients with MS (Enskat et al 2001, Fader et al 2001).

The use of selective neurotoxic vanilloids, which target vanilloid receptors and reduce the number of afferent nerve endings in the suburothelium, has been documented as being effective in reducing the symptoms of neurogenic bladder overactivity. Instillation of intravesical capsaicin has been shown to have good effect; however, it may cause significant discomfort on initial instillation. Resiniferatoxin, which is less pungent, was studied with regard to effect but there were manufacturing difficulties. Work with intravesical capsaicin dissolved in glucidic acid still continues but only in a few centres in France (de Seze et al 2004, Kalsi & Fowler 2005).

Intradetrusor medication Schürch et al (2000) were the first to describe injection of botulinum neurotoxin type A (BoNT/A, Botox) in spinal patients with detrusor overactivity. It has been suggested that BoNT/A temporarily blocks the presynaptic release of acetylcholine from the parasympathetic innervation and this results in a paralysis of the detrusor smooth muscle. Various

studies have shown a significant reduction in urinary urgency, frequency and incontinence. However, as there is a high possibility of incomplete emptying in patients with neurogenic detrusor overactivity, prior to injection the patient must consent freely and be able to intermittently self-catheterise. The average duration for efficacy is 10 months, with a significant improvement in overall quality of life. At present BoNT/A is not licensed for this use, although many centres are offering it as a second line treatment option with local dispensation from their Trusts (Apostolidis et al 2005, Kalsi et al 2006).

Other medication Desmopressin acetate (DDAVP), a synthetic antidiuretic hormone, is used to treat nocturnal enuresis. Antidiuretic hormone causes less urine to be excreted by the kidneys and as a result the volume of urine in the bladder is reduced for some hours. Desmopressin can be administered nasally or taken as an oral tablet. Desmopressin reduces nocturia (passing urine frequently during the night) (Eckford et al 1994) but can also be used during the day to decrease urinary frequency in patients with MS (Hoverd & Fowler 1998). However, it should only be used once in a 24-h period.

Studies carried out using a medical cannabis extract have shown improvement in urinary symptoms of frequency, urgency and incontinence (Brady et al 2004) but at present this has not been licensed for general use in the UK. At this time patients with a diagnosis of MS can request Sativex – an oral spray containing cannabis extract – on a 'named patient' basis at the discretion of their GP.

Neuromodulation/electrical stimulation

This has been shown to be both beneficial in improving symptoms of overactivity and difficulty in voiding. Electrical stimulation of sacral anterior nerve roots, combined with division of posterior sacral nerve roots, was first described by Brindley (1994) and is a method that has been used primarily for spinal cord injured patients to control continence (by eliminating overactivity) and to enable complete voiding. Sacral deafferentation produces an areflexic, low-pressure bladder and voiding is activated by electrical stimulation of the

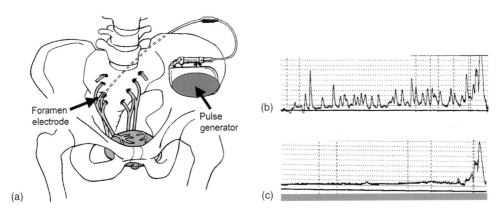

Figure 6.7 (a) Implantable stimulator (using the Medtronic Interstim® stimulator); (b) detrusor instability without stimulation; (c) with stimulation of the S3 sacral nerves.

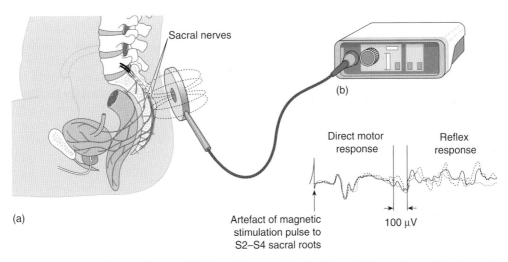

Figure 6.8 Functional magnetic stimulator. (a) Powerful magnetic stimulators with a coil over the sacrum can stimulate deep-lying spinal nerves without causing pain. (b) The neurophysiological record shows five superimposed traces of compound muscle action potentials recorded with electrodes near the striated urethral sphincter following five single pulses of stimulation to the S2–S4 nerve roots. Reproduced with permission from *Urology News*.

anterior roots (Fig. 6.7). This produces contraction not only of the detrusor (to enable voiding) but also of the external sphincter and pelvic floor. Applying stimulation in bursts of a few seconds results in the relaxation of these striated muscles between stimulations, whilst the detrusor contraction is maintained.

Electrical stimulation of the pelvic nerves has also been used successfully for patients with spinal injury as a non-pharmacological method of controlling detrusor hyperreflexia. A small study of

nine patients, five of whom had MS, reported clinical and urodynamic improvement (Emmanuel et al 2000). Sacral nerve stimulation using an implantable device (Fig. 6.8) is an established therapy and has been shown to suppress unstable contractions during urodynamic testing (Jezernik et al 2002).

Magnetic stimulation using brief magnetic pulses to induce electric currents is an alternative and has the very considerable advantage of being able to reach deep into neural structures non-

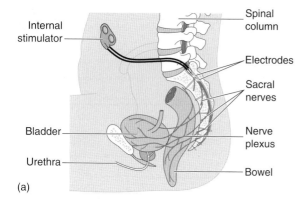

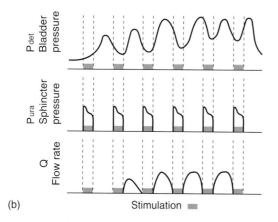

Figure 6.9 (a) Implantable stimulator; (b) bladder/sphincteric pressures and flow rate during stimulation.

to commencing anticholinergic medication. Intermittent catheterisation has the potential to significantly improve continence and reduce the likelihood of upper urinary tract problems by overcoming bladder emptying difficulties. Many patients will require repeated instruction and follow-up as their neurological disabilities progress; however, with perseverance, the majority of patients succeed. Some neurological patients are unable to catheterise themselves, but with the consent of the patient the procedure can be carried out by their caregiver. However, this approach requires a relationship that can cope with the intimacy of the procedure.

Voiding triggers, manoeuvres and aids

Simple methods of triggering bladder contractions such as tapping the abdomen or digital stimulation can prove effective in precipitating voiding and can give the patient some control over continence (although voiding may be incomplete). The Queen Square bladder stimulator is a hand-held vibrating device designed for the same purpose (Dasgupta et al 1997, Prasad et al 2003) although it effectiveness is variable. Methods to aid voiding such as manual expression (the Crede manoeuvre) and the Valsalva manoeuvre are not now generally recommended as it has been reported that the Crede manoeuvre may result in dilatation of the upper tracts (Smith et al 1972) and that the Valsalva manoeuvre may stretch the pelvic floor (Arnold 1999).

Long-term catheterisation

It is important that long-term catheterisation is not perceived as a failure on the part of the patient or caregiver. For those with a progressive neurological disease an indwelling catheter comes as a release from all the worries of various aspects of toileting. With the common catheter-associated problems and the potential for urethral trauma, suprapubic catheters are becoming more widely used and offer some substantial advantages over conventional urethral catheters. Recatheterisation is usually easier, urethral trauma is avoided and sexual activity can take place much more easily (see Ch. 10).

invasively (Fig. 6.9). Direct stimulation of the mixed motor and sensory sacral nerve roots using high frequency magnetic stimulation has been found to inhibit bladder contractions in patients with detrusor hyperreflexia (Craggs et al 1995, Sheriff et al 1996) and detrusor instability (McFarlane et al 1997).

Treatment strategies for voiding problems

Intermittent catheterisation

Clean intermittent catheterisation has been the preferred method of bladder emptying for people with neurogenic voiding problems for many years (see Ch. 10). Patients with a postvoid residual ≥100 ml are advised to learn this procedure prior

Other aids and appliances

Despite the many advances in the treatment of neurogenic bladder problems, incontinence (or the worry of incontinence) commonly persists and some form of containment using aids or appliances may be necessary. For a man there are two main options, a penile sheath or pads and pants; for women, pads and pants are the main method available. A detailed discussion of containment products can be found in Chapter 10 and the following website carries a number of product evaluation reports which may help informed product selection (http://www.medical-devices.gov.uk).

Surgical intervention

With the ongoing improvement in treatment and management options, surgical intervention in neurological disorders has taken a lesser role. However, there remain selective surgical procedures that may be necessary and of benefit to patients, particularly those with stable neurological conditions (SCI, spina bifida). Chapters 3 and 4 provide some discussion of surgical options.

Bowel interventions and management

As stated previously, several neurological diseases cause constipation and/or faecal incontinence which can restrict social activities and reduce quality of life. The aim for the majority of neurologically impaired patients is likely to be planned evacuation, with an individualised bowel programme that reduces constipation without causing faecal incontinence. A combination of the management options may be required as there are few controlled studies available specifically for neurological conditions. The aim – as with all patient groups – is that the programme is tailored to the individual's needs, taking into consideration ability to toilet, carer requirement and daily plan. A predictable bowel habit means that constipation and faecal incontinence can be avoided and daily activities can be organised with greater confidence (Wiesel & Bell 2004).

Boxes 6.10 and 6.11 provide some guidance on assessment and management of the neurogenic bowel.

Box 6.10   Assessment of the neurogenic bowel

ENVIRONMENT ASSESSMENT
- Community and health care (community liaison team, social worker)
- Sociofamilial (general practitioner, social worker)
- Home, workplace (visits)

INDIVIDUAL ASSESSMENT
- Impairment, disability and handicap
- Cognitive function, ability to learn and to direct others
- Mood, coping strategies, compliance, quality of life
- Concomitant diseases and drugs

BOWEL ASSESSMENT
- Past/current gastrointestinal symptoms (questionnaire, bowel diary)
- Past/current bowel programme (relatives, carers)

Motor assessment
- Abdominal wall (physical examination)
- Pelvic floor (physical examination, balloon expulsion, defecography)
- Anal sphincters (physical examination, anorectal manometry, endoanal ultrasonography)

Sensory assessment
- Sacral reflexes (physical examination)
- Anorectal thresholds (balloon distension, mucosal electrostimulation)

Adapted with permission from Wiesel & Bell (2004).

KEY POINTS FOR PRACTICE

- The person with a neurological disability is likely to require long-term continence support with the potential for further neurological and functional deterioration
- Mobility and manual dexterity problems can compound bladder and bowel symptoms as they can make toileting access difficult. Other problems such as visual disturbances, dysphagia and cognition also contribute directly to continence difficulties
- Active management – personalised plan, taking into consideration required assistance, personal needs and goals
- Environmental assessment with the aid of physiotherapist and occupational therapist

---

Box 6.11   Management of the neurogenic bowel

The management of the neurogenic bowel should offer the best method based on the assessment of the patient and their environment (see text for details).

ENVIRONMENT MANAGEMENT
- Community and home (adapted, safe and pleasant, financial support)
- Carers (informed consent, ethical, skilled, empathetic)

INDIVIDUAL MANAGEMENT
- Emotional (carers, relatives, professionals)
- Concomitant diseases, side effects of drugs
- Bladder management (collaboration with urological team)

BOWEL MANAGEMENT
Bowel programme
- Routine (scheduling, gastrocolic response)
- Diet (healthy), fibre, fluid intake (accordance with the bladder)

Bowel care
Assistive methods
- Massage, push-ups, Valsalva manoeuvre, deep breathing and forward-leaning position
- Digital stimulation
- Manual evacuation
- Behavioural methods (biofeedback)

Pharmacological methods
- Laxatives (bulk-forming, faecal softeners, osmotic, stimulant)
- Retrograde colonic irrigation (enema, pulsed irrigation enhanced evacuation)
- Constipating drugs (Loperamide, codeine phosphate)

Surgical methods
- Antegrade continence enema procedure (Malone procedure)
- Stoma (ileostomy, colostomy)
- Sacral nerves neuromodulation (transcutaneous, direct anterior and direct posterior)

Adapted with permission from Wiesel & Bell (2004).

References

Frail elderly

Ancelin M L, Artero S, Portet F et al 2006 Non-degenerative mild cognitive impairment in elderly people and use of anticholinergic drugs: longitudinal cohort study. British Medical Journal 332:455–458

Baltes P B, Smith J 2003 New frontiers in the future of aging: from successful aging of the young old to the dilemmas of the fourth age. Gerontology 49(2):123–135

Bates-Jensen B M, Alessi C A, Al-Samarrai N R et al 2003 The effects of an exercise and incontinence intervention on skin health outcomes in nursing home residents. Journal of the American Geriatrics Society 51:348–355

Baztan J J, Arias E, Gonzalez N et al 2005 New-onset urinary incontinence and rehabilitation outcomes in frail older patients. Age and Ageing 34(2):172–175

Bear M, Dwyer J W, Benveneste D et al 1997 Home-based management of urinary incontinence: a pilot study with both frail and independent elders. Journal of Wound, Ostomy and Continence Nursing 24(3):163–171

Berghmans L, Hendriks H J, de Bie R A et al 1999 Conservative treatment of urge urinary incontinence in women: a systematic review of randomised clinical trials. BJU International 85:254–263

Brandeis G H, Baumann M M, Hossain M et al 1997 The prevalence of potentially remediable urinary incontinence in frail older people: a study using the minimum data set. Journal of the American Geriatrics Society 45:179–184

Bressler R, Bahl J J 2003 Principles of drug therapy for the elderly patient. Mayo Clinic Proceedings 78(12):1564–1577

Brown J S, Vittinghoff E, Wyman J F et al 2000 Urinary incontinence: does it increase risk for falls and fractures? Study of Osteoporotic Factures Research Group. Journal of the American Medical Association 48(7):721–725

Burgio K L, Locher J L, Goode P S et al 1998 Behavioral vs drug treatment for urge urinary incontinence in older women. Journal of the American Medical Association 280(23):1995–2000

Colling J, Owen T R, McCreedy M et al 2003 The effects of a continence program on frail community-dwelling elderly persons. Urologic Nursing 23(2):117–131

Covinsky K E, Eng C, Lui L Y et al 2003 The last 2 years of life: functional trajectories of frail older people. Journal of the American Geriatrics Society 51:492–498

Dallosso H M, McGrother C W, Matthews R J et al 2003 The association of diet and other lifestyle factors with overactive bladder and stress incontinence: a longitudinal study in women. BJU International 92:69–77

Department of Health 2000 Good practice in continence services. TSO, London

Department of Health 2006 Our health, our care, our say: a new direction for community services. TSO, London

Dowd T T, Jones J A 1996 Fluid intake and urinary incontinence in older community-dwelling women. Journal of Community Health Nursing 13(3):179–186

Engberg S, Kincade J, Thompson D 2004 Future directions for incontinence research with frail elders. Nursing Research 53(6S):S22–S29

Eustice S, Wagg A 2005 Nocturia and older people. Nursing Times Supplement 101(29)

Eustice S, Roe B, Paterson J 2006 Prompted voiding for the management of urinary incontinence in adults (Cochrane Review). The Cochrane Library, Issue 3. Update Software. John Wiley, Chichester. Online. Available: http://www.update-software.com/abstracts/ab002113.htm

Ferrucci L, Guralnik J M, Studenski S et al 2004 Designing randomised, controlled trials aimed at preventing or delaying functional decline and disability in frail older persons: a consensus report. Journal of the American Geriatrics Society 52:625–634

Fonda D, Resnick N M, Colling J et al 1998 Outcome measures for research of lower urinary tract dysfunction in frail older people. Neurourology and Urodynamics 17:273–281

Fonda D, DuBeau C E, Harari D et al 2005 Incontinence in the frail elderly. In: Abrams P, Cardozo L, Khoury S, Wein A (eds) Incontinence. Health Publication, Paris, p 1163–1239

Fried L P, Tangen C M, Walston J et al 2001 Frailty in older adults: evidence for a phenotype. The Journals of Gerontology. Series A, Biological Sciences and Medical Sciences 56A:M1–M11

Gammack J K 2004 Urinary incontinence in the frail elder. Clinics in Geriatric Medicine 20:453–466

Gitlin L N, Miller K S, Boyce A 1999 Bathroom modifications for frail elderly renters: outcomes of a community-based program. Technology and Disability 10:141–149

Gnanadesigan N, Saliba D, Roth C P et al 2004 The quality of care provided to vulnerable older community-based patients with urinary incontinence. Journal of the American Medical Directors Association 5(3):141–146

Hanlon J T, Schmader K E, Koronkowski M J et al 1997 Adverse drug events in high risk older outpatients. Journal of the American Geriatrics Society 45:945–948

Holroyd-Leduc J M, Mehta K M, Covinsky K E 2004 Urinary incontinence and its association with death, nursing home admission, and functional decline. Journal of the American Geriatrics Society 52:712–718

Hunskaar S, Burgio K, Diokno A et al 2003 Epidemiology and natural history of urinary incontinence in women. Urology 62(4 Suppl 1):16–23

Johnson T M, Kincade J E, Bernard S L et al 1998 The association of urinary incontinence with poor self-rated health. Journal of the American Geriatrics Society 46:693–699

Keilman L J 2005 Urinary incontinence: basic evaluation and management in the primary care office. Primary Care: Clinics in Office Practice 32:699–722

Kelleher C 1997 Psychiatric aspects of urinary incontinence. In: Cardozo L (ed) Urogynaecology: the King's approach. Churchill Livingstone, Edinburgh, Chapter 33

Kron M, Loy S, Sturm E et al 2003 Risk indicators for falls in institutionalized frail elderly. American Journal of Epidemiology 158(7):645–653

Landi F, Cesari M, Russo A et al 2002 Benzodiazepines and the risk of urinary incontinence in frail older persons living in the community. Clinical Pharmacology and Therapeutics 72(6):729–734

Landi F, Cesari M, Russo A et al 2003 Potentially reversible risk factors and urinary incontinence in frail older people living in the community. Age and Ageing 32(2):194–199

Lekan-Rutledge D 2004 Urinary incontinence strategies for frail elderly women. Urologic Nursing 24(4):281–301

Loeb M, Bentley D W, Bradley S et al 2001 Development of minimum criteria for the initiation of antibiotics in residents of long-term care facilities: results of a consensus conference. Infection Control and Hospital Epidemiology 22(2):120–124

Lundgren R 2004 Nocturia: a new perspective on an old symptom. Scandinavian Journal of Urology and Nephrology 38(2):112–116

McMurdo M E T, Gillespie N D 2000 Urinary tract infection in old age: over-diagnosed and over-treated. Age and Ageing 29:297–298

Madersbacher S, Pycha A, Scatzl G et al 1998 The aging lower urinary tract: a comparative urodynamic study of men and women. Urology 51(2):206–212

Marinkovic S P, Gillen L M, Stanton S L 2004 Managing nocturia. British Medical Journal 328:1063–1066

Miles T P, Palmer R F, Espino D V et al 2001 New-onset incontinence and markers of frailty: data from Hispanic established populations for epidemiologic studies of the elderly. The Journals of Gerontology. Series A, Biological Sciences and Medical Sciences 56A:M19–M24

Mitteness L S 1990 Knowledge and beliefs about urinary incontinence in adulthood and old age. Journal of the American Geriatrics Society 38:374–378

Mitteness L S, Barker J C 1995 Stigmatizing a 'normal' condition: urinary incontinence in later life. Medical Anthropology Quarterly 9(2):188–210

Muller-Lissner S 2002 General geriatrics and gastroenterology: constipation and faecal incontinence. Best Practice & Research. Clinical Gastroenterology 16(1):115–133

Newman D K, Fader M, Bliss D Z 2004 Managing incontinence using technology, devices and products. Nursing Research 53(6S):S42–S48

Nicolle L E 2001 Urinary tract infections in long-term-care facilities. Infection Control and Hospital Epidemiology 22(3):167–175

Nilsson M, Sarvimaki A, Ekman S L 2000 Feeling old: being in a phase of transition in later life. Nursing Inquiry 7(1):41–49

Nordling J 2002 The aging bladder – a significant but underestimated role in the development of lower urinary tract symptoms. Experimental Gerontology 37:991–999

Ostaszkiewicz J, Johnston L, Roe B 2004a Habit retraining for the management of urinary incontinence in adults (Cochrane Review). Cochrane Library, Issue 3. Update Software. John Wiley, Chichester. Online. Available:

http://www.update-software.com/Abstracts/AB002801.htm

Ostaszkiewicz J, Johnston L, Roe B 2004b Timed voiding for the management of urinary incontinence in adults (Cochrane Review). Cochrane Library, Issue 3. Update Software. John Wiley, Chichester

Ouslander J G 2000 Intractable incontinence in the elderly. BJU International 85(supplement 3):72–78

Ouslander J G, Johnson T M 2004 Continence care for frail older adults: it is time to go beyond assessing quality. Journal of the American Medical Directors Association 5(3):213–216

Palmer M 1994 A health-promotion perspective of urinary incontinence. Nursing Outlook 42:163–169

Palmer M H 2005 Effectiveness of prompted voiding for incontinent nursing home residents. In: Melnyk B, Fineout-Overholt E (eds) Evidence-based practice in nursing and healthcare: a guide to best practice. Lippincott Williams & Wilkins, Baltimore

Peet S M, Castleden S M, McGrother C W 1995 Prevalence of urinary and faecal incontinence in hospitals and residential and nursing homes for older people. British Medical Journal 311:1063–1064

Popovich J M, Stewart-Amidei C 1991 Alterations in elimination. In: Bronstein K S (ed) Promoting stroke recovery. Mosby-Year-Book, Missouri

Resnick N M 1996 An 89-year-old woman with urinary incontinence. Journal of the American Medical Association 276(22):1832–1840

Resnick N M, Yalla S V 1987 Detrusor hyperactivity and impaired contractile function. An unrecognised but common cause of incontinence in elderly patients. Journal of the American Medical Association 257(22):3076–3081

Resnick N M, Elbadawi A, Yalla S V 1995 Age and the lower urinary tract: what is normal? Neurourology and Urodynamics 14:577–579

Reuben D B, Roth C, Kamberg C, Wenger N S 2003 Restructuring primary care practices to manage geriatric syndromes: the ACOVE-2 intervention. Journal of the American Geriatrics Society 51:1787–1793

Richards C L 2004 Urinary tract infections in the frail elderly: issues for diagnosis, treatment and prevention. International Urology and Nephrology 36:457–463

Robinson J P 2000 Managing urinary incontinence in the nursing home: residents' perspective. Journal of Advanced Nursing 31(1):68–77

Rochon P A, Anderson G M, Tu J V et al 1999 Age- and gender-related use of low-dose drug therapy: the need to manufacture low-dose therapy and evaluate the minimum effective dose. Journal of the American Geriatrics Society 47:954–959

Rockwood K, Hubbard R 2004 Frailty and the geriatrician. Age and Ageing 33:429–430

Royal College of Physicians 1995 Incontinence: causes, management and provision of services. RCP, London

Royal College of Physicians 2005 Report of the national audit of continence care for older people (65 years and above) in England, Wales and Northern Ireland. Clinical Effectiveness and Evaluation Unit, RCP, London

Schnelle J F, Smith R L 2001 Quality indicators for the management of urinary incontinence in vulnerable community-dwelling elders. Annals of Internal Medicine 135:752–758

Shah R R 2004 Drug development and use in the elderly: search for the right dose and dosing regimen. British Journal of Clinical Pharmacology 58(5):452–469

Shimanouchi S, Kamei T, Hayashi M 2000 Home care for the frail elderly based on urinary incontinence level. Public Health Nursing 17(6):468–473

Siegler E L, Reidenberg M 2004 Treatment of urinary incontinence with anticholinergics in patients taking cholinesterase inhibitors for dementia. Clinical Pharmacology and Therapeutics 75(5):484–488

Simmons S F, Schnelle J F 2004 Effects of an exercise and scheduled-toileting intervention on appetite and constipation in nursing home residents. Journal of Nutrition, Health and Aging 8(2):116–121

Tannenbaum C, Perrin M D, DuBeau C E et al 2001 Diagnosis and management of urinary incontinence in the older patient. Archives of Physical and Medical Rehabilitation 82:134–138

Teunissen T A M, de Jonge A, van Weel C et al 2004 Treating urinary incontinence in the elderly – conservative measures that work: a systematic review. Journal of Family Practice 53(1):25–32

Thom D H, Haan M N, van Den Eeden S K 1997 Medically recognized urinary incontinence and risks of hospitalization, nursing home admission and mortality. Age and Ageing 26:367–374

van Kerrebroeck P, Abrams P, Chaikin D et al 2002 The standardisation of terminology in nocturia. Report from the Standardisation Sub-committee of the International Continence Society. Neurourology and Urodynamics 21:179–183

Weiss J P, Blaivas J G 2000 Nocturia. Journal of Urology 163:5–12

Yoshimura K, Matsui T N, Kinukawa N et al 2004 Prevalence of risk factors for nocturia: analysis of a health-screening program. International Journal of Urology 11:282–287

Mental health needs

Acheson D 1998 Independent inquiry into inequalities in health. TSO, London

Ashworth P D, Hagan T 1993 The meaning of incontinence: a qualitative study of non-geriatric urinary incontinence. Journal of Advanced Nursing 18:1415–1423

Berglund A L, Eisemann M, Lalos O 1994 Personality characteristics of stress incontinent women: a pilot study. Journal of Psychosomatic Obstetrics and Gynaecology 15:165–170

British National Formulary 2004 British National Formulary, British Medical Association & Royal Pharmaceutical Society of Great Britain, London

Department of Health 1999 The National Service Framework for mental health. DH, London

Department of Health 2000a Good practice in continence services. DH, London

Department of Health 2000b No secrets: guidance on developing and implementing multi-agency policies and procedures to protect vulnerable adults from abuse. DH, London

Department of Health 2002 Tackling health inequalities: the results of a consultation exercise. DH, London

Department of Health 2004 Choosing health – making healthier choices easier. DH, London

Department of Health 2005 Chief Nursing Officer's review of mental health nursing: consultation document. DH, London

Dugan E, Cohen S, Robinson D 2000 The quality of life of older adults with urinary incontinence: determining generic and condition specific predictors. Quality of Life Research 7:337–344

Faulkner A, Layzell S 2000 Strategies for living: a report of user-led research into people's strategies for living with mental distress. Mental Health Foundation, London

Fuller M, Pharm D, Borovicka M et al 1996 Clozapine induced urinary incontinence: incidence and treatment with ephedrine. Journal of Clinical Psychiatry 57(11): 514–519

Gardner C, Smith M 2004 Have a heart: awareness of cardiac problems in mental health patients. Mental Health Practice 8(3):28–30

Goffman E 1963 Stigma. Notes on the management of spoiled identity. Prentice-Hall, Englewood Cliffs, NJ

Henderson J S, Kashka M S 1999 Development and testing of the urinary incontinence scales. Urologic Nursing 19(2):109–119

Hunskaar S, Lose G, Sykes D et al 2004 The prevalence of urinary incontinence in women in four European countries. British Journal of Urology 93:324–330

Iqbal M M, Rahman A, Husain Z et al 2003 Clozapine: a clinical review of adverse effects and management. Annals of Clinical Psychiatry 15(1):33–48

Joachim G 2000 Stigma of visible and invisible chronic conditions. Journal of Advanced Nursing 32(1):243–248

Kennedy M 2006 Exploring the education and training needs of mental health nurses caring for clients with urinary incontinence: an action research study. PhD thesis. University of Essex, Essex

Kessler D, Lloyd K, Lewis G 1999 Cross sectional study of symptom attribution and recognition of depression and anxiety in primary care. British Medical Journal 318:436–439

Kitwood T, Benson S (eds) 1995 The new culture of dementia care. Hawker, London

Kitzinger J 1990 Recalling the pain. Nursing Times 86(3):38–40

Koch T, Ashton M, Kelly S et al 2002 Development of a collaborative model of care for long term management of incontinence for people living in the community with mental illness. Port Adelaide Mental Health Service, Australia, Research Unit, Royal District Nursing Service (SA Inc.)

Lloyd K, Jenkins R 1995 The economics of depression in primary care: Department of Health initiatives. British Journal of Psychiatry 166(supplement 27):1110–1116

McNeill A 2001 Smoking and mental health – a review of the literature. Smoke Free London Programme, London

Melville J, Walker E, Katon W et al 2002 Prevalence of co-morbid psychiatric illness and its impact on symptom perception, quality of life, and functional status in women with urinary incontinence. American Journal of Obstetrics and Gynecology 187:80–87

Mental Health Foundation 2000 Pull yourself together: a survey of the stigma and discrimination faced by people who experience mental distress. Mental Health Foundation, London

Mentality 2003 Making it effective: a guide to evidence based mental health promotion, radical mentalities, briefing paper 1. Mentality, London

Mitteness L S 1990 Knowledge and beliefs about urinary incontinence in adulthood and old age. Journal of the American Geriatrics Society 38:374–378

Mitteness L S, Barker J C 1995 Stigmatizing a 'normal' condition: urinary incontinence in later life. Medical Anthropology Quarterly 9(2):188–210

Mowforth G 1999 Power, gender and nursing work. In: Wilkinson G, Meirs M (eds) Power and nursing practice. Macmillan, London, Chapter 3

Nash M 2002 Voting as a means of social inclusion for people with a mental illness. Journal of Psychiatric and Mental Health Nursing 9:697–703

Nash M 2005 Physical care skills: a training needs analysis of inpatient and community mental health nurses. Mental Health Practice 9(4):20–23

National Institute for Clinical Excellence 2002 Schizophrenia. Core interventions in the treatment and management of schizophrenia in primary and secondary care. Clinical Guideline 1. NICE, London. Online. Available: http://www.nice.org.uk/pdf/CG1NICEguideline.pdf

Nolan P, Badger F (eds) 2002 Search of collaboration and partnership. In: Promoting collaboration in primary mental health care. Nelson Thornes, Cheltenham, Chapter 1

Ohlsen R, Peacock G, Smith S 2005 Developing a service to monitor and improve physical health in people with serious mental illness. Journal of Psychiatric Mental Health Nursing 12(5):614–619

Peveler R, Carson A, Rodin G 2002 ABC of psychological medicine: depression in medical patients. British Medical Journal 325:149–152

Phelan M, Stradins L, Morrison S 2001 Physical health of people with severe mental illness. British Medical Journal 322:443–444

Roe B, Doll H 2000 Prevalence of urinary incontinence and its relationship with health status. Journal of Clinical Nursing 9:178–188

Rogers A 1997 Vulnerability, health and health care. Journal of Advanced Nursing 26(1):65–72

Saltmarche A, Gartley C 2001 Communication: the key to effective incontinence assessment, treatment and patient satisfaction. In: Cardozo L, Staskin D (eds) Textbook of female urology and urogynaecology. Isis Medical Media, London

Sells H, McDonagh R 1999 Psychological aspects of incontinence. In: Lucas M, Emery S, Beyon J (eds) Incontinence. Blackwell Science, Oxford

Shaw C 2001 A review of the psychosocial predictors of help seeking behaviour and impact on quality of life in people with urinary incontinence. Journal of Clinical Nursing 10(1):15–24

Singleton N, Bumpstead R, O'Brien M et al 2000 Psychiatric morbidity among adults living in private households. Office of National Statistics, London

Smart L, Wegner D M 1999 Covering up what can't be seen: concealable stigma and mental control. Journal of Personality and Social Psychology 77(3):474–486

Smith C 1998 Attitudes of health workers to incontinence. Journal of Community Nursing 12(4):8–14

Sobieraj M 1998 The impact of depression on the physical health of family members. British Journal of General Practice 48:1653–1655

Valvanne J 1996 Major depression in the elderly: a population study in Helsinki. International Psychogeriatrics 8(3): 437–443

Vinsnes A G, Harkless G E, Haltbakk J et al 2001 Healthcare personnel's attitudes towards patients with urinary incontinence. Journal of Clinical Nursing 10(4):455–461

Warner J, Harvey C, Barnes T 1994 Clozapine and urinary incontinence. International Clinical Psychopharmacology 9:207–209

Wood C, O'Neill J 2005 Global clinic and physical health. Mental Health Nursing 25(4):4–7

Zorn B H, Montgomery K P, Gray M et al 1999 Urinary incontinence and depression. Journal of Urology 162:82–84

Continence problems in neurological disability

Abrams P, Cardozo L, Fall M et al 2002 The standardisation of terminology in lower urinary tract function. Neurology Urodynamics 21(2):167–178

Anderson K E 2001 The basis for drug treatment of the overactive bladder. World Journal of Urology 19:294–298

Andrews K 1994 Bladder disorders in brain damage. In: Rushton D N (ed) Handbook of neuro-urology. Marcel Dekker, New York

Apostolidis A, Dasgupta P, Fowler C J 2005 Proposed mechanisms for the efficacy of injected botulinum toxin in the treatment of human detrusor overactivity. European Journal of Urology 49(4):644–650

Araki I, Kuno S 2000 Assessment of voiding dysfunction in Parkinson's disease by the international prostate symptom score. Journal of Neurology, Neurosurgery and Psychiatry 68:429–433

Arnold E P 1999 Spinal cord injury. In: Fowler C J (ed) Neurology of bladder, bowel and sexual dysfunction. Blue books of practical neurology. Butterworth-Heinemann, Oxford

Bakke A, Myhr K M, Gronniny M et al 1996 Bladder, bowel and sexual dysfunction in patients with multiple sclerosis – a cohort study. Scandinavian Journal of Urology and Nephrology Supplement 179:61–66

Barer D H 1989 Continence after stroke: useful predictor or goal of therapy? Age and Ageing 18:183–191

Baztan J J, Domenech J R, Gonzales M 2003 New-onset fecal incontinence after stroke: risk factor or consequence of poor outcomes after rehabilitation? Stroke 24:101–102

Beck R O, Betts C D, Fowler C J 1994a Genitourinary dysfunction in multiple system atrophy: clinical features and treatment in 62 cases. Journal of Urology 151:1336–1341

Beck R, Fowler C J, Mathias C J 1994b Genitourinary dysfunction in disorders of the autonomic nervous system. In: Rushton D N (ed) Handbook of neuro-urology. Marcel Dekker, New York

Betts C D, D'Mellow M T, Fowler C J 1993 Urinary symptoms and the neurological features of bladder dysfunction in multiple sclerosis. Journal of Neurology, Neurosurgery and Psychiatry 56:245–250

Borrie M F, Campbell A J, Caradoc-Davies T H 1986 Urinary incontinence after stroke: a prospective study. Age and Ageing 15:177

Brady C M, Das Gupta R, Dalton C et al 2004 An open-label pilot study of cannabis-based extracts for bladder dysfunction in advanced multiple sclerosis. Multiple Sclerosis 10:425– 433

Brindley G 1994 The first 500 patients with sacral anterior root stimulation: general description. Paraplegia 32:795–805

Brittain K R, Peet S M, Castleden C M 1998 Stroke and incontinence. Stroke 29:524–528

Brocklehurst K C, Andrews K, Richards B et al 1985 Incidence and correlates of incontinence in stroke patients. Journal of the American Geriatrics Society 33:540–542

Bycroft J, Shergill I S, Choong E A L et al 2005 Autonomic dysreflexia: a medical emergency. Postgraduate Medical Journal 81:232–235

Chandiramani V A, Fowler C J 1999 Urogenital disorders in Parkinson's disease and multiple system atrophy. In: Fowler C J (ed) Neurology of bladder, bowel and sexual dysfunction. Blue books of practical neurology. Butterworth-Heinemann, Oxford

Chandiramani V A, Palace J, Fowler C J 1997 How to recognize patients with parkinsonism who should not have urological surgery. British Journal of Urology 80:100–104

Chia Y W, Fowler C J, Kamm M A et al 1995 Prevalence of bowel dysfunction in patients with multiple sclerosis and bladder dysfunction. Journal of Neurology 242(2):105–108

Craggs M, Vaizey C 1999 Neurophysiology of the bladder and bowel. In: Fowler C J (ed) Neurology of bladder, bowel and sexual dysfunction. Blue books of practical neurology. Butterworth-Heinemann, Oxford

Craggs M D, Sheriff M K M, Shah P J R et al 1995 Responses to multi-pulse magnetic stimulation of spinal nerve roots mapped over the sacrum in man. Journal of Physiology 483:127P

Dasgupta P, Haslam C, Goodwin R et al 1997 The Queen Square bladder stimulator: a device for assisting emptying of the neurogenic bladder. British Journal of Urology 81:234–237

de Seze M P, Wiart L, Soyeur L et al 2004 Intravesical capsaicin versus resiniferatoxin for the treatment of detrusor hyperreflexia in spinal cord injured patients: a double-blind, randomized, controlled study. Journal of Neurology 171:251–255

Di Carlo A, Lamassa M, Pracucci G et al 1999 Stroke in the very old: clinical presentation and determinants of 3 month functional outcome: a European perspective. European BIOMED Study of Stroke Care Group. Stroke 30:2313–2319

Eckford S D, Swami K S, Jackson S R et al 1994 Desmopressin in the treatment of nocturia and enuresis in patients with multiple sclerosis. British Journal of Urology 74:733–735

Emmanuel J, Chartier-Kastler J L, Bosh R et al 2000 Long-term results of sacral nerve stimulation (S3) for the treatment of neurogenic refractory urge incontinence related to detrusor hyperreflexia. Journal of Urology 164:146–148

Enskat R, Deaney C N, Glickman S 2001 Systemic effects of intravesical atropine sulphate. BJU International 87(7):613–616

Fader M, Barton R, Malone-Lee J et al 2001 A new use for an old drug: results of a dose titration study of intra-vesical atropine. International Continence Society (UK) Proceedings, April, Manchester

Fowler C J 1996 Investigation of the neurogenic bladder. Journal of Neurology, Neurosurgery and Psychiatry 60(1):6–13

Gallien P, Robineau S, Nicolas B et al 1998 Vesicourethral dysfunction and urodynamic findings in multiple sclerosis: a study of 149 cases. Archives of Physical Medicine and Rehabilitation 79:255–257

Glickman S, Kamm M A 1996 Bowel dysfunction in spinal-cord-injury patients. Lancet 347:1651–1653

Haboubi N Y, Hudson P, Rahman Q et al 1988 Small intestinal transmit time in the elderly. Lancet 1:933

Harari D, Coshall C, Rudd A G et al 2003 New onset fecal incontinence after stroke: prevalence, natural history, risk factors, and impact. Stroke 34:101–102

Harari D, Norton C, Lockwood L et al 2004 Treatment of constipation and fecal incontinence in stroke patients. Randomized controlled trial. Stroke 35:2549–2555

Hennessey A J, Robertson N P J, Swingler R J, Compston D A 1999 Urinary, faecal and sexual dysfunction in patients with multiple sclerosis. Journal of Neurology 246(11):1027–1032

Horton J A, Chancellor M B, Labatia I 2003 Bladder management for the evolving spinal cord injury: options and considerations. Spinal Cord Injury Rehabilitation 9(1):36–52

Hoverd P A, Fowler C J 1998 Desmopressin in the treatment of daytime frequency in patients with multiple sclerosis. Journal of Neurology, Neurosurgery and Psychiatry 65:778–780

Jawad S H, Ward A B 1999 Study of the relationship between premorbid urinary incontinence and stroke functional outcome. Clinical Rehabilitation 13:447–452

Jezernik S, Craggs M, Grill G et al 2002 Electrical stimulation for bladder dysfunction: current state and future possibilities. Neurological Research 24(5):413–430

Kalsi V, Fowler C J 2005 Therapy Insight: bladder dysfunction associated with multiple sclerosis. Nature Clinical Practice Urology 2:492–501

Kalsi V, Apostolidis A, Popat R et al 2006 Quality of life changes in patients with neurogenic versus idiopathic detrusor overactivity after intradetrusor injections of botulinum neurotoxin type A and correlations with lower urinary tract symptoms and urodynamic changes. European Urology 49(3):528–535

Khan Z, Starter P, Yan W C, Bhola A 1990 Analysis of voiding disorders in patients with cerebrovascular accident. Urology 21:315–318

Krogh K, Nielson J, Dijurhuus J C et al 1997 Colorectal functions in patients with spinal cord lesions. Diseases of the Colon and Rectum 40:1233–1239

Litwiller S E, Froman E M, Kreder K J 1999 Multiple sclerosis and the urologist. Journal of Urology 161:743–757

Liu Z, Sakakibara R, Odaka T et al 2005 Mosapride citrate, a novel 5-HT4 agonist and partial 5-HT3 antagonist, ameliorates constipation in parkinsonian patients. Movement Disorder 20(6):680–686

Lose G, Norgaard J P 2001 Intravesical oxybutynin for treating incontinence resulting from an overactive bladder. BJU International 87:767–773

McFarlane J P, Foley S J, de Winter P et al 1997 Acute suppression of idiopathic detrusor instability with magnetic stimulation of the sacral nerve roots. British Journal of Urology 80:734–741

National Institute for Clinical Excellence 2003 Multiple sclerosis. Management of multiple sclerosis in primary and secondary care. Clinical Guideline 8. NICE, London. Online. Available: http://www.nice.org.uk/pdf/CG008guidance.pdf

Ouslander J G, Morishita L, Blaustein J et al 1987 Clinical, functional and psychological characteristics of an incontinent nursing home population. Journal of Gerontology 42:631–637

Pannek J, Sommerfeld H J, Botel U, Senge T 2000 Combined intravesical and oral oxybutynin chloride in adult patients with spinal cord injury. Urology 55:358–362

Patel M, Coshall C, Lawrence E et al 2001 Recovery from poststroke urinary incontinence: associated factors and impact on outcome. Journal of the American Geriatrics Society 49(9):1229–1233

Podnar S, Fowler C J 2004 Sphincter electromyography in diagnosis of multiple system atrophy: technical issues. Muscle and Nerve 29:151–156

Prasad R S, Smith S J, Wright H 2003 Lower abdominal pressure versus external bladder emptying in multiple sclerosis: a randomized controlled study. Clinical Rehabilitation 17(1):42–47

Raudino F 2001 Non motor off in Parkinson's disease. Acta Neurologica Scandinavica 104(5):312–315

Robain G, Chennevelle J M, Petit F et al 2002 Incidence of constipation after recent vascular hemiplegia: prospective cohort of 152 patients. Revue Neurologique (Paris) 158:589–592

Sakakibara R, Hattori T, Uchiyama T et al 2000 Urinary dysfunction and orthostatic hypotension in multiple system atrophy: which is the more common and earlier manifestation? Journal of Neurology, Neurosurgery and Psychiatry 68:65–69

Sakakibara R, Hattori T, Uchiyana T et al 2001 Videourodynamics and sphincter motor unit potential analysis in Parkinson's disease and multiple system atrophy. Journal of Neurology, Neurosurgery and Psychiatry 71:600–606

Sakakibara R, Odaka T, Uchiyama T et al 2003 Colonic transit time and rectoanal videomanometry I: Parkinson's disease. Journal of Neurology, Neurosurgery and Psychiatry 74:268–272

Schürch B, Stohrer M, Kramer G et al 2000 Botulinum-A toxin for treating detrusor hyperreflexia in spinal cord injured patients: a new alternative to anticholinergic drugs? Preliminary results. Journal of Urology 164:692–697

Sheriff M K M, Shah P J R, Fowler C et al 1996 Neuromodulation of detrusor hyper-reflexia by functional magnetic stimulation of the sacral roots. British Journal of Urology 78:39–46

Smith P, Cook J, Rhine J 1972 Manual expression of the bladder following spinal cord injury. Paraplegia 9:213–218

Stocchi F 1999 Disorders of bowel function in Parkinson's disease. In: Fowler C J (ed) Neurology of bladder, bowel, and sexual dysfunction. Blue books of practical neurology. Butterworth-Heinemann, Oxford, p 255–264

Stocchi F, Badiali D, Vacca L et al 2000 Anorectal function in multiple system atrophy and Parkinson's disease. Movement Disorders 15:71–76

Thomas L H, Barrett J, Cross S et al 2005 Prevention and treatment of urinary incontinence after stroke in adults (Cochrane Review). The Cochrane Library Issue 3. Update Software, John Wiley, Chichester

Vahtera T, Haaranen M, Viramo-Koskela A L et al 1997 Pelvic floor rehabilitation is effective in patients with multiple sclerosis. Clinical Rehabilitation 11(3):211–219

Waldron D J, Horgan P G, Patel F R et al 1993 Multiple sclerosis: assessment of colonic and anorectal function in the presence of faecal incontinence. International Journal of Colorectal Diseases 8:220–224

Wiesel P, Bell S 2004 Bowel dysfunction: assessment and management in the neurological patient. In: Norton C, Chelvanayagam S (eds) Bowel continence nursing. Beaconsfield Publishers, Beaconsfield, p 181–203

Wing K, Rasmussen L, Werdelin L M 2003 Constipation in neurological diseases. Journal of Neurology, Neurosurgery and Psychiatry 74:13–19

Chapter 7

Continence training in intellectual disability

Linda J. Smith and Paul S. Smith

There is a story about Martin Luther seeing what we would now recognise as a multiply handicapped child who 'ate, drooled and defaecated'. At a time when such children were regarded as monsters, Luther's remedy was that the child should be taken to the river and drowned.

INTRODUCTION

The prognosis for incontinence in people with intellectual disabilities has, historically, been pessimistic. Incontinence was formerly a major reason for admission to institutional care (McCoull 1971). Those whose memories of services go back some decades will remember the pervasive smell of urine and faeces on long-stay wards for people with severe and profound intellectual disabilities. At that time, incontinence was perceived as part and parcel of severe intellectual disability. It is really only since the 1970s that remediation has been considered possible, since which time it has become evident that incontinence is not intractable.

It is generally accepted that training for self-help and independence skills in people with intellectual disabilities should adopt a developmental approach. Therefore, before reviewing intervention studies, we shall first consider the evidence regarding the 'normal' development of continence and the implications of this for the field of intellectual disability.

NORMAL DEVELOPMENTAL SEQUENCE OF BOWEL AND BLADDER CONTROL

Continence is generally acquired during the second to third year of life, with modesty training occurring after the acquisition of daytime control. Thus, first we teach children to be proud of their toileting prowess then, shortly after, we teach them to keep quiet about it. The feelings of disgust we associate with urine and faeces are not, however, universal (Smith & Smith 1987). In Western culture, for example, children in the early years regard the smell of urine and faeces as pleasant, although by school age they have learned to regard these as unpleasant. Also, while adults in all societies regard faeces as offensive, this is not universally true of urine. This is important, as cultural taboos surrounding toileting influence the attitudes of carers, both professional and family.

Age of acquisition and sequence of development of bowel and bladder control have been studied in Western children over a number of decades. Largo and Stutzle (1977a,b), for example, found that 78% of 3 year olds had bladder control and 97% had bowel control. A later study (Largo et al 1996) showed that, despite the later onset and less intense nature of toilet training by the 1990s, the age of achievement of full bladder and bowel control was similar.

The most commonly accepted sequence for the acquisition of bowel and bladder control is as follows:

1. bowel control at night
2. bowel control by day
3. bladder control by day
4. bladder control by night.

Some children, however, have a different pattern. Largo and Stutzle (1977a,b), for example, found that the sequence differed in 8% of the children studied. Brazelton (1962), in a sample of over 1000 children, found that 12.3% acquired bowel control first, 8.2% acquired bladder control first, while the majority achieved bowel and bladder control simultaneously. This suggests that, when considering continence training programmes for people with intellectual disabilities, there is no rigid requirement to adhere to a particular developmental sequence. Nowadays, bowel and bladder control often appear to be acquired simultaneously because of the tendency towards late toilet training.

Components of bowel and bladder control

A developmental model of acquisition of daytime bladder control, rooted in the views of Gesell and Armatruda (1941), may be summarised thus:

- *Infancy*: reflex micturition
- *1–2 years*: some awareness of a full bladder and brief holding of urine
- *3 years*: holding urine for prolonged periods, thus increasing bladder capacity
- *3–4 years*: able to initiate urine stream reliably with full bladder when seated on the toilet
- *6 years*: able to commence urine stream without full bladder.

This widely accepted model should not be given too much credence, however, as there is in fact little hard evidence to support it. By contrast, there is evidence (Smeets et al 1985, Yeung et al 1995, Mattson & Lindstrom 1996) to support the following:

- that the concept of reflex micturition is too simplistic and there are in fact wide variations in voiding patterns in infancy
- that babies only a few months old have awareness of bowel and bladder sensations
- that passing urine in the absence of a full bladder is an early rather than a late-acquired component
- that complete bladder emptying may be more difficult than has been thought
- that there are wide variations in the pattern of acquisition of continence components.

> **Box 7.1   Implications of developmental sequences for training strategies in intellectual disabilities**
>
> - Bowel control does not always precede bladder control in 'normal' children. Therefore, for practical reasons, intervention may focus first on bladder training if double incontinence is present: emptying the bladder is a more frequent event, providing more bladder training 'opportunities', particularly if fluids can be increased.
> - The ability to pass urine in the absence of a full bladder is important for fully developed continence. Although believed to be a late-acquired skill, neither the evidence nor the experience of training people with intellectual disabilities supports this belief.
> - Some people with intellectual disabilities experience chronic difficulty with bladder emptying. This is likely to militate against complete dryness (Lindstrom et al 2000).
> - Almost 70% of boys in the general population are trained to pass urine sitting rather than standing (Seim 1989). This is normal, as well as easier, in the early stages of bladder training.

> **Box 7.2   Is continence 'trained' or does it depend on maturation?**
>
> While the basic mechanisms are probably largely innate and continence would eventually be acquired spontaneously, there is evidence of variation in the age at which continence is achieved and clear effects for structured behavioural training. This suggests that some aspects of continence are malleable and open to manipulation by training, but that both maturation and training play a role.

Models of the acquisition of continence need to be more fully researched, for if continence training is predicated on false beliefs, training approaches will not be soundly based and research on the development of bowel and bladder control may pose the wrong questions (Box 7.1).

In the field of intellectual disability, fundamental issues remain to be answered with respect to the development of bowel and bladder control, for example:

- Does continence acquisition in children with an intellectual disability differ from that of normal children and, if so, in what way?
- Does bladder function remain normal for the 'untrained' bladder, given that the bladder did not evolve to function long term in this uninhibited way and the untrained bladder is therefore essentially an abnormal condition?

One study relevant to the issue of long-term consequences of faulty voiding patterns investigated 'bladder dysfunction in the commercial television child . . .' (Vande Walle et al 1995). Although no data are given, the authors noted an increase in children of the 'TV generation' presenting with bladder dysfunction, because they do not empty their bladders regularly or completely. This may explain why continence training tends to present such a challenge in people with intellectual disabilities and incomplete bladder emptying.

Learning or maturation

A fundamental question concerns whether bowel and bladder control are 'trained' or whether they are acquired through a maturational process (Box 7.2). A maturational process implies that control unfolds naturally, independent of environmental factors such as toilet 'training'. If this were the case, bowel and bladder control would be outwith the expectation of profoundly intellectually disabled people who, with a developmental age equivalent of less than 18 months, would fail to reach the widely accepted 'readiness criteria' outlined by Michel (1999). As we shall see later in this chapter, this is not the case.

Training effects

Evidence in favour of training includes studies of toilet training practices in different cultures. In some cultures, such as hunter–gatherers in arctic climates where there is a survival premium attached to being dry, toilet training starts earlier. Conversely, in hunter–gatherer societies in warmer climates, there may be little or no emphasis on toilet 'training'. As well as cultural differences, national and social class differences have been reported in the age at which toilet training begins and is achieved within Western Europe.

The case for toilet 'training' is strengthened by studies involving children and adults with severe intellectual disabilities, children in the general population and infants only a few months old. For example, many studies (discussed later in this chapter) have demonstrated that behavioural training methods are effective for incontinent children and adults with a profound intellectual disability.

Behavioural training approaches have also shown better outcomes than other methods of continence training in normal children (Madsen et al 1969, Butler 1976). For example, Madsen et al's (1969) controlled comparison of different methods of toilet training normal children, over 1 week of baseline and 4 weeks of training, involved five groups:

1. a maturational control group, where parents used no training whatsoever
2. a 'parents' own' control group, where parents used whatever toilet training procedures they would have used normally
3. a reinforcement schedule group, involving contingent reinforcement and other behavioural training strategies
4. a pants alarm group, where parents were given miniature urine alarms and took their children to the toilet when the alarm sounded, but otherwise used their usual training methods
5. a pants alarm plus behavioural methods group.

Analysis of the frequency of continent and incontinent urine showed that results for the two behavioural training groups (3 and 5) were significantly better than those of the other three. Also, although outcome was better for older children, behavioural training was more effective than other methods across all age levels. The latter would not be predicted by maturational theory.

Dramatically accelerated potty 'training' has also been demonstrated by an interesting study of four babies aged between 3 and 6½ months, who were successfully trained in 4–5 months to reach for the potty in response to bladder and bowel sensations, using an intensive, structured behavioural training approach (Smeets et al 1985). Although these babies could not postpone elimination for longer than a few minutes, Smeets et al demonstrated that elimination is not a simple, reflex action at this stage; that babies of only a few months old can be trained to be clean and dry; and that preverbal babies are aware of and can be taught to communicate their bowel and bladder needs.

Thus, studies from a number of sources suggest that 'training' does play a role.

Maturation effects

Largo et al (1996), studying the change in toilet training practices with the introduction of disposable nappies and the consequent tendency to later toilet training, compared over 300 children born in the 1950s to over 300 born in the 1970s and 1980s. Differences were found between the two generations in terms of age at onset of toilet training, intensity of maternal prompting and the degree of the child's involvement in 'training'. Despite these differences, the age of acquisition of independent bowel and bladder control was similar in both groups, particularly with regard to nocturnal bladder control.

In the case of nocturnal continence, strong evidence has recently emerged on the importance of genetic (Eiberg et al 1995) and biological factors such as diurnal variation in vasopressin levels (Rittig 1996).

Readiness for training

Just as there is little evidence to support the widely accepted developmental sequence of acquisition of bladder components, so there is no evidence to support popular criteria for determining readiness for training. Michel (1999), for example, has suggested the following signs of readiness in normal children:

- The ability to ambulate to the potty.
- Stability while sitting on the potty.
- Ability to remain dry for several hours.
- Receptive language skills that allow the child to follow one- and two-step commands.

- Expressive language skills that allow the child to communicate the need to use the potty with words or reproducible gestures.
- The desire to please based on a positive relationship with caregivers.
- The desire on the child's part for independence and control of bladder and bowel function.

According to these criteria, toilet training would be appropriate for a child (or an adult with an intellectual disability) who can walk, understand simple instructions and express basic needs, has an adequate bladder capacity as demonstrated by the ability to remain dry for several hours, is sociable and understands the social consequences of continence.

On the one hand, it is difficult to argue against such plausible criteria, all of which can reasonably be expected to assist the toilet training process. Certainly, in terms of good practice, an incontinent child or adult with an intellectual disability who meets the above criteria and has no evidence of bladder or bowel dysfunction should be provided with toilet training opportunities. On the other hand, many people with a profound intellectual disability will never meet these criteria, but no studies have demonstrated that they cannot be toilet trained, albeit perhaps with more challenges.

PREVALENCE

Children in the general population

There is an impression that the prevalence of continence problems in humans is high compared with other mammals and also compared with other basic independence skills. Largo and Stutzle (1977a,b) found that 5% of 5 year olds and 1% of 10–12 year olds in the general population were still incontinent of faeces; Weir (1982), in a study of over 700 3 year olds in the general population, found that 23% of boys and 12% of girls were still regularly wet by day, of whom the majority were also still wet at night; and in a study of over 2000 children in the general population, Bower et al (1996) found regular nocturnal enuresis in 10% of 5 year olds and 1.4% of 11 year olds and regular

Table 7.1 Diurnal urinary incontinence in children and adults

Survey	Sample	Children (%)	Adults (%)
Thomas 1986	General population	18.5	9.5
DHSS 1972	Mild intellectual disability	25	5
Smith 1979b	Mild intellectual disability	–	6
Von Wendt et al 1990	Mild intellectual disability	16.7	5.6

Table 7.2 Diurnal urinary incontinence by degree of intellectual disability

Degree of disability	Smith 1979b (%)	von Wendt et al 1990 (%)
Borderline	6	–
Mild	6	5.6
Moderate	11	14.7
Severe	18	23.8
Profound	58	64.3

daytime incontinence in 2.1% of 5 year olds and 0.6% of 12 year olds.

People with intellectual disabilities

A number of surveys have studied the prevalence of incontinence in people with intellectual disabilities (e.g. DHSS 1972, Smith 1979b, von Wendt et al 1990) (Table 7.1).

The above surveys support the view that the prevalence of diurnal urinary incontinence in children and adults with a mild intellectual disability is within the range reported for the general population. Smith (1979b) and von Wendt et al (1990) have also provided prevalence of diurnal urinary incontinence by level of intellectual disability (Table 7.2).

These studies, whose findings are remarkably consistent, show that diurnal urinary incontinence increases with degree of intellectual disability and

---

Box 7.3   Prevalence of diurnal urinary incontinence

- There are few prevalence studies in intellectual disability.
- The validity of those involving community samples with low response rates is often unclear. Earlier studies involving institutional populations remain the most informative.
- The evidence supports the view that the prevalence of diurnal urinary incontinence in mild intellectual disability:
  - is within the range reported for the general population
  - increases with increasing degree of intellectual disability
  - is significantly higher for those with a profound intellectual disability.
- Even so, around 40% will have acquired daytime bladder control by adulthood.

---

is significantly higher in people with a profound intellectual disability. Even so, around 40% of those with the most profound intellectual disability will acquire diurnal bladder control by adulthood. Box 7.3 summarises key points.

ENCOPRESIS

Prevalence of constipation

Constipation is believed to be a significant precipitating factor in around 80% of cases of encopresis in the general population (Doleys et al 1981). There is a widespread belief that chronic constipation and faecal impaction are major problems for high-dependency populations in general (von Wendt et al 1990, Agnarsson et al 1993). However, the limited available evidence on the prevalence of constipation in the field of intellectual disability does not support a firm conclusion in this field and the role of constipation as a precipitating factor in encopresis has not been empirically established.

A number of surveys have considered or referred to the prevalence of constipation in people with intellectual disabilities (Ganesh et al 1994, Evenhuis 1997, Bohmer et al 2001). Results have not been wholly consistent, probably due to sam-

pling differences and different definitions of constipation. Nevertheless, the prevalence of constipation in these studies does seem generally high: Bohmer et al (2001) found that 69.3% of a random sample of 215 institutionalised children and adults with an IQ less than 50 were constipated over a 3-month recording period; Ganesh et al (1994), in a study of 38 adults with profound and multiple disabilities, and Evenhuis (1997) in a study of 70 elderly people with mild, moderate or severe intellectual disabilities (no profound disabilities), found that chronic constipation was present in 57% of the participants. However, only 15% of Bohmer et al's constipated participants were encopretic, suggesting that constipation did not represent a high risk factor for encopresis.

If constipation is generally high in the field of intellectual disability, there has been no study of precipitating factors or their relative importance as there has been in the field of the elderly, where insufficient dietary fibre, lack of exercise, low fluid intake and commonly prescribed constipating medications such as major tranquillisers are all considered to contribute to constipation and retentive encopresis (Resnick 1985).

Prevalence of encopresis

Smith (1979b) and Smith et al (1975) have provided figures for daytime soiling in a population of institutionalised (mainly) adults with intellectual disabilities (Table 7.3). Neither of these surveys provides prevalence by degree of intellectual disability. However, von Wendt et al's (1990) survey of community-living 20 year olds supports the view that prevalence of encopresis in those with a mild intellectual disability is within the range reported for the general population; that prevalence increases with degree of intellectual disability; and prevalence is significantly higher in those with a profound intellectual disability (Table 7.4). Nevertheless, approximately half of the latter will have acquired bowel control by adulthood. Box 7.4 summarises the key points.

NOCTURNAL ENURESIS

Von Wendt et al (1990) report the prevalence of nocturnal enuresis at age 7 and 20 (Table 7.5).

Table 7.3   Daytime encopresis

	Daytime soiling				
	n	Daily	Frequently	Sometimes	Never
Smith et al 1975	767	50 (6.5%)	58 (7.5%)	67 (8.7%)	592 (77.3%)
Smith 1979b	1330	142 (10.6%)	115 (8.6%)	189 (14.2%)	884 (66.6%)

Table 7.4   Intellectual disability and encopresis

Intellectual disability level	n	Encopresis at age 7	Encopresis at age 20
Mild	36	1 (2.8%)	0 (0%)
Moderate	34	11 (32.4%)	6 (17.6%)
Severe	21	8 (38.1%)	6 (18.6%)
Profound	14	12 (85.7%)	8 (57.1%)

From von Wendt et al (1990), reproduced with permission of MacKeith Press.

Table 7.5   Nocturnal enuresis by degree of intellectual disability

	Nocturnal enuresis at age 7		Nocturnal enuresis at age 20	
Ability level	n	Percentage	n	Percentage
Mild	4	11.1	0	0
Moderate	15	44.1	6	17.6
Severe	7	33.3	4	19.1
Profound	14	100	11	78.6

Again, it is noteworthy that a prevalence of 11.1% at age 7 and 0% at age 20 for nocturnal enuresis in those with mild intellectual disability is within the range reported for the general population (Box 7.5).

AETIOLOGICAL FACTORS

There has been little study of the factors which contribute to the failure to acquire continence or contribute to the breakdown of continence, in the field of intellectual disability (Box 7.6). Why this

Box 7.4   Prevalence of encopresis

- Fewer studies address the prevalence of encopresis than of urinary incontinence in the field of intellectual disability.
- The available evidence supports the view that the prevalence of encopresis in mild intellectual disability:
  - is within the range reported for the general population
  - increases with increasing degree of intellectual disability
  - is substantially increased in people with a profound intellectual disability.
- Even so, about 50% will have acquired bowel control by adulthood.

Box 7.5   Prevalence of nocturnal enuresis

- Fewer surveys address the prevalence of nocturnal enuresis than either that of diurnal urinary incontinence or encopresis.
- Prevalence of nocturnal enuresis in people with a mild intellectual disability is within the range reported for the general population.
- As before, prevalence increases with increasing degree of intellectual disability and is significantly higher in those with a profound disability.
- Only a quarter will have acquired nocturnal bladder control by adulthood.

is so is unclear, but evidence from other high-dependency fields suggests that incontinence in such fields is often perceived as a 'normal' part of the disabling condition.

Groves (1982) has asserted that, where an incontinent person has an intellectual disability, the

---

Box 7.6   Aetiological factors

- Vulnerability to incontinence in the field of intellectual disability might be increased by a number of factors, of which a profound degree of intellectual disability is likely to be one.
- It is not yet clear which other factors might militate against acquisition of bowel and bladder control in this field:
  - hyperactivity may result in the failure to sit on the toilet, or sit for long enough
  - deficits of attention might reduce awareness of cues of impending evacuation
  - lack of sociability reduces awareness of the social consequences of incontinence
  - severely challenging behaviours, including general non-compliance and anxiety-mediated behaviours such as toilet-related fears, are all likely to militate against the learning of associations between toilet cues and evacuation.
- Other barriers to treatment might include:
  - lack of toilet training opportunities due to negative carer beliefs
  - the ease of availability of free, disposable incontinence pads and other aids/appliances for the easier management of incontinence
  - negative attitudes to investigation and treatment in general hospital settings.

---

intellectual disability is assumed to be *the* causal factor in incontinence. Thus, incontinent people with intellectual disabilities may be assumed to have failed to reach a level of development consistent with the expectation of bowel and bladder control. Such assumptions are implicit, for example, in the 'readiness' criteria outlined by Michel (1999), described earlier. Although few adults with a profound degree of intellectual disability will meet Michel's criteria (with the exception of that relating to gross motor skills), around half do in fact acquire daytime bowel and bladder control by adulthood and one quarter will be dry at night. These findings challenge traditional assumptions about 'readiness' for toilet training.

While studies of children in the general population have indeed shown that incontinence is often associated with general developmental delay, spe-

cific learning and cognitive deficits, speech and language deficits, poor neuromuscular coordination and general neurological immaturity (Stern et al 1988, Madge et al 1993), most incontinent children are not developmentally delayed, nor do they have specific cognitive deficits, but are within the average range of intelligence and neurologically intact (Bellman 1966, Fritz & Armbrust 1982). Furthermore, most people with neurological abnormalities or immaturity, developmental delay or cognitive deficits are, in fact, continent. For example, Roijen et al (2001), in a study of the development of bladder control in children and adolescents with cerebral palsy (CP), found that most children with CP achieve urinary continence and do so spontaneously.

Intellectual disability as such therefore cannot be the sole factor in incontinence, because even where a profound intellectual disability is present, 40–50% of adults have acquired bowel and bladder control (DHSS 1972, Smith 1979b, von Wendt et al 1990). On the other hand, increasing degree of intellectual disability must be a factor because prevalence increases with increasing degree of intellectual disability (Smith 1979b, von Wendt et al 1990, Dalrymple & Ruble 1992) and behavioural continence training, although highly successful even in those with severe intellectual disabilities, may take longer in those with profound intellectual disabilities (Smith & Smith 1977).

If a profound degree of intellectual disability is not of itself an adequate explanation for the failure to acquire bowel and bladder control, what other factors might be implicated? A number of studies suggest that hyperactivity, deficits of attention and various challenging behaviours are likely to militate against the acquisition of control (Spencer et al 1968, Dalrymple & Ruble 1992). For example, Buttross (1999) has suggested that the inattentive child may fail to perceive the call to stool. Two studies have discussed the negative effect of various types of 'challenging behaviour'. These have included anxiety-related behaviours, such as toilet-related fears or adverse reactions to environmental change (Dalrymple & Ruble 1992), and negative or non-compliant behaviour, lack of sociability and lack of social awareness (Spencer et al 1968). These factors, which often coexist, may – in association with a more severe degree of intellectual disability – significantly reduce the likelihood of continence acquisition.

The assumption that the presence of an intellectual disability itself is sufficient to explain the failure to acquire continence has another unacceptable consequence, which is that medical causes of incontinence can be overlooked in people with intellectual disabilities because there can be a reluctance to conduct diagnostic investigations in people with severe and profound intellectual disabilities. Reasons for this might include practical, legal and ethical problems associated with invasive examinations of non-consenting adults. This not only means that medical causes of incontinence in people with intellectual disabilities are less likely to be diagnosed and treated (Groves 1982), it is also a barrier to research into the acquisition and breakdown of continence processes in people with intellectual disabilities.

INTERVENTION

Strategies for different problems

Although there is as yet no consensus on classification or typology in the field of intellectual disability, the following distinctions can be helpful when considering intervention:

- Is incontinence double or single?
- Is encopresis, when associated with constipation, anal poking/smearing or 'spurious' diarrhoea, due to simple constipation, complex faecal impaction or active retention of faeces?
- Is toilet refusal present? This can include elimination under highly specific conditions, such as exclusively into a nappy/pad, and is often associated with obsessional behaviour and general difficulty in adapting to changes in the environment.
- Do accidents occur repeatedly in inappropriate locations, such as in corners or against doors, despite the ability to use the toilet? Is faecal smearing present, but not in association with impaction?
- Do wetting or soiling accidents occur shortly after coming off the toilet?
- Are there repeated small urinary accidents?
- Does the child spray around the toilet or urinate on his clothing at toilet?

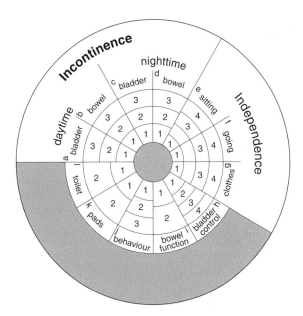

Figure 7.1 Continence skills rating chart. Reproduced with permission from Smith & Smith (1987).

Base-line assessment of continence skills

The rating scale shown in Figure 7.1 offers a quick and easy way to rate some of the components of continence in someone with intellectual disabilities. This ad-hoc rating scale is intended to give an initial overall picture of continence skills for the purpose of planning continence training programmes.

Bladder training

By the late 1960s, the key features of successful behavioural continence training programmes in the field of intellectual disability had been identified (Hundziak et al 1966, Kimbrell et al 1967). Although a number of previous programmes had used behavioural techniques, Azrin and Foxx (1971) combined a number of these in a package. Their study of nine institutionalised adults with profound intellectual disabilities, whose frequency of wetting was reduced by 90% over an average of 4 days despite being regarded at that time as incapable of learning, is seminal (Box 7.7).

The work of these authors stimulated many attempts at replication (e.g. Pfadt & Sullivan 1981,

> **Box 7.7 Main features of Azrin and Foxx's intensive daytime continence training**
>
> - One-to-one training close to the toilet
> - Increased fluid intake to increase the frequency of urination
> - The use of pants and bowl alarms, enabling consistent and immediate detection of inappropriate and appropriate urination
> - Rewards for continent passing urine and remaining dry
> - Punishment for wetting/soiling accidents
> - Prompts to toilet at 30-min intervals
> - Fading of prompts to teach independent toileting
> - Shaping of dressing skills
> - Procedures to generalise skills and maintain progress after completion of training

Averink et al 2005). The work of Pfadt represents the largest reported continence training programme in an institutional setting. Sixty-three clients with severe intellectual disabilities progressed through a series of stages comprising intensive training, maintenance and long-term preservation of skills. One-to-one intensive training, using Azrin and Foxx procedures for bladder training and independence training, was completed after either nine self-initiated toiletings or 4 weeks' intensive training. Of the 63 trainees, eight failed to reach this criterion and 55 (87%) proceeded to the next stage. Maintenance training, involving one trainer per two trainees, aimed to maintain self-initiated toileting, reduce accidents further and teach additional skills, including hand washing and toilet flushing. This stage was completed either after independent toileting was maintained with fewer than two bladder accidents per week for 2 weeks, or after 2 months of training. Of the 55 who entered maintenance, six were still undergoing maintenance training at the time of the report, nine had failed to reach criterion and 40 had progressed to the 'preservation' stage. Preservation aimed to prepare trainees to maintain their skills in their long-term placements. Staffing ratios at this stage were one to three, preservation being completed after two consecutive accident-free weeks, or 2 months of training and an accident rate of one per week or less. Of the 40 trainees who

entered this stage, 31 (77.5%) reached criterion for full continence after 5 months' intervention.

In the UK, Buchan et al (1989) attempted to investigate the feasibility of using structured behavioural continence training with 53 intellectually disabled, community-living adults and children, most of whom were living at home. Although support to parents was described as 'intensive', the parents in fact carried out the training themselves so that Azrin and Foxx's techniques, including urine alarms, were used only 'where possible and appropriate'. Not surprisingly, success was much lower than that reported in any institutional study, leading the authors to conclude that this 'package' was not feasible in the community.

By contrast, Smith and Bainbridge (1991) successfully applied a modified Azrin and Foxx approach to daytime continence training for an 11-year-old boy with a profound intellectual disability and severe behavioural problems living at home. For both ethical and practical reasons, 'punishment' techniques were not used and prompts to toilet and dry pants checks were less frequent. Training was conducted in the home by a trainer 5 days per week from 9.00 a.m. to 4.00 p.m., the parent carrying out a minimum of pants checks and prompts to toilet during the evenings and weekends. Results of this and other community toilet-training programmes implemented by the present authors demonstrate that intensive continence training is feasible in ordinary family homes. Figure 7.2 illustrates an example of five community-living children with severe intellectual disabilities, in which it can be seen that the frequency of continent urine increases while that of incontinence decreases. However, the nature of these training programmes does raise questions about the feasibility of using parents as trainers. In order to achieve success, it may be necessary to modify some aspects of the programme and/or provide training staff for some of the time. Box 7.8 summarises key points.

Maintenance and generalisation

Although acquisition of bladder control using intensive continence training maintains well in the short to medium term (Bettison et al 1976) and in the long term (Hyams et al 1991), preservation of

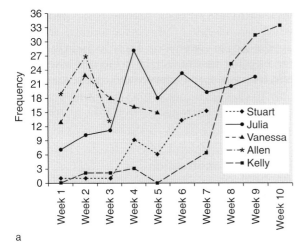

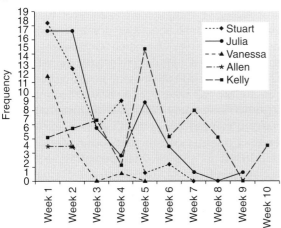

Figure 7.2 (a) Weekly continent passing of urine for five children. (b) Weekly bladder accidents for five children.

newly acquired bladder skills is a key concern, because the impact of initial success can be reduced by environmental conditions which are not conducive to long-term maintenance of newly acquired skills. A number of factors may influence long-term effectiveness of behavioural continence training approaches (Box 7.9).

Hyams et al (1991) followed up 15 children with severe intellectual disabilities, who were by then between 18 and 29 years, 10 years after continence training. Ten had received one-to-one, structured behavioural continence training, while five had received structured continence training as a group.

Recording established that continence had maintained substantially, but independence at toilet less so. A major reason for this seemed to be the fact that staffing changes in the intervening years meant that current care staff were unaware that these residents had previously been independent at toilet and had, since then, reverted to prompting them along with other residents. Despite this, intensive training was still more cost-effective, the extra investment of resources being quickly repaid in terms of the greater reduction in care costs. In fact, over a 10-year period, the total savings in carer time for the 10 individually trained residents was calculated to be over 50 000 staff hours.

Box 7.10 emphasises the importance of generalising the training setting.

Training principles

Continence training programmes should always be designed to meet individual needs and circumstances. One of the great strengths of behavioural

---

Box 7.9   Maintenance factors

- Less intensive training, although on the face of it cheaper and easier to implement, may be less cost-effective in the long term than intensive, one-to-one training (Hyams et al 1991).
- Shutting/locking doors between classrooms, living rooms and toilets and the use of clothing with difficult fasteners, all militate against the maintenance of continence and independence skills.
- If self-initiated toileting has been established, self-initiations reduce and dependency on prompts increases if carers revert to prompting trainees to toilet (Foxx & Azrin 1973, Hyams et al 1991).
- Studies of continence retraining in the elderly with dementia show that close monitoring and supervision, regular group and individual feedback and staff motivational systems are more effective in changing staff attitudes and practices in the long term than staff training alone (Burgio et al 1990).
- A full discussion of factors affecting long-term maintenance is provided by Pfadt and Sullivan (1981) and Bettison (1982). Some factors may present fewer problems in community settings.

Box 7.10   Generalising training across different settings

- The importance of generalising training across different settings has been demonstrated in early studies (Baumeister & Klosowski 1965, Dunlap et al 1985).
- If intensive training is carried out in a specialist training facility (Baumeister & Klosowski 1965), a sudden return to the regular daytime situation can erase progress if generalisation training is not carried out.
- This also applies in community settings where clients trained in one situation then access new environments without generalisation training.

---

training approaches is their flexibility – their capacity to be adjusted to meet the specific goals, specific learning requirements and environmental circumstances of the individual. However, although this avoids a 'block' treatment approach,

there are nevertheless certain basic principles which underpin all behavioural training approaches to continence. These include the need for baseline assessment by which to assess the effectiveness of the intervention, definition of the objectives, ongoing recording to evaluate success or failure, and the use of rewards to motivate learning.

Systems of motivation

Some people express concern about the use of rewards. Professional and family carers may have a negative view of rewards as 'bribes', or may worry that rewards will 'spoil' the child ('Why should I give him/her an extra treat for doing something he/she should be doing anyway?') or be difficult to stop. One parent expressed concern that the 'reward' of music, which played when the child urinated into the musical potty, would teach the child to wet whenever he heard the same tune in other situations. Parents with more negative parenting approaches which focus on reprimands or other punishments for 'bad' behaviour can find it difficult to change their parenting style and reward positive behaviour. Such parents may hold negative attributions of their child's incontinence, believing it to be due to laziness or defiance (especially if the child can eliminate on the toilet at times and is sometimes dry/clean). Other parents firmly believe that the problem is outwith the child's control, even where investigations have ruled out medical causes.

In fact, the evidence shows that rewards, carefully chosen and used consistently, speed up the learning process in people with severe intellectual disabilities by helping them to differentiate between the desired and the undesired behaviour (Box 7.11). In order to be effective, however, rewards must be given consistently on every occasion and immediately upon occurrence of the desired behaviour and not, for example, 5 min later. Rewards must also be maintained until the desired behaviour has been reliably established. Once the goals of training have been achieved, rewards should be phased out gradually rather than discontinued abruptly. Some parents stop rewards as soon as the ability to eliminate in the toilet has been demonstrated but before conti-

Box 7.11   Flexible rewards

Rewards should be flexible and may include the following:

- Praise – talking about how pleased other people, such as family members, teacher, will be.
- Physical contact – hugs, tickling (unless 'giggle micturition' is a problem), rough and tumble play, or other physical contact such as stroking cheek or head.
- A brief period of exclusive parent/care staff attention.
- Access to a favourite toy, object, game, music or computer games.
- Primary reinforcers, i.e. rewards based on biological needs such as food and drink, should be small, easy to administer and quickly consumed. They can include small segments or pieces of fresh or dried fruit, small savoury items such as crisps or savoury biscuits, or small sweets. A variety of drinks may be used.
- A wide range of rewards should be used in order to avoid satiation. A small 'goody' bag containing a selection of small sweet or savoury items, small/inexpensive collectible toys (those marketed as 'pocket money' toys are often suitable) or stickers/cards which can be collected to form sets, allow more able children to make a choice (always provided choice is not stressful and does not provoke a tantrum). Small amounts of money such as 10 or 20 pence pieces or 'tokens' that can be saved for larger rewards are often popular with older or more able children. (It is reasonable to conclude that items which are repeatedly left in the bottom of the bag are not rewarding and should be discarded.)
- Star charts, although easy to administer, are somewhat 'one size fits all' and tend to quickly lose their reward value with longer-term use. The concept is also too abstract for children with more severe disabilities, who require more individualised, 'concrete' reinforcement.
- 'Social' reinforcement is appropriate for most but not all children.

Box 7.12   Objectives

Example of a badly defined objective:
At the end of training John will be toilet trained.

Example of a well-defined objective:
At the end of training, John will be dry by day, with no more than one accident per week, and will pass urine on the toilet when prompted every 2 h. He will be able to lower and raise his pants, but will still need prompts to the toilet and supervision in the toilet area.

This specifies more clearly:

- the aims of the programme
- positive skills/behaviours to be taught
- the degree of success expected
- the support/supervision ultimately expected, which may reflect his general ongoing degree of dependency
- standards by which to evaluate the outcome.

imagination. What is rewarding to one person may be punishing to another. For example, 'social reinforcement' such as praise or a hug, while rewarding to most people, can be punishing to those with sensory abnormalities or people with autism. When identifying suitable rewards, it is important not only to ask what a person likes, but also how they choose to spend their time.

Defining objectives

Clear definition of goals is important for training and essential for evaluation (Box 7.12). The term 'toilet training' is vague: are we talking about bladder or bowel, day or night? Do we expect the participant to be fully independent at toilet or to require help and supervision; to go to the toilet without the need for prompting, or be dry and use the toilet by means of prompting at regular intervals? Objectives should be stated in an unambiguous form that can be clearly understood by everyone involved, as different people may have a different understanding of 'toilet training'.

Objectives are important at a practical level. Once objectives are properly formulated, the outline of the programme should follow and outcomes are set by which the effectiveness, or otherwise, of the programme can be evaluated. Rather

nence skills are reliable. Such parents may say that when they saw that the child could do it, they did not believe rewards were needed any longer.

Identifying what is rewarding to the individual and suitable for the needs of the programme can be difficult and sometimes calls for a degree of than formulating objectives in terms of behaviour(s) to be decreased, it is better to turn the formulation round to reflect the behaviour you wish to increase in order to emphasise the positive side of training. For example, if the problem relates to daytime urinary incontinence, the objectives should be to increase the frequency of dryness and continent passing of urine by day.

Next, consider the aspect of continence on which you wish to focus: bladder or bowel training, or both? Does it include handling clothes and going to toilet independently? The degree of success expected and how much help, if any, the individual is expected to require when the objective is reached should be included in the statement of objectives.

Training procedures

Assessment determines the current level of an incontinent person's bladder and bowel control; objectives specify the goals to be achieved. Having assessed and rated current toileting skills, having determined the objectives clearly and having identified appropriate rewards, the methods of teaching these new skills can now be considered.

The task is to break down the distance between the observed and the desired skills into a series of steps. The structured teaching methods used to teach toileting skills are the same as those used to teach other self-help skills. Two of the key techniques for teaching new skills are known as 'prompt and fade' and 'backward chaining'.

Prompt and fade

There are three types of prompts: physical prompts, verbal prompts and gestural prompts.

- A physical prompt consists of any prompt involving physical contact. A major physical prompt might consist of physically guiding the trainee to the toilet, positioning him in front of the toilet and physically guiding him to sit. Physical prompts range from this extreme, to holding the hand lightly or even simply 'shadowing' the trainee's back or elbow with your hand.
- A verbal prompt consists of any spoken prompt to the child such as: 'John, go to the toilet.'

- A gestural prompt consists of any other form of prompt in which the trainer prompts the trainee non-verbally, without touching or verbally instructing him. At one extreme, a gestural prompt can involve an elaborate mime whereby the trainer makes eye contact then looks at the toilet, points to the trainee and then, with a sweeping wave of the arm, points to the toilet, gestures the trainee to move to the toilet, then pats the toilet seat and gestures to the trainee to sit on the toilet. At the other extreme, a gestural prompt can consist of a very small point with one finger, or a small head nod. Ultimately, establishing eye contact and following this with a movement of the eyes towards the toilet is the smallest gestural prompt possible.

The prompting procedure Having established the minimum type and level of prompt required to get the trainee to go to the toilet from a few feet away, the prompts are then broken down into their physical, verbal and gestural components and a series of steps determined to systematically fade these out. Prompts to toilet are always faded in order from physical to verbal to gestural. As physical prompts represent the highest level of prompt/dependence on others to go to the toilet, they are faded first. Verbal prompts are faded next because, in practice, they are the most difficult to fade: the smallest verbal prompt of just one word spoken softly – 'toilet' – is impossible to fade further. As there is more scope for fading gestural prompts completely, these are faded last.

Fading In order to facilitate the correct sequence for fading prompts, the prompts are given in the reverse order: the lowest level of prompt (gestural) is given first. If this is not sufficient, a verbal prompt is given next, accompanied by a gestural prompt. If the trainee does not move towards the toilet in response to either of these, the highest level of prompt (a physical prompt) is given last, accompanied by a verbal prompt. These are tried, in the order referred to, with a gap of a second or so in between in order to give the trainee the opportunity to respond to a lower category of prompt first. Thus, whenever a prompt is given, a lower level than was successful on the previous occasion is always tried first. As soon as the trainee responds to a lower level of prompt, subsequent prompts should never go back up beyond that category or level.

Fading whole categories of prompts is accomplished using the correct sequence of prompts described above, but procedures for facilitating the process further have developed from experience of these programmes. For example, it is possible to fade directly from physical to gestural prompts without the intervening step of verbal prompts. This can be done by first fading the physical prompt to the point where the trainee is held lightly by the hand. The trainer then prompts the trainee from in front, rather than from the side, by reaching out to hold the trainee's hand. The trainer then moves their hand away just as the trainee is about to touch it. If the trainer's hand is moved away, the trainee is likely to step forward to try to hold it. The trainer then points dramatically to the toilet. In this way, fading gestural prompts is achieved more rapidly. Seated close to the toilet and going back and forward to the toilet every half hour or so, with substantial reinforcement for using the toilet and for having dry pants, self-initiated toileting (i.e. going without a prompt) is a relatively easy step to make.

If prompts have been faded to the lowest possible gestural prompt and the trainee has still not self-initiated, the following procedure may be useful. A few minutes before a prompt is due, the trainee should be casually manoeuvred to stand close to the toilet without any overt prompting. Standing next to the toilet, the chances are that after a few minutes the trainee will sit down on the toilet. When this happens and is followed by successful passing of urine, the trainee should be praised lavishly and rewarded, and training should proceed from there.

Prompts to toilet are reduced as soon as self-initiations appear and discontinued completely when the trainee can self-initiate consistently. After an initial low level prompt on the first occasion in the morning, two or three self-initiations during the day should be sufficient to warrant the complete termination of prompts thereafter that day. However, because of individual differences, it is impossible to set an exact criterion for terminating prompts. It is unwise to stop prompts altogether after the first self-initiated toileting unless self-initiations are occurring very frequently.

When prompts to toilet have been stopped and the trainee has been self-initiating successfully for a few days from close to the toilet, the trainee can be moved gradually away from the toilet and back towards the classroom or sitting room, a few feet each day, always ensuring that self-initiations have been established consistently at each point. It is especially important to train from corners, doors or any point where there is a choice of direction or a barrier on the way to the toilet.

Chaining

Chaining is when a skill is broken down into small steps and taught one step at a time. In 'forward chaining', step 1 is taught first. When this can be executed without assistance, step 2 is added. When steps 1 and 2 can be executed without help, step 3 is added, and so on. 'Backward chaining', by contrast, teaches the last step in the chain first. This step, being closest to the goal to be achieved, is closest to the reward to be earned and is hence, in learning terms, the step most easily learned. Thus, when the last step can be executed without assistance, the second last step is added, and so on. For example, the objective might be to teach lowering pants at toilet without help. Using backward chaining, first the hands are held and guided through the entire procedure, for which the child is rewarded at the end. Once this sequence can be executed with assistance, the trainer guides the trainee through the sequence leaving the last step, the relatively easy one of lowering the pants from below the knees, to be completed by the trainee without assistance. When this can be completed without assistance, the trainee is required to lower the pants from above the knees without help, then from the hips and finally the waist. Smaller steps than this may be required, but the concept behind backward chaining involves teaching skills in small steps from the goal backwards.

Fluid intake

In contrast to the long-standing tradition of restricting fluid to incontinent people, increased fluid is common in behavioural continence training programmes. The purpose of increased fluid is to increase training opportunities and thereby

---

Box 7.13   Fluid intake

- Increased fluids for training purposes should be carefully monitored
- Candidates for behavioural continence training programmes involving augmented hydration should be medically screened
- Hydration should not be used with those being treated simultaneously with medication known to increase urinary retention
- Hydration should not be used in those with pre-existing epilepsy, a history of spinal injury or impaired cerebrospinal fluid such as hydrocephalus
- Fluid intake should be limited to 85–125 ml/h for children weighing between 60 and 100 lbs (27 and 45 kg) and 165 ml/h for adolescents and adults weighing between 100 and 150 lbs (45 and 68 kg), for no more than 12 h per 24 h.

---

speed up training by increasing the frequency of passing urine (Box 7.13). Although advice to restrict fluid is still found, a number of studies have established a positive role for increased fluid in bladder function (Smith & Wong 1981, Spangler et al 1984). For example, Smith and Wong studied bladder function data over several weeks in 10 children with severe intellectual disabilities undergoing intensive behavioural continence training utilising increased fluid intake. When daily frequencies and volumes of continent and incontinent urine were analysed in relation to fluid intake, no association was found between increased fluid intake and incontinence, but a positive association was found with continent passing urine and with increased functional bladder capacity.

Concern has been expressed about the risk of overhydration where fluid intake is increased in association with structured behavioural continence training (Thompson & Hanson 1983). 'Normal' fluid intake is difficult to define because of cultural differences and environmental factors such as ambient temperature and humidity (Vande Walle et al 1995). Increased fluid in conjunction with intensive behavioural continence training is demonstrably successful (as compared with fluid restriction, in which there has traditionally been a popular belief but for which there is no evidence) in people whose incontinence was formerly con-

sidered untreatable. There have been no reports of adverse effects of increased fluid intake during structured bladder training programmes. The success of intensive behavioural continence training programmes does not, however, justify risk to the trainee. Therefore, the following recommendations have been made by Thompson and Hanson (1983) as shown in Box 7.13.

Regular prompting versus timing

One major difference in continence training approaches is that of 'regular prompting' versus 'timing'. In the former, the trainee is prompted to toilet at regular, set intervals of time, regardless of whether the bladder is full; the latter approach involves prompting at the time an accident occurs, or attempting to predict when the bladder is likely to be full and prompting just before an accident is likely to occur. Although timed voiding allegedly based on bladder filling cycles appears common in clinical practice, the timing of prompts is usually based simply on visual inspection of base-line data. However, as has already been discussed, there is strong evidence that the bladder does not in fact operate in a simple, reflexive, filling–emptying cycle. This means that predicting when the bladder is about to empty is, in practice, difficult and explains why this common approach often fails to keep the incontinent person dry and why prompts may then become progressively more frequent, as frustrated carers and support staff attempt to get the client to the toilet in time.

In the field of intellectual disability, a small comparison of these two approaches was undertaken by Smith (1979a,b). Five children with profound intellectual disabilities were intensively trained using regular prompts (based on Azrin and Foxx) and five intensively trained using a timing approach (Van Wagenen et al 1969). Although both methods were equally effective, timing was more complicated in practice. Furthermore, the training situation in this project, which took place in an institutional setting, was more 'artificial' than most community settings: trained within sight of the toilet and with 'pants alarms' to detect the onset of urination, the 'timing' group could be prompted as soon as a wetting accident began, enabling them to reach the toilet, which was

Box 7.14   Case study 1

Fiona is a young adult with a severe intellectual disability who lives at home. She has some speech (two-word combinations) and challenging behaviours, including occasional tantrums. She can pass urine on the toilet when taken, but still has accidents and her mother complains that Fiona's incontinence has destroyed a new settee. Fiona is described as being wet 'all the time' and her mother thinks she is doing it deliberately to 'get at' her.

	Time of day												
Time	9am	10	11	12	1pm	2	3	4	5	6	7	8	9
Day													
Mon	PU	D	D	D	PU	D	D	PU	D	D	PU	D	D
Tues	D	PU	D	D	NPU	PU	D	D	W	D	NPU	PU	D
Wed	NPU	D	PU	D	PU	D	D	PU	D	D	PU	D	D
Thur	PU	D	D	D	D	PU	D	D	D	W	D	PU	D
Fri	D	PU	D	D	PU	D	D	PU	D	D	PU	D	D
Sat	PU	D	D	D	NPU	PU	D	PU	D	D	PU	D	D
Sun	NPU	D	D	D	PU	D	D	PU	D	D	NPU	D	D
Mon	NPU	D	PU	D	D	PU	D	PU	D	D	PU	D	D
Tues	PU	D	D	D	PU	D	D	D	D	W	D	PU	D
Wed	PU	D	D	D	PU	D	PU	D	D	D	PU	D	D
Thur	NPU	D	D	D	D	PU	D	D	W	D	NPU	PU	D
Fri	D	PU	D	D	PU	D	D	PU	D	D	PU	D	D
Sat	D	PU	D	D	PU	D	D	PU	D	D	PU	D	D
Sun	PU	D	D	D	PU	D	D	PU	D	D	NPU	PU	D

Recording key: D, dry; W, wet; PU, prompted to toilet and passed urine; NPU, prompted to toilet and did not pass urine.

Two weeks' base-line recording of frequency and times of passing continent and incontinent urine show that:
- Fiona is not wetting all of the time but only twice a week
- these accidents occur when Fiona has not been prompted to toilet early in the evenings.

Discussion of base-line records established that missed prompts coincided with mother's favourite TV programmes. The problem was solved by adjusting the times of prompts on those evenings.

immediately to hand, in time. As this is not generally the case in everyday community settings, the bladder has often emptied before the child reaches the toilet. Indeed, regardless of whether timing involves prompting when an accident is predicted or after an accident has started, timing is more complicated in practice. Regular prompting avoids the above problems. It also enables the essential skill of passing urine in the absence of a full bladder to be acquired quickly. There can be exceptions to this rule, however, as demonstrated by the case studies in Boxes 7.14 and 7.15.

DOUBLE INCONTINENCE

Before discussing encopresis intervention, it is appropriate first to consider intervention for double incontinence. It might be assumed that the rational approach would be to start with bowel training, as bowel control is generally acquired first. However, where someone with a severe or profound intellectual disability is doubly incontinent, bladder training carried out first often results in associated improvement in bowel control, as demonstrated in Figure 7.3.

Box 7.15   Case study 2: Developing an intensive daytime bladder training programme

Stewart is an incontinent teenager with a profound intellectual disability. He has a degree of cerebral palsy but is ambulant. He has single words of speech and can comprehend simple instructions. He can feed with a fork and drink from a cup. His play tends to involve manipulation of objects rather than imaginative or constructive play. He has no serious behaviour problems but can have temper tantrums when frustrated. He is affectionate and responsive to attention.

Stewart does not communicate the need to eliminate and has frequent diurnal bladder and bowel accidents, is often wet but never soiled at night, can sit unaided on the toilet, assists with lowering his underpants, passes urine on the toilet occasionally and has regular bowel movements. The priority is daytime bladder control. The objectives are to teach him to remain dry and to pass urine on the toilet every time when toileted on a 2-hourly basis.

Before bringing together the points covered above, we need to consider:
1. fluid intake
2. urine-sensitive alarms
3. clothing
4. the environment in which the training is to be implemented
5. training procedures.

FLUIDS
Increasing fluid for the first part of the training day in accordance with the recommendations discussed above will help increase bladder capacity and will increase the number of training opportunities by increasing the frequency of urination.

EQUIPMENT
Two types of continence-training alarms are available: toilet bowl alarms and pants alarms. The toilet bowl alarm attaches to the toilet and signals immediately urine is passed on the toilet.[1] The pants alarm is a small device attached to the underpants which signals the occurrence of a wetting accident. Body-worn nocturnal enuresis alarms are suitable.[2]

[1] Toilet bowl alarms are available from:
- BIME, Wolfson Centre, RUH, Combe Park, Bath BA1 3NG, UK.
- TFH, 76 Barracks Road, Sandy Lane Industrial Estate, Stockport on Severn, Worcester, DY12 9QB UK.

[2] A number of companies supply enuresis alarms, including:
- ERIC, 34 Old School House, Britannia Road, Kingswood, Bristol BS15 2DB, UK.
- Ferraris Medical, Ferraris House, Aden Road, Enfield, Middlesex EN3 7SE, UK.
- Malem Medical, 10 Willows Holt, Lowdham, Nottingham NG14 7EJ, UK.

Pants and bowl alarms, used as part of a well-designed training programme, both aid immediate detection of urination and hence immediate and consistent reinforcement. Bowl alarms, which emphasise the positive side of training, are more important than pants alarms as well as being more reliable and easier to use in practice. Musical potties are available for smaller children and musical toilet targets for boys who stand,[3] although it is often simpler to train boys seated first. Do not worry that using a musical potty will 'condition' a child to pass urine in response to this tune later in life – this does not happen.

CLOTHING
Extra clothing should be organised in advance. If a pants alarm is to be used, underpants should be close-fitting and made of cotton. Trousers should have elastic waists for easy handling. Dresses or skirts should not be too long. Incontinence pads, tights, dungarees or anything with belts, buttons, clips or zips should be avoided.

THE TRAINING ENVIRONMENT
As Stewart is beyond the age where spontaneous remission is likely, he may require more intensive, structured training. This means that, in the early stages at least, training may have to be carried out close to the toilet. If this is the case, the toilet area should be made as pleasant and comfortable as possible. Although school and day centre toilets are often more spacious, they are usually less pleasant than toilets at home. If so, the décor, heating, lighting and ventilation should be improved where possible and soft furnishings introduced. A variety of toys or appropriate activities should be available. The trainer should have a chair, radio, access to coffee and a clock. Although intensive toilet training is hard work, it need not be unpleasant. At home, it may be necessary to leave the door open if the bathroom is small, but the space outside the bathroom may be used as the training area provided the toilet is within sight.

TRAINING PROCEDURES
Following the work of Foxx and Azrin, the aspects of training for which we need separate procedures are

[3] The Aaronshield toilet target was originally designed to teach boys who spray around the toilet to aim accurately. When the urine hits the bull's eye, a tune is played. The target can be ordered with or without the musical movement, but the music represents an important and 'fun' reward for boys with intellectual disabilities. From Masters Instruments, Dorset Ave, Thornton Cleveleys, Lancashire FY5 2DB, UK.

Box 7.15 *Continued*

bladder training, dry pants training, accident training and independence training.

Bladder training

- Engage Stewart in play within sight of the toilet.
- Every 30 or 45 min, prompt him to sit on the toilet.
- Let him sit on the toilet until he passes urine or for a maximum of 10 min.
- Immediately he passes urine and activates the bowl alarm, reward him with praise and a small reward. A small 'goody bag' containing a selection of inexpensive rewards can be kept out of sight and quickly brought in when the bowl alarm is activated. Reward Stewart while he is still on the toilet and when he starts to pass urine, not when he finishes (this procedure can be reviewed if Stewart stops the urine stream as soon as he is rewarded, or begins to stop and start in the expectation of earning further rewards).

Dry pants training

Teaching Stewart to discriminate between dry and wet pants through feedback and social consequences is an important part of training which is usually insufficiently emphasised. It is important to remember that children who wear disposable incontinence pads with 'stay-dry' liners do not experience 'feedback' in the form of the feeling of wetness when incontinent.

- Dry pants checks are carried out between prompts to toilet. Every 15 min throughout the training day, guide Stewart's hand to check his underpants and praise/reward him for being dry.
- Also do this before any activity he enjoys, such as before meals, drinks and activities, or other enjoyable and hence rewarding social interactions. It is not necessary to give an additional reward at this time – the meal, drink, activity will serve the purpose.

The purpose of bladder training and dry pants training is to increase Stewart's motivation to pass urine on the toilet and remain dry, respectively. Remember that, even if he rarely passes urine on the toilet before training, with increased fluids and regular prompts to toilet, he will pass urine on the toilet at some point.

Wetting accident procedure

- When a wetting accident occurs and the pants alarm (if used) is triggered, immediately guide Stewart's hand to feel his wet pants. Ensure that you have his attention and say 'No, your pants are wet'. This should be said in a clear but neutral voice. Do not shout – this would be unacceptable and it is important to remember that the purpose of this procedure is not to administer a reprimand but to

assist Stewart to discriminate between wet and dry pants.

- Switch the pants alarm off, but do not prompt him to the toilet or change his clothes immediately, as this would afford him one-to-one attention for wetting.
- Quietly withdraw eye contact, praise and attention for a few minutes.
- After a few minutes, change him into dry clothes in a neutral manner with a minimum of fuss. Then assist Stewart to check his (now) dry pants and praise him for having dry pants. Recommence the bladder training procedure as above.

Training independent toileting

We have trained Stewart to remain dry and pass urine consistently on the toilet. If the aim of training had been to teach him to initiate going to the toilet himself, an additional procedure would be required which is more complex and requires more intensive training. If Stewart's comprehension is limited, the procedure is as follows:

1. Establish the type and level of prompt required to get Stewart to go to the toilet, then systematically fade, i.e. phase out, prompts. For example, does he require to be physically guided? If so, does he need to be guided with an arm around the shoulders, led by the hand or does he only require the presence of a light touch on his back? Or will he go in response to a verbal prompt only such as 'Stewart, toilet', without the need for any physical prompting?
2. Start training close to the toilet, then when prompts have been faded and Stewart can self-initiate from close to the toilet, gradually move him backwards from the toilet to all the rooms from which he will be expected to self-initiate.

Relapses in independent toileting

A clear definition of a relapse should be established beforehand, for example, two full days without a self-initiated toileting, or when wetting accidents are daily or if Stewart starts to follow others when they are prompted to toilet.

Organisational issues

A well-designed but badly organised or inconsistently implemented programme will have little effect. A little prior planning and organisation can pre-empt many of the common problems that affect the integrity of the programme. These include:

- responsible staff
- generalisation and maintenance
- the evaluation of training
- the length of the training programme.

Box 7.15 *Continued*

Responsibility for training. Consistent training is achieved more easily if one person has responsibility for coordinating the programme. Those carrying out the training will need training and practice in the procedures involved. It can be useful to enact the training procedures using a simulated training situation and role playing. Daily support is also very important, as intensive, structured continence training is tiring. Clear feedback and close supervision should be provided. Whether Stewart lives at home or in supported living, he is likely also to attend school or access day services.

Generalisation and maintenance. It is essential that training is generalised to all settings and that everyone who comes into contact with Stewart is familiar with the programme (Box 7.16). Maintenance refers to sustaining progress once the objectives have been achieved. As maintenance and generalisation can present problems for people with more severe degrees of intellectual disability, the likelihood that problems will arise should be considered in advance (Box 7.17).

Evaluation. Evaluating the effects of training is important. A baseline or pretreatment measure of the

behaviour should be obtained. Simple but accurate records of the frequency of continent and incontinent urine enable success to be evaluated and decisions to be made about whether to continue the programme unchanged or to modify it.

Length of training. The base-line period must be long enough to establish that the behaviour is stable. There should be evidence that the behaviour is neither increasing nor decreasing in frequency, otherwise it will be difficult to establish conclusively whether change was due to treatment or some other factor. If incontinence is already reducing, introducing a new training programme may not be necessary or desirable. A base-line period of 3 weeks is preferable to 2.

A bladder training programme can be expected to last for several weeks, so that there may be little point in starting if Stewart is about to go on holiday. A period should be chosen in which few interruptions are expected. It is important also to specify achievable objectives if there is a time limit on training. If progress is slow and time is limited, objectives may need to be redefined. Progress should be evident in 4 weeks, even though training takes longer to complete.

Box 7.16   Generalisation

- Training should be generalised both to different places and to different people.
- If possible, train initially in one location only (e.g. at home) and with one trainer. When some progress has been made, extend training to other environments in which the trainee uses the toilet regularly. Finally, extend training to include toilets used less frequently, such as on trips or outings, arranging some trips specifically for the purpose of training in these situations.
- Similarly, start with one trainer conducting most of the training, then introduce others to the programme when progress is underway. The first person should be present until Stewart can perform equally for different people.

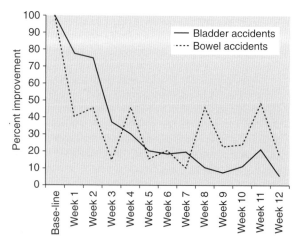

Figure 7.3 Reduction in bowel accidents during intensive bladder training for 10 children with profound learning disabilities. Reproduced with permission from Smith (1979b).

Box 7.17 Maintenance

Maintenance of a newly learned skill is achieved as follows:

- Do not terminate the programme abruptly, phase it out gradually. Reduce the amount of extra attention given during the training period as gradually as possible. Continue to reinforce the desired behaviour with extra rewards for some time after the objective is reached, then phase them out by dropping them intermittently at first. For example, from rewarding the desired behaviour on every occasion, reward on four out of five occasions, then three, two and one out of five occasions, until rewards for passing urine and for dry pants are completely phased out. Social reinforcement, usually praise, should continue indefinitely.
- Ensure that everyone in contact with Stewart knows how to strengthen and support the new behaviour and that no-one reverts to previous toileting procedures. Ensure that old behaviours are not inadvertently rewarded, e.g. attention given contingent upon a wetting accident.
- If a relapse occurs, briefly reimplement the original training procedures as quickly as possible.
- Consider carefully the environment(s) where the new skills or abilities are to be maintained indefinitely.

Bowel training

Treatment for encopresis in the field of intellectual disability has received relatively little attention. Treatment approaches to encopresis in children within the general population have included psychoanalytic psychotherapy, family therapy, hypnotherapy, biofeedback and behavioural therapy. However, with a success rate of 70% or better reported for children within the general population (Kaplan 1985, Bosch 1988, Dawson et al 1990), behavioural approaches, which focus on the appropriate and inappropriate eliminatory behaviours themselves, represent the treatment of choice.

In the field of intellectual disability, because encopresis is often attributed to the intellectual disability, treatment for encopresis is rare and there is no consensus on treatment guidelines (Groves 1982). Bowel managem[e] issue in people with intellectua[l] 1994), particularly those with a s[] level of disability.

RETENTIVE ENCOPRESIS

Treatment of retentive encopresis has traditionally depended heavily on the use of laxatives and enemas (Kobak et al 1962). Other approaches in this field have included abdominal massage, use of fibre and behavioural training.

Abdominal massage

At a clinical level, there is an interest in the use of abdominal massage for constipation and retention in the field of intellectual disability. The idea is that the faecal mass is helped to move along the ascending, transverse and descending colon by stimulating peristalsis. The method of massage involves a combination of effleurage (stroking) and petrisage (kneading).

Emly (1993) reported the use of abdominal massage in a young man with a history of constipation and high impacted faeces. Thrice-weekly abdominal massage was reported to stimulate regular spontaneous bowel movements. Furthermore, although his communication skills were limited, he was able to indicate when a bowel movement was imminent and could be placed on the toilet.

In an unpublished trial with which one of the present authors was associated, several adults with multiple handicaps and severe intellectual disability received regular abdominal massage for constipation. Although some people showed no improvement, others appeared to benefit, such as a multiply handicapped woman, in the middle years of life, whose results are shown in Figure 7.4. By contrast, however, in a small trial to investigate the effects of abdominal massage in nine elderly constipated patients and seven healthy young adult volunteers in the general population (Klauser et al 1992), neither stool frequency nor colonic transit time changed significantly in either group.

Thus, although two single case studies found an improvement with the use of abdominal

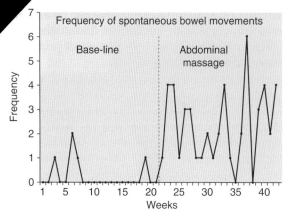

Figure 7.4 Spontaneous bowel movements in one woman with profound and multiple handicaps following abdominal massage.

massage, the effectiveness of this technique in the treatment of constipation has not yet been clearly demonstrated. The potential advantages of abdominal massage, if proven effective, are fairly obvious for a client group whose bowel problems can be difficult to treat. In addition, abdominal massage is believed to be a pleasant sensory experience for many people with physical disabilities.

Fibre

Increased fibre and proprietary bulking agents have been demonstrated to increase the urge to defecate in a natural way in the general population (see Ch. 8). Studies adding bulk to the diets of people with severe intellectual and physical disabilities have shown more variable results (e.g. Fischer et al 1985, Capra & Hannan-Jones 1992). This may be due to differences in the type of fibre and quantities used.

Capra and Hannan-Jones (1992) studied the effects of an added 7 g of fibre for a period of 2 weeks in a random 25% of 36 inpatients, 22 of whom had severe/profound intellectual disabilities together with physical handicaps, while 15 had severe intellectual disabilities but no physical disability. None of the 36 was impacted, due to the 'regular' (unspecified) use of suppositories and enemas. The authors identified three different outcomes within the experimental group: those whose bowel function remained unchanged; those for whom the texture of stools improved, but the frequency of stools and use of elimination aids remained unchanged; those for whom frequency and texture of stools improved and use of elimination aids reduced.

A number of points are worth making in relation to these studies. Read et al (1986) have concluded that constipation is probably part of a diverse group of disorders with a common presenting symptom (Box 7.18). As no reference is made to gastroenterological investigation, participants in these studies may have represented different subgroups, some of whose constipation may have represented a relatively simple problem. Problems easily remedied by the simple addition of fibre to the diet might include constipation due to medication such as major tranquillisers and some anticonvulsants commonly used in 'high-dependency' populations, or a low fibre diet. Constipation in others may have represented a range of other, more complex disorders less easily remedied. At present, as there have been few studies of constipation in the field of intellectual disability (e.g. Bohmer et al 2001), its prevalence and aetiology are still unclear. Constipation in people with severe/profound intellectual disability and/or those with severe physical handicaps should initially address quality of care issues such as fluid intake and dietary fibre.

Some authors, however, have expressed concern about the routine use of increased fibre in high-dependency, immobile or cognitively less able groups. Indeed, the use of increased fibre or bulking agents of any type is not without risk in such populations: phytobezoars (food ball), although uncommon, have occurred in institutionalised people or those with acute psychotic mental disorder (Sroujieh 1988). Furthermore, the addition of large amounts of uncooked bran to the diet can compromise the uptake of vitamins and minerals (Agnarsson et al 1993) in those whose diet may already be poor. By contrast, other authors in such fields recommend routine increases in fibre to counteract the constipating effects of certain commonly used tranquillisers (de Silva et al 1992, Bohmer et al 2001).

Behavioural approaches

Reports of behavioural approaches to encopresis in intellectual disability are few in number and largely confined to secondary (previously clean) soiling (Chopra 1973, Jansson et al 1992) and to those with mild rather than severe intellectual disability (Carpenter 1989, Smith et al 2000). It may be that it is assumed that the chances of success are greater in those with a mild intellectual disability or those who were previously continent. Behavioural training programmes for both retentive and non-retentive encopresis in the field of intellectual disability have used rewards for clean underwear and for continent elimination and punishment for soiling, these techniques being used either singly or in combination.

Retentive encopresis

There are only a small number of published studies which have addressed retentive encopresis, two of which are illustrated here. Piazza et al (1991) successfully treated primary retentive encopresis over 14 weeks in a 15-year-old boy and a 5-year-old girl with profound intellectual disabilities. Regular toilet sits, rewards for appropriate elimination, punishment for soiling, increased fibre and the use of elimination aids had all been tried previously but had failed. The programme for both children involved rewarding all stools initially, both continent and incontinent, with praise, snacks and preferred objects, in order to increase the frequency of defecation and thus decrease retention. It was intended to follow this with a discrimination training procedure to teach elimination on the toilet, involving leading the children to the toilet, placing the incontinent stool down the toilet, assisting them to sit on the toilet for 30 s, then praising them for the stool. However, rewarding all stools resulted in a significant increase in continent bowel evacuation as well as total evacuations.

This multiple-phase study makes an important contribution to the literature. Although limited to two cases, it raises questions about the necessity and effectiveness of punishment procedures, which in these cases had previously exacerbated retention, and also about the use of artificial elimination aids. The authors suggest that punishment for soiling and elimination aids may both reduce the likelihood of continent stools, the latter because the individual's control over elimination is reduced and the former because punishment may decrease not only incontinent but also continent evacuation in people with severe or profound intellectual disability.

Smith et al (1994) describe the treatment of chronic faecal impaction and faecal incontinence in four young people aged from 13 to 23 years, three of whom had a severe or profound intellectual disability. The programme involved supervised, prompted toilet sits after meals for a maximum of 10 min, with praise and rewards for appropriate elimination. Neither punishment techniques for soiling nor rewards for clean pants were used lest these should aggravate retention in an effort to keep clean. Artificial elimination aids were stopped or phased out as quickly as possible and replaced with bulk-forming agents such as Normacol or Fybogel. Enemas or suppositories were used only after abdominal examination. Diet was changed to include high fibre foods or the addition of bran. Stool size and frequency increased, consistency improved, soiling decreased and the use of artificial elimination aids was discontinued in all cases. Improved perception of the need to evacuate was demonstrated by the increased frequency of self-initiated toiletings. Additionally, retraining of the gastrocolic reflex appeared to occur for three participants. Treatment times were, however, long, ranging from 56 to 132 weeks. Results also indicated a continuing, somewhat erratic pattern of bowel function. Smith et al, like Piazza et al, found little evidence to support a major role for artificial elimination aids in conjunction with a behavioural training approach.

Non-retentive encopresis

There are few published reports on behavioural treatment of non-retentive encopresis, two of which are considered here. Lyon (1984) reduced primary non-retentive encopresis to zero in 5 weeks in an 8-year-old boy with a mild intellectual disability, using praise and rewards for cleanliness and appropriate evacuation and 'correction' for soiling. Treatment involved four daily underwear checks, with praise and stickers for cleanliness and appropriate toilet use, stickers being exchanged for individual staff time. 'Correction' for soiling involved assuming responsibility for cleaning and changing himself and washing soiled clothing. Results showed that frequency of encopresis reduced from eight in 10 base-line days to zero by the end of 20 days' intervention.

Smith (1996) used praise and edible rewards for clean pants and appropriate toilet use in the successful treatment of primary non-retentive encopresis in five males between the ages of 18 and 37 years, four of whom had severe intellectual disabilities. The participants were prompted to the toilet for 10 min after each main meal or snack in the hope that an association might develop between the gastrocolic reflex, defecation and the toilet. In addition, underwear was checked at set points throughout the day: on waking, before leaving home, on arrival at school or day centre, mid-morning, before and after lunch, mid-afternoon, before transport home, on arrival home, after tea and before bed. Soiling was briefly drawn to the attention of the participants and minimum assistance given for cleaning and changing. Punishment techniques were not used. Large soilings reduced to zero over periods ranging from 44 to 144 weeks. Underwear checks and rewards were gradually phased out. Stainings or very small bowel accidents continued to occur in some cases.

Long-term maintenance

Huntley and Smith (1999) followed up 9 out of 10 cases of successful treatment for retentive or non-retentive encopresis reported by Smith (1994, 1996) and Smith et al (1994). Results showed that treatment effects had largely endured over periods ranging from 5 to 17 years. Six of the nine were free of major soiling accidents, although one continued to have minor stainings in connection with imperfect wiping. Of the three still experiencing major soiling accidents, one had relapsed completely a few weeks prior to follow-up after remaining continent for 8 years, in association with a major deterioration in physical health; one experienced one full-sized soiling in 21 consecutive days, but also passed 22 continent stools; and one had experienced a partial relapse which had already responded to retraining and was currently averaging one soiling per 2 months. Of interest and perhaps surprisingly, those whose encopresis was previously retentive in nature maintained more successfully than those with previously non-retentive encopresis.

OTHER TOILETING PROBLEMS

Not all continence problems are due to 'skills' deficits, i.e. a simple failure to establish the link between bowel and bladder sensations and the toilet. Functional toileting problems include:

- urinating repeatedly in inappropriate locations such as against doors or in corners
- faecal smearing
- eliminating only under highly specific circumstances such as into an incontinence pad/nappy
- fear or avoidance of toilets other than one specific toilet, usually that at home
- urinating messily around the toilet
- failing to pass urine on the toilet but then passing urine shortly after coming off the toilet.

Some of these behaviours are better explained in terms of anxiety-related or challenging behaviour as opposed to a lack of continence skills as such. In these cases, the approach should initially involve a functional analysis, as with any chal-

Box 7.19   Urinating in inappropriate places

Where bowel or bladder accidents occur repeatedly in particular locations, despite ability to use the toilet:

- reward elimination in the toilet to increase motivation for continent elimination
- record accidents and, if these can be predicted from body postures or locations, divert to the toilet at these times and reward continent elimination
- consider the possibility of scent marking and introducing an acceptable scent to replace the inappropriate use of urine (Siegel 1977, Smith 1988, 1989).

lenging behaviour, in order to elucidate the function, purpose or meaning of the behaviour before attempting to change it.

Urinating repeatedly in inappropriate locations

The function or purpose of behaviour is an important issue when considering some of the more unusual toileting behaviours which present in the field of intellectual disability (Box 7.19). It is widely assumed that the main purpose of micturition is simply to discharge urine clear of the skin although this may be only part of the story. A major function of passing urine in mammals is scent marking for the purpose of chemical communication but the question of whether scent marking occurs in humans is unanswered. However, Smith (discussed in Smith & Smith 1987) describes a young man with a profound intellectual disability and incontinence, whose habit was to wet and then sniff his clothing, despite being able to pass urine on the toilet.

Faecal smearing

Faecal smearing is found in a small number of people with severe intellectual disabilities, although its prevalence and aetiology are not well established. A number of factors may be associated with faecal smearing, including sensory play, deprivation, boredom, protest and constipation.

Faecal smearing can, however, also be seen in favourable living situations. An example is provided here of faecal smearing in a man with a profound intellectual disability in his early 50s, who had been resettled in a small residential home. Having lived most of his life in a large institution, he had a long history of ritualised toileting behaviours including smearing faeces after stooling. Functional analysis of such behaviour may suggest a relationship to anxiety reduction and the demarcation of personal space. A treatment plan to help this previously institutionalised, middle-aged man to feel secure in his new community placement was designed to make toileting a more pleasant experience, and to reward him for continent stools and also for not smearing after defecation. This resulted in a marked reduction in faecal smearing over a period of months (Fig. 7.5).

Transfer of stimulus control

Where a child or adult will urinate/defecate only under specific conditions such as into a nappy or incontinence pad, elimination is said to be under the stimulus control of the pad. Thus, the eliminatory response is stimulated by (i.e. is under the control of) the sensation of the nappy rather than cues associated with the toilet. Quite often such behaviour may be associated with the presence of obsessional behaviours such as are commonly found in autism and fragile X syndrome. In these cases, the solution is to gradually transfer control from the pad to the toilet (Taylor et al 1994, Smith et al 2000). This is done initially by rewarding elimination into the pad, then rewarding elimination into the pad progressively closer to the toilet until the child can eliminate into the pad while sitting on the toilet. Finally, either a hole of increasing size is cut in the crotch of the pad, or the pad is more gradually dismantled by progressively removing the wadding and then cutting strips off the outer edges, until elimination takes place without a pad. A similar explanation may apply to people who can only defecate into a particular toilet, most usually the home toilet. Although such people will usually withhold defecation until their return from school or day service, this does not necessarily present a problem unless respite care

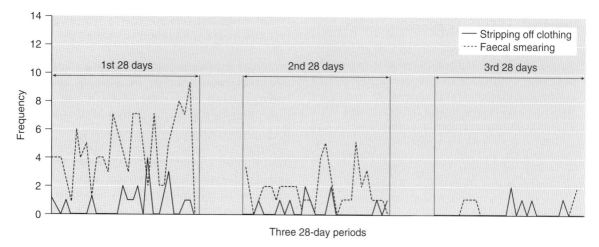

Figure 7.5 Challenging toileting behaviours: reduction in stripping off clothes and in faecal smearing at toilet, over three 28-day periods, in a 52-year-old man with profound learning disabilities.

services away from home are accessed, when they may retain for the duration of the stay.

Avoidant paruresis

Avoidant paruresis refers to the inability to, or difficulty in, passing urine in toilets other than one particular toilet, usually that at home. It is deemed to be anxiety based and may be associated with body shyness. There are no reports of paruresis in people with autism or intellectual disability, although this phenomenon is common in the general population. The treatment of choice is based on behavioural approaches such as paradoxical intention and in vivo desensitisation, which are commonly used to treat phobic anxiety (Timms 1985, McCracken & Larkin 1991, Jaspers 1998, Watson & Freeland 2000).

Urinating messily around the toilet

This is a common problem in males in the general population as well as those in the field of intellectual disability. It occurs when the urine stream is not directed accurately when standing. Research has shown that males have a natural tendency to direct the urine stream at objects. One solution is to float a target in the toilet. For adult males with intellectual disabilities, a coloured table tennis ball or one which is painted half red and which spins when hit, is an ideal target and will not flush

---

Box 7.20 Wetting shortly after coming off the toilet

- This is a common phenomenon in this field. If the client is in the middle years of life or this is a problem of recent onset, refer for medical investigation before considering possible behavioural causes.
- Where accidents are occurring shortly after unsuccessful prompts to toilet, the client may be experiencing 'performance anxiety', i.e. when 'trying' on the toilet, is tensing and thus inhibiting passing urine.
- Take the emphasis off passing urine on the toilet by occupying the client while on, or close to the toilet, in order to relax him and divert him from his purpose. Do not leave and come back later to see if he has performed. Play, read, sing or occupy him with a favourite activity or even favourite food. When relaxed, the probability is that he will pass urine successfully.
- Ensure continent urine is rewarded.

---

away. Whether the problem is due to poor motor control or to poor motivation, this device, which has been empirically validated by Siegel (1977), will greatly improve accuracy. For male children, the Aaronshield toilet target is ideal and fun.

Wetting shortly after coming off the toilet is another common occurrence (Box 7.20).

KEY POINTS FOR PRACTICE

- The presence of an intellectual disability should not, of itself, be regarded as an adequate explanation for the failure to acquire bowel and bladder control
- There has been little study of factors which are likely to militate against the acquisition of continence in people with intellectual disabilities. Degree of intellectual disability is likely to be one factor. Other factors might include the presence of hyperactivity, deficits of attention and challenging behaviours
- Incontinent people with intellectual disabilities have a right to access appropriate medical diagnostic investigations
- Although intervention approaches to incontinence in people with intellectual disabilities have traditionally focused on management rather than training, the evidence supports the success of behavioural training approaches to both urinary and faecal incontinence in this field
- The needs of carers, as well as their beliefs about and attitudes towards incontinence in people with severe and profound intellectual disabilities, may influence the choice of management or training
- Ethical issues must always be considered when caring for, or supporting, clients who are unable to consent to treatment. People with intellectual disabilities, as with other disabled client groups, have the right to treatment to enable them to achieve dignity and independence through validated, non-punitive teaching strategies. Continence training should be a positive experience for all concerned
- Intervention studies tend to involve single cases or small samples. There is a need to progress to larger, controlled trials

References

Agnarsson U, Warde C, McCarthy G et al 1993 Anorectal function of children with neurological problems II: cerebral palsy. Developmental Medicine and Child Neurology 35:903–908

Averink M, Melein L M, Duker P C 2005 Establishing diurnal bladder control with the response restriction method: extended study on its effectiveness. Research in Developmental Disabilities 26:143–151

Azrin N H, Foxx R M 1971 A rapid method of toilet training the institutionalised retarded. Journal of Applied Behavior Analysis 4:89–99

Baumeister A, Klosowski R 1965 An attempt to group toilet train severely retarded patients. Mental Retardation 3:24–26

Bax M 1994 Editorial: Bladder and bowel. Developmental Medicine and Child Neurology 36:1–2

Bellman M M 1966 Studies on encopresis. Acta Paediatrica Scandinavica 56(supplement 170):1–151

Bettison S 1982 Toilet training to independence for the handicapped. C C Thomas, Springfield, ILL

Bettison S, Davison D, Taylor P, Fox B 1976 Longterm effects of a toilet training programme for the retarded. Australian Journal of Mental Retardation 4:28–35

Bohmer C J M, Taminiau J A J M, Klinkenberg-Knol E C et al 2001 The prevalence of constipation in institutionalised people with intellectual disability. Journal of Intellectual Disability Research 45:212–218

Bosch J D 1988 Treating children with encopresis and constipation: an evaluation by means of single case studies. In: Emmelkamp P, Everaerd W, Kraimat F R, Van Son M J M (eds) Advances in theory and practice in behaviour therapy. Swets & Zeitlinger, Amsterdam

Bower W F, Moore K H, Shepherd R et al 1996 An epidemiological study of enuresis in Australia. In: Norgaard J P, Djurhuus J C, Hjalmas K et al (eds) Proceedings of the Third International Children's Continence Symposium. Wells Medical, Kent

Brazelton T B 1962 A child oriented approach to toilet training. Pediatrics 29:121–128

Buchan L, Chow S, Stoddart A 1989 A one-year continence project for people with mental handicaps. Mental Handicap 17:162–167

Burgio L D, Engel B T, Hawkins A et al 1990 A staff management system for maintaining improvements in continence with elderly nursing home residents. Journal of Applied Behavior Analysis 31:111–118

Butler J F 1976 Toilet training a child with spina bifida. Journal of Behavior Therapy and Experimental Psychiatry 7:63–65

Buttross S 1999 Encopresis in the child with a behavioral disorder: when the initial treatment does not work. Pediatric Annals 28:317–321

Capra S M, Hannan-Jones M 1992 A controlled dietary trial for improving bowel function in a group of training centre residents with severe or profound intellectual disability. Australian and New Zealand Journal of Developmental Disabilities 18:111–121

Carpenter S 1989 Development of a young man with Prader–Willi syndrome and secondary functional encopresis. Canadian Journal of Psychiatry 34:123–127

Chopra H D 1973 Treatment of encopresis in a mongol with operant conditioning. Indian Journal of Mental Retardation 6:43–46

Dalrymple N J, Ruble L A 1992 Toilet training. Journal of Autism and Developmental Disabilities 22:265–270

Dawson P M, Griffith K, Boeke K M 1990 Combined medical and psychological treatment of hospitalised children with encopresis. Child Psychiatry and Human Development 20:181–190

Department of Health and Social Security 1972 Census of mentally handicapped people in hospital in England and Wales at the end of 1970. Statistical and Research Report, Series 3. HMSO, London

De Silva P, Deb S, Drummond R D Rankin R 1992 A fatal case of ischemic colitis following long-term use of neuroleptic medication. Journal of Intellectual Disability Research 36:371–375

Doleys D M, Schwartz M S, Ciminero A R 1981 Elimination problems: enuresis and encopresis. In: Mash E J, Terdal L G (eds) Behavioral assessment of childhood disorders. Guilford Press, New York

Dunlap G, Koegel R L, Koegel L K 1985 Continuity of treatment: toilet training in multiple community settings. Journal of the Association for Persons with Severe Handicaps 9:134–141

Eiberg H, Berendt I, Mohr J 1995 Assignment of dominant inherited nocturnal enuresis (ENUR1) to chromosome 13q. Nature Genetics 10:354–356

Emly M 1993 Abdominal massage. Nursing Times 89:34–37

Evenhuis H M 1997 Medical aspects of ageing in a population with intellectual disability: III. Mobility, internal conditions and cancer. Journal of Intellectual Disability Research 41:8–18

Fischer M, Adkins W, Hall L 1985 The effects of dietary fibre in a liquid diet on bowel function of mentally retarded individuals. Journal of Mental Deficiency Research 29:373–381

Foxx R M, Azrin N H 1973 Toilet training the retarded: a rapid programme for day and night-time independent toileting. Research Press, Champaign, ILL

Fritz G K, Armbrust J 1982 Enuresis and encopresis. Psychiatric Clinics of North America 5:283–296

Ganesh S, Potter J, Fraser W 1994 An audit of physical health needs of adults with profound learning disability in a hospital population. Mental Handicap Research 7:228–236

Gesell A, Armatruda C S 1941 Developmental diagnosis: normal and abnormal child development. Harper, New York

Groves J A 1982 Encopresis. In: Hollis J H, Meyers C E (eds) Life-threatening behavior: analysis and intervention. American Association of Mental Deficiency Monograph 5, Washington DC, p 279–327

Hundziak M, Maurer R A, Watson L S 1965 Operant conditioning in toilet training of severely retarded boys. American Journal of Mental Deficiency 70:120–124

Huntley E, Smith L 1999 Long term follow-up of behavioural treatment for primary encopresis in people with intellec-tual disability in the community. Journal of Intellectual Disability Research 43:484–488

Hyams G, McCoull K, Smith P S et al 1991 Behavioural continence training in mental handicap: a 10-year follow-up study. Journal of Intellectual Disability Research 36:551–558

Jansson L M, Diamond O, Demb H B 1992 Encopresis in a multihandicapped child: rapid multidisciplinary treatment. Journal of Developmental and Physical Disabilities 4:83–90

Jaspers J P 1998 Cognitive-behavioral therapy for paruresis: a case report. Psychological Reports 83:187–196

Kaplan B J 1985 A clinical demonstration of a psychobiological application to childhood encopresis. Journal of Child Care 2:47–54

Kimbrell D L, Luckey R E, Barbuto P et al 1967 Operation dry pants: an intensive habit training programme for severe and profound retardation. Mental Retardation 5:32–36

Klauser A G, Flaschentraeger J, Gehrke A et al 1992 Abdominal wall massage: effect on colonic function in healthy volunteers and in patients with chronic constipation. Zeitschrift für Gastroenterologie 30:247–251

Kobak M W, Jacobson M A, Sirca D M 1962 Acquired megacolon in psychiatric patients. Diseases of the Colon and Rectum 5:373–377

Largo R H, Stutzle W 1977a Longitudinal study of bowel and bladder control by day and night in the first six years of life II: the role of potty training and child's initiative. Developmental Medicine and Child Neurology 19:606–613

Largo R H, Stutzle W 1977b Longitudinal study of bowel and bladder control in the first six years of life I: epidemiology and the interrelations between bowel and bladder control. Developmental Medicine and Child Neurology 19:598–606

Largo R H, Molinari L, Von Siebenthal K et al 1996 Does a profound change in toilet training affect development of bowel and bladder control? Developmental Medicine and Child Neurology 38:1106–1116

Lindstrom T C, Baerheim A, Flatass A S 2000 Behaviour modification group-treatment of children with recurrent lower urinary tract infections. Scandinavian Journal of Caring Science 14:259–267

Lyon M A 1984 Positive reinforcement and logical consequences in the treatment of classroom encopresis. School Psychology Review 13:238–243

McCoull G 1971 Newcastle-upon-Tyne Regional Aetiological Survey (Mental Retardation), 1966–1971. Northern Regional Health Authority, Newcastle

McCracken L M, Larkin K T 1991 Treatment of paruresis with in vivo desensitization: a case report. Journal of Behavior and Experimental Psychiatry 22:57–62

Madge N, Diamon J, Miller D et al 1993 The National Childhood Encephalopathy Study: a 10-year follow-up. A report on the medical, social, behavioural and education outcomes after serious, acute, neurological illness in early childhood. Developmental Medicine and Child Neurology 68(supplement):1–118

Madsen C H, Hoffman M, Thomas D R, Koropsak E, Madsen C K 1969 Comparison of toilet training techniques. In: Gelfand D M (ed) Social learning in childhood. Brookes-Cole, Pacific Grove, CA

Mattson S, Lindstrom S 1996 How representative are frequency/volume charts? In: Norgaard J P, Djurhuus J C, Hjalmas K et al (eds) Proceedings of the Third International Children's Continence Symposium. Wells Medical, Kent

Michel R 1999 Toilet training. Pediatrics in Review 20:240–245

Pfadt A, Sullivan K 1981 Issues in the generalization and long-term maintenance of the treatment gains achieved by the Foxx–Azrin self initiation training procedure. Paper presented at the Eastern Psychological Association Annual Meeting, New York

Piazza C C, Fisher W, Chinn S et al 1991 Reinforcement of incontinent stools in the treatment of encopresis. Clinical Pediatrics 30:28–32

Read N W, Timms J M, Barfield L J et al 1986 Impairment of defecation in young women with severe constipation. Gastroenterology 90:53–60

Resnick B 1985 Constipation: common but preventable. Geriatric Nursing 6(4):213–215

Rittig S 1996 Enuresis research: current status and future prospects. In: Norgaard J P, Djurhuus J C, Hjalmas K et al (eds) Proceedings of the Third International Children's Continence Symposium. Wells Medical, Kent

Roijen L E G, Postema K, Limbeek V J et al 2001 Development of bladder control in children and adolescents with cerebral palsy. Developmental Medicine and Child Neurology 43:103–107

Seim H 1989 Toilet training in first children. Journal of Family Practice 29:633–636

Siegel R K 1977 Stimulus selection and tracking during urination. Journal of Applied Behavior Analysis 10:255–265

Smeets P M, Lancioni G E, Ball T S et al 1985 Shaping self-initiated toileting in infants. Journal of Applied Behavior Analysis 18:303–308

Smith L J 1994 A behavioral approach to the treatment of non-retentive nocturnal encopresis in an adult with a severe learning disability. Journal of Behavior and Experimental Psychiatry 25:81–86

Smith L J 1996 A behavioural approach to the treatment of non-retentive encopresis in adults with learning disabilities. Journal of Intellectual Disability Research 40:130–139

Smith L J, Bainbridge G 1991 An intensive toilet training programme for a boy with a profound mental handicap living in the community. Mental Handicap 19:146–150

Smith L J, Franchetti B, McCoull K et al 1994 A behavioural approach to retraining bowel function after longstanding constipation and faecal impaction in people with learning disabilities. Developmental Medicine and Child Neurology 36:49–57

Smith L J, Smith P S, Lee S K Y 2000 Behavioural treatment of urinary incontinence and encopresis in children with learning disabilities. Developmental Medicine and Child Neurology 42:276–279

Smith P S 1979a The development of urinary continence in the mentally handicapped. University of Newcastle, Newcastle upon Tyne

Smith P S 1979b A comparison of different methods of toilet training the mentally handicapped. Behaviour Research and Therapy 17:33–43

Smith P S 1988 Can scent marking occur in humans? 18th Annual Meeting of the International Continence Society, Oslo

Smith P S 1989 Education, effects, environmentaux et ethologiques sur l'incontinence associes a un mental handicap. Premier Symposium International Approche Multidisciplinnaire de l'Incontinence de l'Adulte, Paris

Smith P S, Smith L J 1977 Chronological age and social age as factors in daytime toilet training of institutionalised mentally retarded individuals. Journal of Behavior Therapy and Experimental Psychiatry 8:269–273

Smith P S, Smith L J 1987 Continence and incontinence: psychological approaches to development and treatment. Croom Helm, London

Smith P S, Wong H 1981 Changes in bladder function during toilet training of mentally handicapped children. Behaviour Research and Severe Developmental Disabilities 2:137–155

Smith P S, Britton P G, Johnson M et al 1975 Problems involved in toilet training profoundly mentally handicapped adults. Behaviour Research and Therapy 15:301–307

Spangler B F, Risley T R, Bilyew D D 1984 The management of dehydration and incontinence in non-ambulatory geriatric patients. Journal of Applied Behavior Analysis 17:109–112

Spencer R L, Temerlin M, Trousdale W W 1968 Some correlates of bowel control in the profoundly retarded. American Journal of Mental Deficiency 72:879–882

Sroujieh A S 1988 Phytobezoars of the whole gastro-intestinal tract: report of a case and review of the literature. Dirasat 15:103–109

Stern H P, Prince M T, Stroh S E 1988 Encopresis responsive to non-psychiatric interventions. Clinical Pediatrics 27:400–402

Taylor S, Cipani E, Clardy A 1994 A stimulus control technique for improving the efficacy of an established toilet training program. Journal of Behavior Therapy and Experimental Psychiatry 25:155–160

Thomas T M 1986 The prevalence and health service implications of incontinence – a study in progress. In: Mandelstam D (ed) Incontinence and its management, 2nd edn. Croom Helm, London

Thompson T, Hanson R 1983 Overhydration: precautions when treating urinary incontinence. Mental Retardation 21:139–145

Timms M W H 1985 The treatment of urinary frequency by paradoxical intention. Behavioural Psychotherapy 13:76–82

Van Wagenen R K, Meyerson L, Kerr N J et al 1969. Field trials of a new procedure in toilet training. Journal of Experimental Child Psychology 8:147–159

Vande Walle J, Theunis M, Renson C et al 1995 Commercial television bladder dysfunction. Acta Urologica Belgica 63:105–111

von Wendt L, Simila S, Niskanen P et al 1990 Development of bowel and bladder control in the mentally retarded. Developmental Medicine and Child Neurology 32:515–518

Watson T S, Freeland J T 2000 Treating paruresis using respondent conditioning. Journal of Behavior Therapy and Experimental Psychiatry 31:155–162

Weir K 1982 Night and day wetting among a population of children. Developmental Medicine and Child Neurology 245:479–484

Yeung C K, Godley M L, Ho C K W et al 1995 Some new insights into bladder function in infancy. British Journal of Urology 76:235–240

Chapter 8

Bowel care

Gaye Kyle and Phil Prynn

Those, whose intestines are relaxed, if they are young, get over their illnesses better than those who are constipated, but worsen with age. It is a general rule that the intestines tend to become sluggish with age.

Hippocrates of Cos

INTRODUCTION

Disorders of the bowel encompass a wide range of problems; this chapter will discuss constipation and faecal incontinence with particular reference to establishing best practice in the prevention and treatment of these conditions. There is reluctance in the general population to discuss bowel problems as it is considered an unacceptable topic of conversation. This leads to hesitancy by people to admit to and discuss bowel dysfunction. By understanding the functions of the bowel and the need for appropriate assessment, healthcare professionals can begin to positively help patients with bowel disorders.

BOWEL DISORDERS

Constipation

Constipation is an unpleasant and often distressing symptom that can happen to anyone at any time. Its severity may vary from the slight, causing no disruption to life, to the severe, impacting upon an individual's physical, psychological and social well-being.

Definition and classification of constipation

Constipation is multifactorial, and can be influenced by physical, psychological, physiological, emotional and environmental factors. Many of the underlying reasons for constipation remain poorly understood. Constipation is largely a subjective sensation with the consequence that it has no universally accepted definition (Richmond 2003). Thompson et al (1999) suggest that constipation is characterised by persistent difficult or seemingly incomplete defecation. However, even this definition can be difficult to use in practice because of the wide variation in bowel habits in the population and in what patients (and professionals) consider to be 'normal'. Many people still hold to the belief that daily evacuation is necessary although there is no physiological or epidemiological evidence that this is true. Most definitions now include such symptoms as frequency of defecation, hardness of stool, abdominal fullness or bloatedness and abdominal pain (Petticrew et al 1997). Patients with constipation continue to emphasise symptoms such as pain and straining rather than frequency of defecation (Romero et al 1996). The Rome II Criteria (Box 8.1) provide the most commonly accepted definition of constipation. However, they are mainly used as inclusion criteria for research purposes since, in practice, many patients develop and require treatment for constipation before 12 weeks. The American College of Gastroenterology Chronic Constipation Task Force (2005) support this view, stating that the widespread use of the Rome II Criteria is

impractical, as observation studies indicate that most patients who report constipation do not fulfil the criteria.

Individual bowel habits vary from one person to another and this makes it particularly difficult to agree any one definition that is both easy to use in clinical practice and can be applied to all patients. This lack of clarity on what constitutes constipation could be one reason why constipation is seldom attended to until it has become a significant problem (Ross 1998). A lack of consensus on diagnostic criteria is a factor which undoubtedly contributes to the variable prevalence figures quoted for constipation. In the UK it is thought that around 10% of the population regularly experience constipation but figures for the USA may be between 12 and 19% of the population (Higgins & Johanson 2004). It is certainly true that a large amount of nursing time and resources are channelled into the management of constipation and it is estimated that £46M are spent on laxatives per year in England alone (Petticrew et al 2001).

Constipation affects both genders but there is a higher prevalence amongst females (Campbell et al 1993, Thompson et al 1999). Females of all ages are more at risk of developing constipation than their male counterparts (Harari et al 1996, Richmond & Wright 2004) due to a slower colonic transit time (Taylor 1990). It is argued that the higher propensity for constipation in older women reflects changes in musculature following childbirth, attributed in part to an inability to relax the pelvic floor (Campbell et al 1993, Ross 1995). In younger women, an imbalance of hormones, progesterone and motolin has been suggested as a common cause of constipation (Heaton et al 1992). Petticrew et al (1997) speculate that the higher reported prevalence of constipation may be due, in part, to the fact that women tend to seek medical advice more often than men.

For some people, constipation can represent a major healthcare issue, especially for many older patients and/or those with neurological problems (see Ch. 6). The increased prevalence of constipation in older people probably reflects changes due to reduced mobility, polypharmacy, poor diet and chronic illness (Campbell et al 1993, Petticrew et al 1997, Harari 2004). Many patients with a chronic illness have a prolonged total gut transit time,

Box 8.1

The Rome II Criteria require two or more of the following symptoms to be present for at least 12 weeks out of the preceding 12 months:
- Straining at defecation for at least a quarter of the time
- Lumpy and/or hard stools for at least a quarter of the time
- A sensation of incomplete evacuation for at least a quarter of the time
- Three or fewer bowel movements per week.

Thompson et al (1999).

with evacuation being delayed through the sigmoid colon and the rectum (Abrams et al 1995, Talley et al 1996, Walton & Miller 1998), leading to difficulty in bowel evacuation rather than a decline in bowel movement frequency.

Constipation can be clinically classified into three categories: primary, secondary and iatrogenic. Primary constipation is associated mainly with lifestyle characteristics and where there is no underlying pathophysiology causing the constipation. Table 8.1 outlines the more common factors attributed to primary, secondary and iatrogenic

constipation (Moriarty & Irving 1992, Richmond 2003).

Slow transit constipation

A small number of patients, usually women, have chronic constipation that does not respond to either a change in lifestyle or laxative therapy. These patients have no structural abnormality or underlying pathology but bowel transit time is slow. The effect of slow transit constipation may be sufficiently severe to require surgical interven-

Table 8.1 Common factors causing constipation

Type of constipation	Factor	Example
Simple (idiopathic/primary): no underlying causative illness	Lifestyle	Reduced dietary fibre, reduced fluid intake, reduced mobility, environmental changes (e.g. hospitalisation)
	Old age	Often the result of reduced mental and physical function
Secondary: results from physiological diseases or conditions that affect bowel function	Endocrine disorders	Hypothyroidism, diabetes mellitus, pregnancy, childbirth and the puerperium, Addison's disease, hyperparathyroidism
	Metabolic	Hypercalcaemia
	Neurological and neuromuscular	Cerebrovascular accidents, spinal cord lesions/injury, multiple sclerosis, autonomic neuropathy (e.g. Hirschsprung's disease, Parkinson's disease)
	Psychiatric	Dementia, depression, learning difficulties, anorexia nervosa/bulimia nervosa
	Physiological (pelvic disorders)	Pregnancy, old age
	Colonic disorders	Irritable bowel syndrome, diverticular disease, cancer, idiopathic slow transit constipation, haemorrhoids, rectal prolapse, rectocele
Iatrogenic: induced as a consequence of pharmacological agents	Usually as a result of taking medication for the alleviation or prevention of another pathophysiological condition. Five or more medications are a particular risk (Potter et al 2002)	Opioids Diuretics Non-steroidal anti-inflammatory drugs Anticholinergics (e.g. tricyclic antidepressants, antihistamines, antipsychotics) Antacids (containing aluminium or calcium) Amiodarone Antidiarrhoeals Antiparkinsonian drugs Calcium channel blockers Calcium supplements Clonidine Disopyramide Iron preparations Lithium

tion, usually a total colectomy and anastomosis of the ileum to the rectum. Results are not always satisfactory.

Faecal impaction

Faecal impaction describes the condition when constipation has become so severe that a large mass of faeces cannot be passed. Faeces then accumulate in the rectum and may back up in the sigmoid colon and even as far as the transverse and ascending colon. Occasionally impaction of the rectum may be due to soft, poorly formed faeces as a consequence of too much osmotic laxative. In an attempt to soften hard impacted faeces the bowel produces mucus and this can result in faecal impaction with overflow, known as spurious diarrhoea.

Faecal incontinence

There are a variety of definitions of faecal incontinence including 'the involuntary or inappropriate passage of liquid or solid stool' (RCP 1995) or the International Continence Society definition: 'the involuntary loss of liquid or solid stool that is a social or hygienic problem' (Norton et al 2005). Anal incontinence is the term used to describe any involuntary leakage of faeces or flatus from the anus (Chelvanayagam & Norton 1999). The true prevalence of this symptom is unknown due to a lack of standard definitions in terms of severity, frequency and populations sampled. Perry et al (2002) found that faecal incontinence affects over 1% of the population, although this is probably an underestimate since embarrassment and shame are certainly likely to lead to underreporting of the condition. The overall prevalence rate for faecal incontinence in the general population as a whole is widely accepted as between 2 and 5% (Kenefick 2004).

Diarrhoea

A pragmatic definition of diarrhoea is the abnormal passage of watery stools more than three times a day. The stool volume is usually greater than that considered normal for those consuming a normal Western diet. Imbalances in water and electrolytes are likely to occur if diarrhoea is not treated. As symptoms persisting for longer than 4 weeks suggest a non-infectious origin, investigation of functional bowel disorders such as irritable bowel syndrome should follow (Thomas et al 2003).

Diarrhoea may be caused by disease of the small or large intestine or the stomach or indeed by any of the conditions listed in Box 8.2.

It is to be expected that a compromised anal sphincter will be overwhelmed by resulting intestinal hurry and faecal incontinence is likely to occur as a consequence.

Overenthusiastic use of laxatives may cause diarrhoea, which in turn can lead to faecal incontinence, especially if there is anal sphincter incompetence, poor mobility or compromised cognitive function. Misuse of laxatives may be seen as a means of purging by those with an eating disorder – for example, in conditions such as anorexia nervosa and bulimia. These are complex disorders which are symptomatic of underlying emotional or psychiatric issues, linked with general feelings of low self-esteem. Laxatives are also used by some people in attempts to lose weight. This is not an effective or sustainable way to lose weight, although loss of water and essential minerals from the body will give an initial sensation of weight loss. Careful assessment of bowel dysfunction, including unambiguous questioning about eating disorders and laxative use, will help to identify diarrhoea resulting from self-induced causes of this kind.

The main causes of acute diarrhoea, which is usually self-limiting, are bacteria and viruses. As transmission is by ingestion and through faecal contamination of food, proper attention to food hygiene and storage as well as thorough hand washing before food preparation, after handling raw foods such as meat, fish and poultry, and after using the lavatory, is essential. It is estimated that up to 50% of travellers from industrialised to developing countries will encounter travellers' diarrhoea and the following advice is strongly recommended: *Boil it, peel it or forget it.*

Advice on management of acute diarrhoea depends on the severity of the symptoms and the general health of the sufferer. Simple rehydration is adequate for mild diarrhoea in a healthy adult,

Box 8.2 Causes of diarrhoea

Condition	Symptoms
Irritable bowel syndrome ('syndrome' refers to a collection of symptoms)	Abdominal pain and cramps, irregular bowel habit, incomplete emptying, mucus, constipation and diarrhoea
Inflammatory bowel disease refers to ulcerative colitis, which usually affects the large bowel, or Crohn's disease, which can affect any part of the digestive tract	Diarrhoea, bleeding per rectum, abdominal pain, bloating, stricture formation and bowel obstruction, weight loss, fistulae, fatigue and passing mucus
Food poisoning (bacteria gain entry via contaminated food or drink)	Diarrhoea, vomiting, fever, abdominal pain, blood in the stool
Malabsorption, i.e. coeliac disease and lactose intolerance	Diarrhoea, vomiting, bloating, abdominal colic, anaemia and osteoporosis, the last due to poor absorption of iron, calcium, etc.
Carcinomas	A change in bowel habit, bleeding from the bowel, lethargy, diarrhoea, constipation, mucus in the stool, pain, bloating, obstruction
Diarrhoea viruses: astrovirus, calcivirus, reovirus	Prodromal symptoms of low-grade fever, malaise, fatigue
Travellers' diarrhoea, usually from ingesting faecally contaminated food or water	Gastrointestinal pain, nausea, vomiting, fever, cramps, bleeding per rectum, mucus in the stool and faecal urgency
Antibiotic-associated diarrhoea	Frequent watery bowel movements, usually mild, without pain; clears up once antibiotics are discontinued. Sometimes colitis can occur causing abdominal pain, fever and bloody diarrhoea
HIV/AIDS; opportunistic viral infections in the immunosuppressed	Watery diarrhoea, stomach cramps, fever, dehydration

antimotility and perhaps antimicrobial drugs for mild-to-moderate diarrhoea, whilst for severe symptoms a full course of an appropriate antimicrobial drug will be needed.

Abdominal bloating

Bloating is usually absent on awakening and worsens during the day. It may be intermittent and related to eating specific foods. Excessive burping and farting may be present, but are not necessarily related to the bloating (Thompson et al 1999). There is no proven therapy for abdominal bloating as its cause is unknown but education and support aimed at dietary modification are recommended. The practice of restricting certain 'gas-forming' foods may be beneficial and this can be facilitated with the use of food diaries to record the effect of removing and then gradually reintro-

ducing particular 'gas-forming' food. Bloating may be associated with rich fatty meals which delay gastric emptying. Lying down or contracting the abdominal muscles may relieve the discomfort.

Flatus

Flatus or 'bowel wind' is derived from either swallowed air or through bacterial fermentation of food matter. Over 90% of flatus is made up of five gases – nitrogen, oxygen, carbon dioxide, hydrogen and methane; the remaining 10% is made up of other gases. Nitrogen and oxygen come from the air, which is swallowed. The carbon dioxide is produced as a result of the interaction between the stomach, bile and pancreatic fluids. These gases enter the small intestine where most of the oxygen and carbon dioxide are absorbed into the body.

The nitrogen passes into the large bowel where it mixes with the gases produced from bacterial fermentation of food residue. The body passes flatus via the rectum on average 15 times a day (ranging between 3 and 40 times). A high fibre diet produces more flatus than a low fibre diet; however, it is possible to reduce flatus production on a regime rich in fibre. The big gas producers are carbohydrates called oligosaccharides. These include cabbage, Brussels sprouts, cauliflower, turnips, onions, garlic and leeks. Intake of such foods should be reduced if flatus becomes an embarrassing complaint. Charcoal tablets are sometimes advocated but there is little evidence to support their use.

Irritable bowel syndrome

Current figures suggest that as many as 15% of the population may suffer from irritable bowel syndrome (IBS) and it is the most common condition currently seen by gastroenterologists in the Western world (Madden & Hunter 2002). The term IBS is employed to describe a set of symptoms in those with an abnormal bowel habit, including intermittent abdominal discomfort, pain or cramps which opening the bowels often relieves. Other symptoms embrace a fluctuation between constipation and diarrhoea, a sensation of incomplete emptying, faecal urgency and the passage of mucus per rectum (CORE 2005a). Trigger factors for IBS may be unidentified but they are sometimes attributed to psychological influences (e.g. following a major life event) or subsequent to an episode of bacterial gastroenteritis (Rodriguez & Ruigomez 1999).

Treatments include identifying and then excluding foods which trigger a recurrence of symptoms, or increasing the fibre intake and, if necessary, adding a bulking agent to the diet if the main symptom is constipation.

Inflammatory bowel disease

Ulcerative colitis

Ulcerative colitis is a chronic inflammatory bowel disease that causes ulceration of the bowel mucosa, usually in the rectum and sigmoid colon. The mucosa becomes hyperaemic and may appear dark and velvety; small erosions form and develop into ulcers. Oedema and thickening of the muscularis may then narrow the lumen of the bowel. The lesions appear in individuals between 20 and 40 years of age. There is a higher prevalence amongst white populations and additional risk factors include family history and Jewish descent. However, the cause of the disease remains unknown. Patients present with urgency, obviously bloody stools and abdominal cramps and, in severe cases that involve a large portion of the bowel, fever, raised pulse and frequent diarrhoea (10–20 times per day). Complications include anal fissures, haemorrhoids and perirectal abscess.

Treatment needs to be tailored to the individual and depends on the severity of the symptoms, but is usually in the form of anti-inflammatory medication. Broad-spectrum antibiotics may be used if bacterial infection is suggested. The risk of colon cancer increases significantly in ulcerative colitis that persists beyond 10 years.

Crohn's disease

Crohn's disease, named after an American physician, is a chronic inflammatory disorder which can affect both the large and small bowel. The ascending and transverse colon are the most common sites of inflammation; the rectum is rarely involved. The inflammation can affect some segments of the bowels while not affecting others, creating 'skip lesions', i.e. one side of the bowel may be affected but not the other. Of affected individuals, 10–20% have a positive family history. Immunological factors such as increased suppressor T cell activity, alterations in immunoglobulin A (IgA) production, macrophage activation, luminal flora and antigen factors are associated with Crohn's disease.

The inflammatory process begins in the bowel submucosa and spreads inwards and outwards to involve the mucosa and serosa. Activated neutrophils and macrophages cause the tissue injury. The ulceration of Crohn's disease produces fissures that can extend the inflammation into the lymphoid tissue of the bowel wall. It is a debilitating condition characterised by abdominal pain, weight loss and non-bloody diarrhoea. If the ileum is involved the patient may be anaemic as a result of malabsorption of vitamin B_{12}. There is an increased risk of colon cancer in patients with long-standing disease and smoking increases the risk of developing severe disease (Thomas et al 2000).

Diverticular disease

Diverticulae are herniations or sac-like outpouchings of the mucosa through the muscularis, usually in the wall of the sigmoid colon. Diverticular disease is most common amongst the older population, but the incidence is increasing in younger people, possibly as a result of a diet rich in refined foods. The diverticulae form weal points in the bowel wall, usually where arteries penetrate the tunica muscularis to nourish the mucosal layer. A common associated finding is thickening of the circular and longitudinal (taenia coli) muscles surrounding the diverticulum. When diverticulae become infected or irritated, diverticulitis develops. Diverticulitis can cause abscess formation resulting in peritonitis, which can be life threatening.

Meckel's diverticulum is a congenital abnormality and only requires attention if symptoms present. Symptoms of diverticular disease may be vague. Abdominal cramps of the lower abdomen may accompany constriction of the hypertrophied bowel muscles. Diarrhoea, constipation, abdominal bloating or flatulence may all present. An increase in dietary fibre may relieve these symptoms. Occasionally surgical resection may be required to remove damaged sections of the bowel caused by severe diverticulitis.

Coeliac disease

Coeliac disease, or gluten-sensitive enteropathy, is a condition of the small intestine. It is reported that approximately 1% of people in the UK have this condition (CORE 2005b). Gluten is found in wheat, barley and rye, and in coeliac disease it reacts with the small bowel causing damage by activating the immune system to attack the delicate lining of the bowel and thus interfering with the absorption process. Symptoms can be subtle, with patients complaining of feeling unwell for no particular reason, lack of energy, weight loss and depression. The stools may be pale and malodorous. The treatment is to avoid all foods containing gluten whilst maintaining a healthy balanced diet.

Lactose intolerance

According to Crotty (2003), 'Lactose intolerance is a device of nature to expedite weaning and to ensure that mothers, having fed their offspring in infancy, are then set free to re-engage in their natural task of reproduction'.

Lactose intolerance is the inability to absorb the predominant sugar in milk, resulting in symptoms of abdominal pain, a sensation of bloatedness, flatulence and diarrhoea. Lactose is a disaccharide which is split by the enzyme lactase in the small intestine. However, if the levels of lactase are deficient then that splitting does not occur; the lactose is then fermented by bacteria in the large intestine and the symptoms described above occur. A temporary intolerance may occur following an episode of diarrhoea or bowel or stomach surgery. The only treatment is to reduce or avoid foods containing lactose (dairy milk products). Soy milk is often advocated as an alternative.

PHYSIOLOGY OF THE LARGE BOWEL

An understanding of normal bowel function, fluid absorption and the mechanisms involved in defecation are required to assess a patient with a bowel disorder. The overall function of the large bowel is to mix and propel its contents and to absorb water and electrolytes. It takes approximately 6 h for food to progress from the mouth to the large bowel; it can then take any time up to 72 h for food matter, now referred to as faecal matter, to travel from the caecum to the rectum. Constipation can therefore be considered primarily as a large bowel phenomenon. A slow bowel transit time and/or impairment of rectal emptying will result in dry hard stools and difficulty with defecation resulting in the physiological characteristics of constipation. Colonic activity (peristaltic action) is stimulated by faecal content but may also be influenced by emotional state. Regulation is by the sympathetic, parasympathetic and enteric nervous systems. The longer faeces remains in the colon, the more water will be reabsorbed, with the consequence that the faeces become hard and dry. This suggests that there should be an optimum bowel transit time, yet currently there is no research to support this hypothesis.

The large bowel has five main functions:

1. Storage
2. Absorption
3. Secretion
4. Synthesis of vitamins
5. Elimination.

Storage

The colon stores unabsorbed food matter; the longer the residue remains, the more water is reabsorbed, leading to firmer faeces.

Absorption

Between 600 and 1000 ml of watery stool, called chyme, flows into the caecum from the small bowel (ileum) every 24 h; approximately 90% is then reabsorbed into the body. Aldosterone, a steroid hormone, regulates the sodium and potassium in the blood. In the large bowel aldosterone increases membrane permeability to sodium, thereby increasing the diffusion of sodium into the cell and its active transport to the interstitial fluid. Some medications are absorbed through the colonic membrane – for example, some steroids, aspirin and some anaesthetics.

Secretion

Mucus is secreted from goblet cells in the mucosal layer of the bowel wall. The secretory capacity of the colon is controlled by cholinergic nerves and mediated through changes in the intracellular calcium concentrations. Mechanical stimulation can further promote mucus production. Mucus lubricates the faecal matter, thereby protecting the intestinal wall against the abrasive action of faecal bulk. In addition, some potassium and hydrogen carbonate ions may be secreted. It is the hydrogen carbonate that is responsible for the alkaline pH of the mucus and in turn the colonic contents.

Synthesis of vitamins

The colon is colonised by 'friendly' bacteria, such as *Escherichia coli* and *Streptococcus faecalis*. These bacteria, although harmful if they gain access to other parts of the body, perform two important functions in the bowel:

1. They play a role in the synthesis of vitamin K, thiamine, folic acid and riboflavin in small amounts.
2. They are responsible for the bacterial fermentation of food, producing large amounts of gas. The gas consists of nitrogen, carbon dioxide, hydrogen, methane and hydrogen sulphide and it augments the faecal bulk.

Depending on the food eaten, between 500 and 700 ml of gas is produced daily. Bacterial fermentation is responsible for faecal smell and contributes to one-third of the bulk of faeces. Bacterial activity and decomposition continue on impacted or constipated faeces, giving rise to a characteristic offensive smell. There are 10 times more bacteria in the bowel than cells in the entire human body and it is thought that the total bacterial weight equals 1 kg! There is evidence implicating these bacteria in the development of IBS as patients with IBS have higher concentrations of mucosal bacteria than control groups (Swidsinski et al 2002). It is suggested that healthy mucosa is capable of controlling the bacteria whereas in patients with IBS this function is compromised (Sartor 1997, Shanahan 2000).

Elimination

The large bowel is responsible for the elimination of food residue as faeces through the physiological process of defecation. This is considered in further detail below.

The bowel wall

The large bowel is a hollow muscular tube lined by a mucous membrane. The bowel wall consists essentially of four layers which extend through the large bowel from the caecum to the sigmoid colon:

1. Mucosa
2. Submucosa
3. Muscularis propria
4. Serosa.

Mucosa

The mucosa consists of epithelial and inflammatory cells, and is supplied by capillaries and some lymphatics.

Submucosa

This layer is loose connective tissue with capillaries and lymph vessels.

Muscularis propria

This is the thickest layer of the bowel wall. There is an inner circular layer of smooth muscle and an outer layer of three bands of longitudinal smooth muscle (taenia coli). In between the two muscular layers lies the myenteric nerve plexus of Auerbach. Associated with the myenteric plexus are the interstitial cells of Cajal. These cells have a pacemaker function; they facilitate active propagation of electrical events and mediate neurotransmission within the smooth muscle, thus regulating peristaltic action.

Serosa

This is the outermost layer of the bowel wall and comprises a single layer of flat, mesothelial cells attached to fibroelastic tissue.

Blood supply of the large bowel

The superior mesenteric artery and its branches supply blood to the caecum, ascending colon and the transverse colon to the splenic flexure. The inferior mesenteric artery supplies the remainder of the colon, the rectum and the upper half of the anal canal. The superior, middle and inferior rectal arteries and veins supply blood circulation to the rectum.

The hepatic portal vein system carries nutrients from the bowel in deoxygenated blood to the liver via the superior mesenteric vein; it also drains

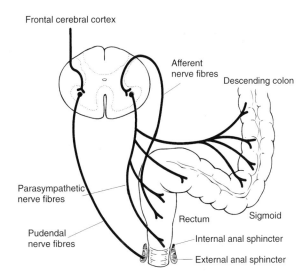

Figure 8.1 Innervation of the lower bowel. Adapted with permission from Popovich & Stewart-Amidei (1991).

blood from the spleen, pancreas and gallbladder. Hepatic veins then convey the blood to the heart by way of the inferior vena cava. The hepatic portal circulation begins as a capillary bed in the bowel, or in the other organs it drains. It empties its blood into the sinusoids within the liver without passing through the heart.

Nerve supply to the large bowel

The sympathetic and vagal nerves, through the superior mesenteric plexus, innervate the proximal two-thirds of the large bowel (Fig. 8.1). Sympathetic and parasympathetic pelvic splanchnic nerves, through the inferior mesenteric plexus, innervate the distal third of the bowel.

The pudendal nerve is a branch of the sacral nerve plexus, sacral nerves 2, 3 and 4, and – by means of its branches – supplies the external anal sphincter.

Parts of the large bowel

The large bowel extends from the ileocaecal valve to the junction of the rectum and anal canal. The colon averages 150 cm in length and is divided

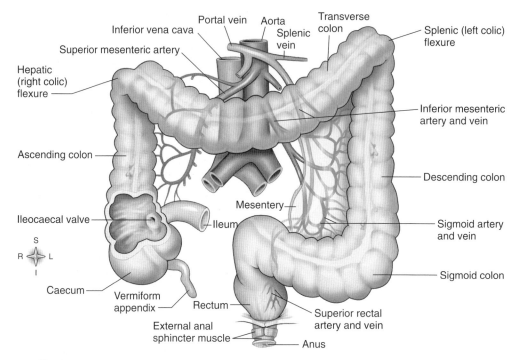

Figure 8.2 Division of th

into four segments: the ascending colon (20 cm), the transverse colon (46 cm), descending colon (31 cm) and sigmoid colon (46 cm). There are two flexures: the hepatic flexure, where the colon turns below the right lobe of the liver to form the transverse colon, and the splenic flexure, where the transverse colon merges into the descending colon (Fig. 8.2).

The caecum is the first part of the large bowel and is joined to the ileum by a sphincter muscle called the ileocaecal valve. This valve is normally constricted, preventing the contents of the small bowel entering the large bowel, and preventing the contents of the large bowel backing up into the ileum. Following the gastrocolic reflex, peristalsis in the ileum is increased, forcing the contents of the small bowel through the ileocaecal valve into the caecum.

Absorption occurs in the ascending, transverse and descending colon, returning useful products to the tissues and blood circulation. By the time faecal matter enters the sigmoid colon it consists entirely of the body's waste products, now called faeces. Faecal content consists of food residue, unabsorbed gastrointestinal secretions, shed epithelial cells and bacteria. The brown colour of faeces is caused by stercobilin and urobilin, which are derivatives of bilirubin.

Constipation can result from faeces being lodged in any part of the large bowel but it is most frequently experienced in the sigmoid colon and rectum (Fig. 8.3). The sigmoid colon is an S-shaped curve prior to the rectum. The rectum is the last 15–17 cm of the large bowel. The rectum lies next to the sacrum and generally follows its curvature. It is attached to the sacrum by the peritoneum and ends about 5 cm below the tip of the coccyx where it becomes the anal canal, often referred to collectively as the anorectum. The rectum is commodious, having a larger diameter than the rest of the colon, with the consequence that it has the ability to stretch easily to accommodate its contents. The anal canal begins at the anorectal junction, passes through the levator ani of the pelvic floor muscles and ends at the anus. Another muscle of the pelvic floor, the puborectalis muscle, forms a sling around

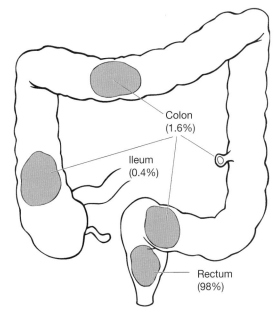

Colon
(1.6%)

Ileum
(0.4%)

Rectum
(98%)

Figure 8.3 Sites and frequency of faecal impactions. Reproduced with permission from Dresden & Kratzer (1959); © American Medical Association.

the anorectal junction (Fig. 8.4). The muscle is normally contracted, pulling the anorectal junction upwards and forwards, thus preventing faeces from entering the anal canal during normal daily activity. The pelvic floor muscles play an important role in the maintenance of faecal continence and successful defecation.

The distal end of the anal canal opens to the outside as the anus and is guarded by two sphincter muscles, the internal and external anal sphincters. The internal anal sphincter is formed by a thick circle of smooth muscle surrounding the anal canal and is not under voluntary control. The external anal sphincter is formed by striated muscle and therefore is under voluntary control. It surrounds the bottom of the internal sphincter, overhanging slightly (Fig. 8.5).

The mucous membrane of the anal canal is folded into a series of six to eight longitudinal anal columns, each column containing a branch of the rectal vein. If these veins are put under pressure they become engorged with blood. If pressure continues, the wall of the vein then stretches and such a distended vessel is known as an internal

haemorrhoid. Haemorrhoids may ooze blood and stretching of the vein can favour clot formation, which results in further swelling and discomfort. External haemorrhoids are covered by the mucous membrane of the lower end of the anal canal and are innervated by the inferior rectal nerves. This explains why external haemorrhoids tend to be so painful. Accumulated faeces or repeated straining during defecation can be responsible for forcing blood into the rectal veins and increasing the pressure within them. Haemorrhoids occurring in pregnancy are due to pressure on the superior rectal veins by the gravid uterus.

DEFECATION

Defecation is the process of rectal emptying and is usually initiated voluntarily, leading to a sequence of coordinated events which are incompletely understood. Defecation is subject to emotional influences or stressors which can produce increased intestinal motility and cause psychosomatic diarrhoea. Movement of faeces into the rectum causes rectal distension. This evokes the desire to defecate, sometimes referred to as the 'call to stool'.

Faeces do not enter the rectum on a continuous basis but as a result of an episodic mass peristaltic movement, travelling the entire length of the colon. Unlike the small bowel that has peristaltic movement on a 1–2-hourly basis, the large bowel has a peristaltic action only five or six times a day. These movements are called gastrocolic reflex actions. They are triggered by distension of the stomach and it is thought that gastrin, a hormone secreted by the mucosa of the stomach, has an action in stimulating the gastrocolic reflex. The most powerful of these reflexes usually occurs in the morning, after breakfast. This is attributed to the bowel being jolted into action following night-time bowel inertia by getting out of bed, and then stimulating the stomach further with a drink or something to eat after a night's sleep. As the rectum expands, the internal anal sphincter relaxes, thus reducing anal pressure. This is known as the *inhibitory reflex*.

Nerve endings on the dentate line of the rectum are able to 'sample' the content of the distended rectum. These 'sampling cells' inform the cortical centre of the brain as to whether the rectal content

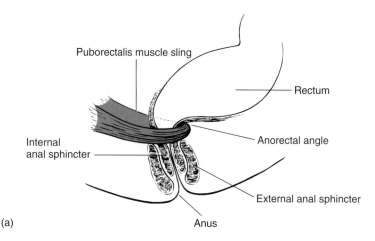

Puborectalis muscle sling

Rectum

Internal
anal sphincter

Anorectal angle

External anal sphincter

(a)   Anus

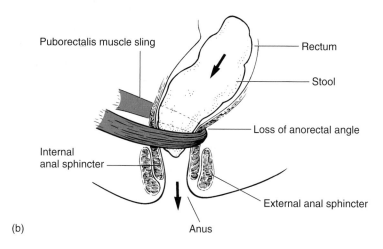

Puborectalis muscle sling

Rectum

Stool

Loss of anorectal angle

Internal
anal sphincter

External anal sphincter

(b)   Anus

Figure 8.4 The anal sphincter mechanism: (a) with the rectum empty; (b) during defecation.

is stool, flatus or liquid. If a normal stool is sensed but it is not convenient to defecate, defecation can be delayed by voluntary contraction of the external anal sphincter. As the rectum becomes accustomed to its new size it no longer inhibits contraction of the internal anal sphincter and the sphincter is able to return to its contracted state, thus restoring anal pressure. The puborectalis muscle contracts, decreasing the anorectal angle. This is known as the *inflation reflex* (Fig. 8.6). Voluntary inhibition or facilitation of defecation is mediated from the cortical projections onto the medulla region of the brain and down the spinal thalamic tract.

Under ideal circumstances, adopting the correct posture for defecation raises the intra-abdominal pressure through contraction of the diaphragm and abdominal muscles. Intra-abdominal pressure can be further increased by initiating the Valsalva manoeuvre, which involves inhaling and forcing the diaphragm and chest muscles against a closed glottis to increase both the intrathoracic and intra-abdominal pressure which is transmitted to the rectum. Raised intra-abdominal pressure causes the pressure in the rectum to rise. The pressures exerted by the internal and external anal sphincters decrease. This mechanism is important, as rectal pressure must be higher than anal pressure for defecation to be effective (Fig. 8.7). Relaxation of the puborectalis muscle then occurs. Relaxation of this muscle allows for widening and lowering of the anorectal angle, with perineal descent allowing faeces to pass more easily into the anal canal.

Coordination between the abdominal contraction and pelvic floor relaxation is vital to the process of defecation. Any abnormality or impairment of the neural input to the colon and pelvic

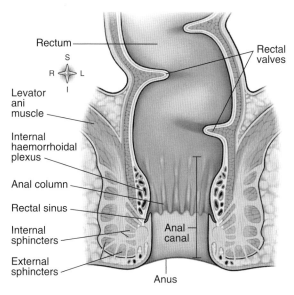

Rectum

S
R ✛ L
I

Levator
ani
muscle

Internal
haemorrhoidal
plexus

Anal column

Rectal sinus

Internal
sphincters

External
sphincters

Rectal
valves

Anal
canal

Anus

Figure 8.5 Rectum and anus. Reproduced from Thibodeau & Patton (1993).

floor will lead to a reduction in colonic propulsion or poor pelvic floor coordination, resulting in decreased defecation or excessive straining.

SYMPTOMS AND FEATURES OF CONSTIPATION

A patient with constipation may experience a variety of symptoms. These can range from headache and fatigue, to feelings of bloatedness, or to loss of appetite leading to nausea and vomiting. Constipation affects the overall well-being of a patient, with symptom severity correlating negatively with perceived quality of life (Glia & Lindberg 1997). Patients experiencing difficulty with defecation may complain physically of a 'full bottom' and an inability to have their bowels opened. The consequence of persistent or poorly managed constipation can lead to disabling complications for the patient. Such complications may

Figure 8.6 How to know when it's time to 'go'.

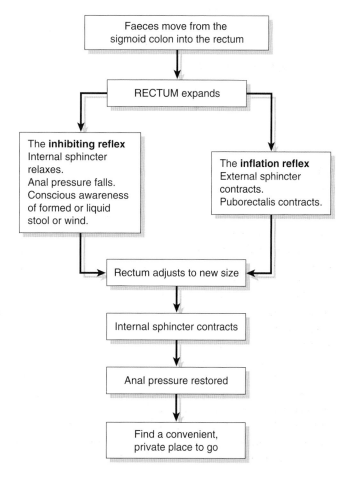

Faeces move from the sigmoid colon into the rectum

RECTUM expands

The **inhibiting reflex**
Internal sphincter relaxes.
Anal pressure falls.
Conscious awareness of formed or liquid stool or wind.

The **inflation reflex**
External sphincter contracts.
Puborectalis contracts.

Rectum adjusts to new size

Internal sphincter contracts

Anal pressure restored

Find a convenient, private place to go

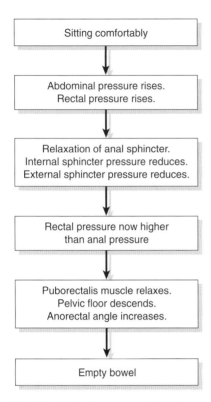

Figure 8.7   How to 'go' at a convenient time.

include haemorrhoids, faecal impaction, faecal impaction with spurious diarrhoea, urinary incontinence, urinary tract infection, rectal bleeding, general weakness and psychological disorders (Prodigy Guidance 2004). Persistent straining at stool leads to increased intrathoracic pressure which can give rise to a reduction in coronary and peripheral circulation leading to other possible complications – development of hernias, worsening of gastro-oesophageal reflux and transient ischaemic attacks (Prodigy Guidance 2004).

Clinical signs of a patient with constipation are a distended abdomen, reduction in bowel sounds and on digital rectal examination a gaping anus or an impacted rectum.

ASSESSMENT OF CONSTIPATION

The assessment of constipation is based on a consideration of all the possible causes, checking in particular that the constipation is not caused by an underlying undiagnosed medical condition. Box 8.3 identifies the assessment criteria that should be

considered. Care pathways for bowel care have been developed and are used in many places (Bayliss et al 2000). Following a training programme, the nurse completes an initial assessment using the care pathway incorporating a bowel habit diary and a 1-week record of dietary intake.

After initial assessment a general physical examination should look for evidence of abdominal distension, pain and tenderness. A digital rectal examination (DRE) may be required to assess rectal loading/faecal impaction and the consistency of the faecal material (which may be hard or soft). Nurses should have received suitable training before performing DRE or manual evacuation of faeces (RCN 2000). The Royal College of Nursing publication, *Digital Rectal Examination and Manual Removal of Faeces: Guidance for Nurses*, is a helpful source of instruction. Any abnormalities of the perineal or perianal area should first be observed – for example, rectal prolapse, haemorrhoids, anal skin tags, anal lesions, gaping anus, general skin condition, bleeding, faecal soiling, infestation or foreign bodies. A DRE should only be used to establish the presence of stool in the rectum and should not be seen as part of the primary assessment (RCN 2000). As the normal state of the rectum is empty, a lack of faecal matter on DRE does not necessarily signify the absence of constipation. Smith and Lewis (1990) found through X-ray that 30% of patients with an empty rectum had a large amount of faeces in the sigmoid colon.

MANAGEMENT OF CONSTIPATION

If there are no underlying conditions, a stepped approach should be used in the management of constipation (Bayliss et al 2000, Prodigy Guidance 2004). The first step should be appropriate dietary and lifestyle advice, the second step the use of a laxative.

Dietary and lifestyle advice

Exercise

All patients experiencing constipation should be encouraged to exercise and increase the range of

Box 8.3   Assessment criteria for constipation

Question	Rationale
Age and gender of patient	
If appropriate, ask about any incontinence following childbirth	Optimum time for nerve and muscle recovery is up to 24 weeks postpartum (Fynes et al 1999)
General health	Severity of illness is a major factor related to constipation (Ross 1995)
Previous laxative use?	Excessive use of stimulant laxatives in younger life may result in secondary changes to the mesenteric plexus resulting in a reduction of peristalsis leading to a slower bowel transit time (Campbell et al 1993)
Description of problem, sensation, wind, feelings of discomfort or incomplete evacuation. If the problem is straining at defecation, is it painful or painless?	
Frequency of normal and current bowel movement? Ask the patient to complete a bowel diary for at least 1 week	
Ask the patient to complete a dietary and fluid intake diary for at least 1 week	
Are there any changes to normal diet or fluid intake?	Any change to dietary pattern may increase the risk of constipation, as does a reduction in normal fluid intake
Any change in mobility?	Decreased physical activity, bed rest or hospitalisation are recognised causes of constipation in adults, especially the older person
Is the patient able to prepare food, or are they reliant on others for shopping and food preparation?	
Check condition of tongue and breath for signs of dehydration	
Check for poorly fitting dentures or bad teeth	Lack of teeth, poorly fitting dentures and reduction of saliva production can make chewing and swallowing more difficult and may contribute to a reduction of fresh fruits and vegetables, thus limiting dietary fibre intake
Check medication	Medication has been found to be a risk factor in more than 50% of constipated patients (Kamm 1994)
	Sheehy & Richards-Hall (1998) state that all medications can affect normal bowel function in a variety of ways. They can: • decrease gastric motility • decrease absorption rates • limit general personal mobility Potter et al (2002) from case controlled trials identify the taking of five or more medications as a particular risk 50% of patients receiving palliative care have constipation and 80% of these patients will require laxatives due to the use of analgesics (Fallon & O'Neill 1997)

Box 8.3 *Continued*

Description of stool – colour, mucus, etc.

Type (consistency) of stool – use Bristol Stool Form Scale (Fig. 8.8)

Any pain/bleeding on defecation

May be suggestive of local injury (e.g. haemorrhoids/anal fissure) or underlying pathology (e.g. rectal cancer)

Any unexplained change in bowel habit

May be suggestive of underlying pathology; constipation may be a risk factor for the development of colorectal cancer in middle-aged patients (Jacobs & White 1998)

Is the patient experiencing any new urinary problems?

Constipation is associated with bladder instability and urinary tract infections

Ask the patient how they usually cope with the problem – do they use over-the-counter preparations? Check any therapeutic regimes already tried; it may be that the patient uses digital stimulation

Psychological aspects need to be explored but require sensitive handling (e.g. was the patient sexually abused in childhood?)

Confused and depressed patients may ignore the sensation of stool in the rectum and this leads to constipation

---

their mobility, especially if housebound. Bed rest or a period of immobility is thought to result in a weakening of the abdominal wall muscles leading to difficulty in raising the intra-abdominal pressure sufficiently for defecation. Alessi and Henderson (1988) found that physical activity increased abdominal muscle tone promoting more efficient defecation.

A large study by Kinnunen (1991) found a statistically significant increased risk of constipation for people walking less than 0.5 km daily. The study also identified risks associated with patients walking with help, being chairbound or bedbound. The results of a study by Ross (1995) found that both mobility and diet play a greater role in changes to bowel elimination in the elderly population than for middle-aged patients. Read et al (1995), after reviewing Kinnunen's research, suggest that walking 0.5 km is sufficient to prevent constipation amongst the older population. De Schryver et al (2005) state that it is advisable to promote regular exercise in inactive patients who are suffering from constipation although they caution that further research is required to understand the underlying mechanisms linking physical exercise and bowel motility.

Posture and timing

As well as encouraging mobility and exercise, nurses should ascertain that patients are sitting correctly on the lavatory in order to raise their intra-abdominal pressure during defecation (Fig. 8.9). The addition of footstools can help patients who have raised lavatory seats or who are wheeled on a commode over the lavatory to sit in the correct position. Patients can be encouraged to take advantage of the morning gastrocolic reflex by having a hot drink soon after waking and sitting on the toilet around 20 min later.

Dietary factors

It has been suggested that constipation, occurring at any age, can be associated with low calorific intake (Sheehy & Richards-Hall 1998), but may be a particular risk factor for older patients (Towers et al 1994). Towers et al reported that constipated older patients consumed fewer meals and tended to consume fewer calories than the general population, and Cope (1996) considered that around 20% of older people skip at least one meal per day. Consumption of fruit, vegetables and bread have

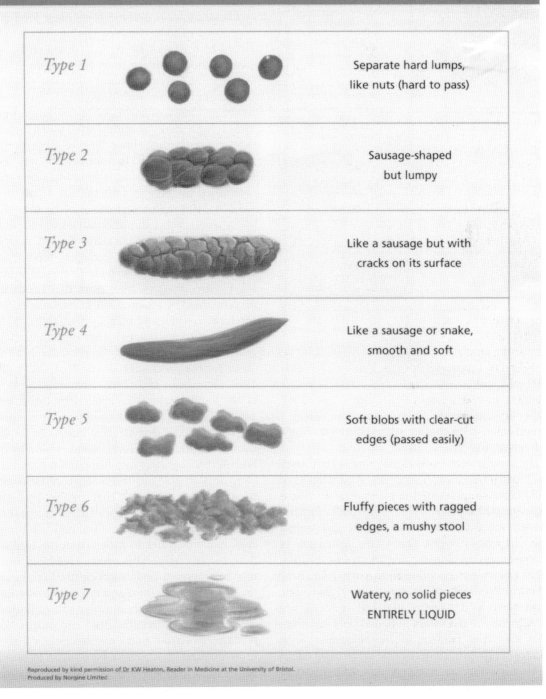

Figure 8.8   The Bristol Stool Form Scale. Reproduced by kind permission of Norgine Ltd from Heaton et al (1992).

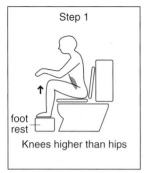
Step 1

foot
rest

Knees higher than hips

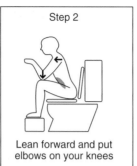
Step 2

Lean forward and put
elbows on your knees

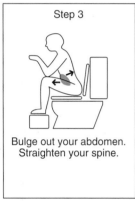
Step 3

Bulge out your abdomen.
Straighten your spine.

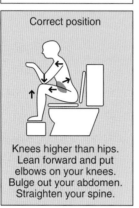
Correct position

Knees higher than hips.
Lean forward and put
elbows on your knees.
Bulge out your abdomen.
Straighten your spine.

Figure 8.9 *Correct position for opening your bowels.*
Reproduced by kind permission of Ray Addison, Nurse
Consultant in Bladder and Bowel Dysfunction, and
Wendy Ness, Colorectal Nurse Specialist.

all been shown to decline significantly with age
(Bennett et al 1995).

The link between bowel movement frequency
and dietary fibre is well recognised (Burkitt et al
1972, Cummings 1984, Maestri-Banks & Burns
1996). In healthy individuals there is a relationship
between dietary fibre intake, whole gut transit
time and faecal weight. During the formation of
faeces, fluids are drawn from the colon into the
faecal matter by insoluble fibre particles. These
fibres can swell up to 20 times their original size,
resulting in bulky faeces that can move easily
through the colon. Dietary fibre and bulk laxatives
have also been shown to be associated with
decreased abdominal pain and improved stool
consistency compared with placebo (Tramonte et
al 1997). However, patients with a slow transit
time tend to show the least effect with a high
fibre diet and Spiller (1990) suggests that a slow

transit time seems to favour a more complete
bacterial degradation of fibre in the ascending
colon, thus reducing the effect of fibre on faecal
output.

Dietary fibre is derived from plant food and is
composed of long complex chains of polysaccharide which cannot be broken down in humans.
Instead they maintain their bulk and in doing so
'stretch' the bowel wall and stimulate peristalsis.
Interestingly, Nair and Mayberry (1994) found a
lower incidence of constipation amongst vegetar-
ians. It is generally recommended that a high fibre
diet, consisting of about 30 g of fibre per day,
should be encouraged to minimise the risk of constipation and that the daily fibre intake should be
consumed in three to four regular meals during
the day. Although the effects may be seen within
a few days, such a diet should be tried for at least
a month before its effects are evaluated. A table of
dietary fibre content of common foods can be
found on the MeReC website (National Prescribing Centre 2004). A high fibre diet needs to be
accompanied by adequate fluid intake in order for
the fibre to swell and bulk up the faeces.

There is conflicting evidence regarding the adequate quantities of fluid required for health, let
alone for the prevention of constipation (Sullivan
1999, Grandjean et al 2003, Richmond & Wright
2004). Fluid intake is controlled by thirst, which
signals the need for more fluid. Elderly people are
at greater risk of dehydration due to an impaired
thirst mechanism (Reedy 1988), especially those
with severe cognitive impairment (Hoffman 1991).
Dehydration leads to the water content of blood
plasma being reduced. This creates an osmotic
gradient between the capillaries in the bowel
mucosa and the interstitial fluid between mucosal
cells, causing water to move from the interstitial
fluid to capillaries. This process leads, in turn, to
the development of an osmotic gradient between
the interstitial cell fluid and the fluid in the lumen
of the bowel. Water then moves out of the bowel
lumen into the interstitial fluid and mucosal cells,
resulting in harder and drier faeces.

Inadequate fluid intake is thought to be a risk
factor for constipation (Richards-Hall et al 1995,
Maestri-Banks & Burns 1996) which may be exacerbated when older people drink less in an attempt
to avoid urinary incontinence. Klauser et al (1990),

in a small study of healthy young men, found that fluid reduction changed bowel frequency and stool weight considerably; however, bowel transit time was not changed significantly. This seems surprising as faecal weight is thought to affect bowel motility, i.e. bulky faeces promotes quicker bowel transit time. These results led Klauser et al (1990) to hypothesise that a low fluid intake could be a risk factor for constipation in some patients and increasing fluids may be a reasonable way of treating constipation. Certainly an increase in fluid is a widely recommended treatment for constipation, based on the assumption that additional fluid leads to an increase in colonic activity. Chung et al (1999) investigated this hypothesis in a small study which looked at the effect of increased fluid on stool output in normal healthy adults. The study showed that increased fluid intake did not produce a significant change in stool weight. What is clear from the work of Chung et al (1999) and Klauser et al (1990) is that fluid deprivation may decrease stool output and lead to constipation but it is less clear what the optimum fluid intake may be.

Daily fluid intake will vary from one person to another due to different body mass index, exercise capability and willingness and/or ability to mobilise, but there is a general consensus in the literature that 1.5 litres/24 h is recommended to maintain good health (Norton 1996a,b, Morrison 2000). Richmond and Wright (2004) propose that 1.5 litres/day is the minimum fluid intake recommended for the prevention and treatment of chronic constipation. This equates to about eight cups or mugs of fluid (capacity 180–200 ml). When advising patients on fluid intake, it is important to be aware that excessively hot weather, alcohol consumption and pyrexia all indicate a need to increase fluid requirements. Nurses can suggest foods that contain large quantities of water in order to increase fluid intake such as jelly, yoghurt, soup, mousses, whipped milk-based puddings, rice pudding and other milky puddings and sauces (Leech & McDonnell 1999). It has been suggested that drinking coffee instead of tea may be helpful for constipation as coffee (not caffeine) appears to stimulate colonic activity (Brown et al 1990), whereas tea in large quantities may lead to constipation (Hojgaard et al 1981); however, there is a lack of robust research evidence to confirm this observation.

Laxatives

Constipation, fear of constipation and possible lack of guidance are all possible reasons for the widespread use and high expenditure on laxatives, whether prescribed or bought over the counter. Yet there is no reliable evidence that laxatives prevent constipation, especially amongst older patients. The recommendation to 'start with a clean bowel' (Weeks et al 2000) proposes that laxatives may be a necessary treatment option for severe constipation. However, a recent audit demonstrates that bowel care problems can be linked to ineffective and/or inappropriate prescribing of laxatives (Addison et al 2003). The audit outcomes indicated that many patients received a combination of laxative regimens, which suggests that treatment was poorly planned and treatment guidelines for constipation were not followed.

It is important for nurses to understand the mode of action of laxatives since they are the most commonly prescribed pharmacological intervention for the management of constipation. (Laxatives are also considered, more briefly, in Chapter 9.) The main types currently used regularly in practice are listed below:

- Bulk-forming
- Stimulant
- Osmotic
- Softeners.

Bulk-forming laxatives

Bulk-forming laxatives are least harmful and can be used in conjunction with the lifestyle advice of increasing fibre in the diet. The most commonly used preparations are from ispaghula husk (Fybogel) and sterculia (Normacol). These preparations should be taken with plenty of water and not immediately before going to bed as there is then insufficient time to drink enough water. An inadequate fluid intake will result in hard desiccated faeces and the possible complication of intestinal obstruction. Evidence from recent trials suggests that bulk-forming laxatives may be better tolerated than other laxatives. However, there is little comparative evidence of differences between bulk and other laxatives in terms of frequency or symptoms (NHS Centre for Reviews and Dissemination 2001).

Stimulant laxatives

These laxatives stimulate an increase in colonic motility and mucus secretion when the laxative or its breakdown products come into contact with the intestinal mucosa, intramural nerve plexus or intestinal musculature (Shafik 1993). The most commonly used are anthraquinones (senna and dantron) and diphenylmethane cathartics (bisacodyl). Anthraquinones may discolour urine as a result of the metabolites excreted. Senna is the most powerful of the anthracene purges and is an effective short-term remedy for acute constipation. It is usually effective within 6–12 h of administration and is therefore best given at bedtime. There is no evidence to suggest that one stimulant laxative is more effective than another (Petticrew et al 1997). Dantron-containing laxatives are subject to licence limitations (terminally ill patients only) following evidence from studies on rodents that in high doses it could be carcinogenic (BNF 2005).

Bisacodyl may be given in suppository form and may be effective within 15–60 min. Glycerine suppositories may also act as a rectal stimulant by virtue of the mildly irritant action of glycerol (BNF 2005). Glycerine suppositories must be moistened prior to insertion and then placed alongside the bowel wall. All bowel care suppositories need body heat in order to dissolve so that the content can act as a bowel irritant. If suppositories are placed in the middle of faecal matter they will remain intact and useless. Mallet and Dougherty (2005) advocate the insertion of suppositories blunt end first for bowel care, using the research of Abd-El-Maeboud et al (1991) to substantiate this viewpoint. However, Abd-El-Maeboud et al's study makes no particular reference to the insertion of suppositories for bowel care, so arguably their research can be interpreted for either systemic or local action of suppositories, or both. Furthermore, analysis of the research uses simple descriptive statistics, which brings into question the robustness of conclusions drawn and implications for practice, although the work is cited in many commonly used clinical nursing textbooks. A review of available evidence by Bradshaw & Price (2007) suggests best practice is a common sense attitude, particularly as pharmaceutical companies make suppositories with a blunt end to push against.

Osmotic laxatives

This group of laxatives includes mixed electrolyte solutions containing polyethylene glycol and non-absorbable sugars such as lactulose and sorbitol. Their action is to retain fluid in the bowel by osmosis. The National Prescribing Centre (2004) states that lactulose may take up to 2–3 days to have an effect and is therefore not suitable for the rapid relief of constipation. Osmotics are not appropriate for prevention and treatment of constipation where gut motility is impaired (Abrams et al 1995). Prodigy Guidance (2004) further emphasise that lactulose should not be regarded as first-choice therapy in the management of constipation. Interestingly, despite lactulose's popularity through prescription, it remains one of the most expensive forms of laxative therapy.

Macrogols (Movicol and Idrolax) are relatively new laxatives. They are inert polymers of ethylene glycol. There is now limited evidence from several trials that polyethylene glycol is a safe and effective alternative in the management of constipation (Attar et al 1999, Corazziari et al 2000). Movicol is the only laxative currently recommended for faecal impaction.

Rectal preparations such as phosphate enemas and microenemas are useful for bowel clearance. However, there is a lack of evidence in the published literature to support the use of phosphate enemas in the management of constipation (Davies 2004). Indeed, Davies suggests that nurses should be aware of the risks involved with the use of phosphate enemas and should be conversant with alternative treatments that are evidence based. The risks identified by Davies (2004) are:

- possible rectal injury by the enema tip, with any damage being exacerbated by the phosphate solution

- phosphate absorption from pooling of the enema, due to incomplete evacuation of enema or due to altered bowel anatomy of the patient
- hyperphosphataemia in patients who are unable to excrete phosphate adequately, such as those with some degree of renal impairment or reduced renal clearance.

Softeners

These laxatives act by lowering surface tension, thereby allowing penetration of hardened faeces by water and fats. The most commonly used softener is docusate sodium, which also has weak stimulant properties. Liquid paraffin is a stool softener/lubricant but it can cause anal seepage and irritation, lipoid pneumonia (rarely) and malabsorption of lipid-soluble vitamins. It is not recommended for use in clinical practice (Prodigy Guidance 2004) but is still available over the counter.

Retention enemas containing arachis oil both lubricate and soften impacted faeces. Arachis oil enemas should be warmed to body temperature before use and if possible given last thing at night. Patients should be asked if they have a nut allergy as arachis oil contains nut oils.

Digital removal of faeces

In most cases the need for the digital removal of faeces is preventable (Addison 1996, Bayliss et al 2000). Powell and Rigby (2000) suggest that the digital removal of faeces is a last resort procedure and should only be practised when all other methods of bowel evacuation have failed. However, for some patients, such as those with spinal cord injury (SCI), cauda equina, spina bifida and multiple sclerosis, digital removal of faeces is an integral part of their routine bowel management. This essential routine is often interrupted when these patients are admitted into a hospital that does not specialise in treating spinal injuries (National Patient Safety Agency 2004) because nurses lack knowledge and expertise to competently perform a digital removal of faeces.

Box 8.4 sets out the procedure for digital removal of faeces (Kyle et al 2005). Practitioners should also adhere to the guidance provided by the Royal College of Nurses in the *Digital Rectal Examination and Manual Removal of Faeces: Guidance for Nurses* (RCN 2000), with particular reference to Sections 8 and 9. It is recommended that only a competent practitioner should carry out this procedure and to ensure competence the nurse should have successfully completed a Digital Rectal Examination course based on the recent Royal College of Nursing publication. Nurses undertaking the procedure must also be aware of their Trust/organisation's policies and protocols. In some situations digital removal of faeces can be considered a form of patient abuse and nurses must be aware of this risk.

CAUSES OF FAECAL INCONTINENCE

Faecal incontinence is not only an extremely unpleasant symptom but it can also contribute to medical morbidity such as urinary tract infections (UTIs) and decubitus ulcers (Madoff et al 2004), as well as emotional, psychological and financial worries, often leading to self-imposed lifestyle restrictions. Bowel dysfunction (with or without bladder dysfunction) is a well-recognised factor which may precipitate the requirement for institutionalised care and one which incurs great costs in terms of medication, containment equipment and care (DH 2000a). Similarly, Madoff et al (2004) suggest that families simply cannot manage faecal incontinence at home and its development is instrumental in securing care home placement.

Faecal incontinence is likely to be a significant factor in child abuse and bullying (Lukeman 2003), as well as in elder abuse (Bradley 1996), as illustrated by Department of Health guidance on developing and implementing multiagency policies and procedures to protect vulnerable adults from abuse (*No Secrets*, DH 2000b)

Faecal incontinence may result from a single straightforward cause, but more often it follows a cumulative, multifactorial process, and a combination of factors may give rise to the symptoms of faecal incontinence (Norton & Chelvanayagam 2004). An accumulation of triggers such as postnatal anal sphincter injury and chronic constipation may lead to the development of faecal incontinence later in life when other conditions such as IBS or diabetes may emerge. Some of the

---

Box 8.4   Digital removal of faeces: the four DOs, DON'Ts and THINK TWICE

DOs
1. DO complete a full bowel assessment (Bayliss et al 2000).
2. DO consider treatment options with your team (Powell & Rigby 2000, NMC 8.1 2002).
3. DO inform the patient of treatment options and the risks involved (NMC 3.1, 4.3 2002).
4. DO gain valid consent (written, verbal or implied) from the patient (Willis 2000, DH 2001, NMC 2002).

DON'Ts
1. DON'T proceed if there is a lack of consent (written, verbal or implied) or if the patient refuses.
2. DON'T proceed if the patient's doctor has given specific instructions not to undertake the procedure.
3. DON'T proceed if the patient has recently undergone rectal/anal surgery or trauma.
4. DON'T proceed if you *do not* feel competent (NMC 6 2002).

THINK TWICE
If the patient has the following diseases and/or conditions:
1. Active inflammatory bowel disease
2. Rectal pain
3. Obvious rectal bleeding or the patient is taking anticlotting medication (new SCI patients will be anticoagulated to prevent deep vein thrombosis but still require digital removal of faeces (DRF) – see local policy)
4. Spinal injury at T6 or above. Remember that allowing constipation to occur leads to a greater risk of autonomic dysreflexia developing.

Action	Rationale
Complete bowel assessment with the patient (Bayliss et al 2000)	To ascertain the need for digital removal of faeces: • all other bowel empting techniques have failed • faecal impaction/loading • incomplete defecation • inability to defecate • neurogenic bowel dysfunction (e.g. multiple sclerosis) • patient with spinal injury (RCN 2000)
Check the *Dos, Don'ts and Think Twice* section at the beginning of this document	To identify exclusions and contraindications or circumstances when extra caution is required (RCN 2000)
Discuss treatment with the patient and the team. *Justify the need for this procedure and document*	To allow the patient choice and to ensure optimum treatment option (NMC 3.1, 4.3 2002)
Explain procedure and potential risks to the patient. Document consent given	To gain the patient's consent and cooperation, you must ensure that the patient has the mental ability to give consent and that the patient has been given sufficient information about the risks involved (NMC 3.3 2002) to either consent or refuse (NMC 3.2 2002) Digital removal of faeces entails the possible risk of damage to the anal and rectal mucosa and of stretching the anal sphincter The patient needs to consent freely and voluntarily without coercion or manipulation (DH 2001)
Document if the patient is unable to give valid consent, i.e. the patient has lost the capacity to consent to or to refuse the procedure due to, for example, unconsciousness, sedation or confusional state. Why the procedure is in the patient's best interest *must be documented*	As this is an invasive procedure and may be harmful in certain circumstances, you must ensure your professional accountability is maintained (NMC 3.6, 3.8 2002)

Box 8.4 *Continued*

Ensure privacy	To help the patient relax and minimise embarrassment (NMC 2.2 2002)
Take the patient's pulse at rest prior to the procedure	To obtain a base-line of the patient's condition prior to the procedure as vagal stimulation can slow the heart rate
Assess the risk of autonomic dysreflexia of SCI patients with injury at T6 or above (see also Ch. 6)	Autonomic dysreflexia is a sudden and exaggerated autonomic response to an unpleasant stimulus, e.g. a full rectum or digital stimulation of the rectum during bowel evacuation It occurs in spinal injuries at T6 or above (Ahrens & Prentice 1998) Patients present with marked hypertension and complain of headaches
Record BP if the patient has an SCI at T6 or above	To obtain a base-line BP
Has the patient recently had an autonomic episode? Is the patient constipated?	Yes to either of these questions signifies a risk of autonomic dysreflexia but this risk must be balanced against the risk of constipation leading to dysreflexia secondary to not emptying the bowel
Place a protective pad under the patient and ensure a suitable receiver is to hand	To protect bedding from faecal matter
Assist the patient to adopt, if possible, the left lateral position with knees flexed	To expose the anus and allow easy insertion of finger
A sitting position should be avoided	To prevent overstretching of the anal sphincter and discomfort for the patient
Individual assessment of each patient's DRF regime is required	Independent SCI patients may prefer to conduct DRF over a toilet
Observe the perineal and perianal area. Document and report any abnormalities	To check for rectal prolapse, haemorrhoids, anal skin tags, wounds, discharge, anal lesions, gaping anus, bleeding, infestation, foreign bodies
Wash hands, put on disposable apron and non-latex gloves of a suitable thickness	To minimise cross-infection and to protect your hands
For patients undergoing this procedure on a *regular* basis, place water-based lubricating gel on gloved index finger	To facilitate easier insertion of index finger
As an *acute* procedure, a local anaesthetic gel may be applied topically to the anal area	To reduce sensation and discomfort for the patient
Read contraindications, warnings, precautions and interactions of the anaesthetic gel you propose to use	Lidocaine is a topical local anaesthesia and is absorbed via the anal mucous membrane
Do not apply if you have documented evidence of anal damage or bleeding	Lidocaine may cause anaphylaxis, hypotension, bradycardia or convulsions if applied to damaged mucosa
Inform the patient of imminent examination	To ensure the patient is ready and relaxed
Insert non-latex gloved, lubricated index finger slowly and gently, encouraging the patient to relax. Use one finger only	To avoid trauma to the anal mucosa and prevent forced overdilation of the anal sphincter
In scybala type stool (Bristol Stool Form Scale type 1) remove one lump at a time until no more faecal matter can be felt	To relieve patient's discomfort

Box 8.4 *Continued*

In a solid faecal mass, push finger into the middle of the mass, split it and remove small pieces with hooked finger until no more faecal matter can be felt	To relieve patient's discomfort
If faecal mass is too hard or larger than 4 cm across and you are unable to break it up, *stop* and refer to medical team for DRF under general anaesthetic	To avoid considerable pain and trauma (anal sphincter damage) to the patient
Proceed with caution with SCI patients; those patients with a reflex bowel may require a further rectal stimulant	Most SCI patients will not experience any pain
As faecal matter is removed it should be placed in a suitable receiver	To facilitate appropriate disposal of faecal matter
Encourage patients who receive this procedure on a *regular* basis to have a period of rest or to assist, if appropriate, with Valsalva manoeuvre. Patient and nurse education is required to safely use this manoeuvre Extra lubrication may be required	To allow further faecal matter to descend into the rectum Correct breathing technique will prevent raised intracranial pressure Use of the Valsalva manoeuvre in an upright position may result in increased hydrostatic pressure in perirectal blood vessels, thereby increasing the likelihood of haemorrhoids (Menter et al 1997) SCI patients may assist with evacuation by using the Valsalva manoeuvre; however, excessive straining should be discouraged for the reasons above NB: For some SCI patients, raising intra-abdominal pressure does not result in relaxation of the sphincter or excessive pressures may be required, therefore the Valsalva manoeuvre should be used with caution and its effects evaluated for each patient Valsalva manoeuvre is not recommended for patients with intrathecal baclofen pumps
Observe the patient throughout the procedure: • *Stop* if there is anal area bleeding • *Stop* if pain persists • *Stop* if the patient asks you to stop	To note signs of distress, pain, bleeding and general discomfort
Check the patient's pulse. *Stop* if heart rate drops or rhythm changes	Vagal stimulation can slow heart rate and alter heart rhythm
Stop at the first sign of autonomic dysreflexia. Nurses must respond immediately to any signs of autonomic dysreflexia	Symptoms include headache, blurred vision, nausea, sweating, bradycardia, respiratory distress, pupil constriction and flushing above the lesion with pallor below (Walker 2002)
Take BP if an SCI patient becomes distressed or feels the onset of an autonomic episode – compare with baseline BP	BP is always raised during an autonomic episode
If possible, sit the patient up, give the patient's prescribed medication for autonomic dysreflexia and reassure. If concerned, contact the local Spinal Cord Injury Centre	To reduce hypertension and the patient's apprehension. If it is inadequately treated, the patient can become sensitised and then develop autonomic dysreflexia with the minimum of stimulus (Grundy & Swain 1996)
When the procedure is complete, wash and dry the patient's buttocks and anal area	To leave the patient comfortable and clean

Box 8.4   *Continued*

Inform the patient of the outcome and ensure procedure and outcome are documented	Documentation should provide clear evidence of care planned, decisions made and care delivered (NMC 4.4 2002)

- Remember bowel management strategies must be continually reviewed and assessed.
- Effective bowel management strategies for patients with a spinal cord injury at any level is extremely important and at T6 or above is the best proactive measure for preventing autonomic dysreflexia.
- Be proactive, not simply reactive.

causes of faecal incontinence are listed in Box 8.5.

Anal sphincter or pelvic floor muscle damage

Childbirth, particularly instrument assisted or vacuum extraction vaginal delivery, is a major factor in faecal incontinence for women although vacuum extraction is associated with fewer third/fourth degree tears than forceps (Norton et al 2002). Pollack et al (2004) concluded that anal incontinence at 9 months postpartum is a significant forecast that persisting symptoms and anal incontinence among primiparous women will increase over time and will be affected by further childbirth. Risk factors for damage to the pudendal nerve, the inferior aspects of the levator ani muscle and fascial pelvic organ supports also include attempted vaginal delivery, a long second stage of labour and macrosomia (Dietz & Wilson 2005). The importance of pudendal nerve damage in the aetiology of postpartum faecal incontinence is gaining increasing attention and although prevention of such injury may not always be possible, Fitzpatrick and O'Herlihy (2005) advise that adequate treatment and management options must be explored in order to prevent an increased prevalence of later-onset symptoms.

Sultan and Stanton (1996) found that the demand for elective caesarean section was on the increase. This preference, in order to preserve the pelvic floor musculature, may be seen as a reliable option; however, discussion around cost as well as associated morbidity and mortality will influence obstetricians, midwives and women in their decision making. MacArthur et al (1997) found that elective caesarean section without attempted vaginal delivery was effective in preventing anal incontinence. Patrick et al (2005) suggested that following ultrasound at 39 weeks' gestation and assessment of individual risk, a caesarean section may well be clinically justified to prevent, among other symptoms, the development of anal incontinence. This view is supported by Dietz and Wilson (2005) who conclude that since delivery-related pelvic floor trauma is a reality, not a myth, preventative intervention by elective caesarean section must be preceded by identifying those women most at risk.

There is disagreement regarding the benefits of routine episiotomy (Taskin et al 1996). Midline episiotomy is described as not protective to the perineum and sphincters during childbirth and may impair anal continence (Signorello & Repke 2000); however, mediolateral episiotomy is associated with lower rates of significant perineal tears (Eogan et al 2006). Restraint in the use of episiotomy has not resulted in increased anal sphincter breach and, when it is considered necessary, then the rate of episiotomy ideally should not exceed 30% (Abrams et al 2002). Overt rectal sphincter injury is relatively rare in women who have not undergone episiotomy or instrumental delivery (Zetterstrom et al 1999); however, occult damage to the anal sphincter anatomy may occur. As this can be identified by endoanal ultrasonography, there should be no delay in diagnosis and implementing prompt treatment in order to minimise the risk of bowel problems at a later date. Meas-

Box 8.5 Common causes of faecal incontinence in adults

Causes of faecal incontinence	Resulting from:
Constipation leading to impaction and spurious diarrhoea	Diarrhoea and stool leakage around the impacted faeces
Chronic constipation causing pelvic floor muscle damage	Incompetent anal sphincters; unable to arrest incontinence of faeces
Anal sphincter or pelvic floor muscle damage	Obstetric trauma, radiation injury, anal surgery or direct violation
Laxative abuse	Prescribed and over-the-counter laxatives leading to diarrhoea
Diarrhoea (especially combined with pelvic floor muscle weakness)	Loose stool is more difficult to contain than formed stool
Intestinal hurry	Inflammatory bowel disease, colitis and irritable bowel syndrome aggravate the sensitive bowel and may result in diarrhoea
Muscle/nerve damage due to neurological disease or insult	Diabetes Multiple sclerosis Parkinson's disease (usually secondary to constipation) Secondary to degenerative neurological disease (e.g. dementia) Spinal cord injury, lesion or tumour Cerebrovascular accident Spina bifida
Congenital rectal malformation	Anal sphincter incompetence
Anorectal pathology	Rectal prolapse, anal or rectovaginal fistula
Post surgery	Post haemorrhoidectomy Sphincterotomy Fissure repair
Environment and immobility	Inadequate support and poor toilet facilities
Idiopathic	No discernible aetiology; unknown cause
Food intolerance or allergies	Lactose and gluten intolerance can lead to diarrhoea

ures to prevent obstetric anal sphincter lacerations including avoidance of liberal use of instrumental delivery and episiotomy are advisable. First or second degree tears are regarded as mild whilst third or fourth degree tears are considered severe (Box 8.6; see also the case study in Box 8.7).

Investigations for bowel disorders

Following assessment of bowel dysfunction, further investigations may be required for those patients with new or severe symptoms. Various degrees of bowel preparation are carried out in readiness for any bowel investigations. For bowel investigations to be effective it is essential to have clear images of the bowel mucosa as this improves the chances for a clear diagnosis. Patients, particularly the frail elderly, may find bowel preparation very distressing as the urgency evoked by the bowel cleansing can cause further problems such as faecal incontinence. Depending on the specific investigation, a variety of either oral or rectal preparations may be used. An important deciding factor when choosing the type of bowel preparation is the patient's tolerance and symptoms (Bulmer 2000).

Radiology

A plain X-ray is useful in assessing the general health of the colon, particularly the presence of faecal matter. If a primary structural anorectal or colonic abnormality is suspected, a double con-trast barium enema will be suggested. A series of X-rays are then taken with the patient lying in various positions. Patients should be advised to drink plenty of water following a barium enema because of the constipating effect of the barium and the possible dehydrating effects of a bowel cleansing preparation.

Rigid sigmoidoscopy, flexible sigmoidoscopy, colonoscopy

All these investigations assess the pathology of the bowel. Rigid sigmoidoscopy is a quick, effective method of evaluating the rectum. However, a sig-nificant amount of pathology lies out of view of the rigid sigmoidoscope. Colonoscopy provides a good view of most of the colon and offers the

---

Box 8.6   Obstetric tears

- First degree: Vaginal mucosa
- Second degree: Vaginal fascia and perineum
- Third degree: External anal sphincter (EAS)
  (partial or
  complete)
- Fourth degree: EAS, internal anal sphincter (IAS)
  and rectal
  mucosa

Box 8.7   Case study

Emma, 27 years old, was referred to the continence clinic by her obstetrician/gynaecologist 6 months after the birth of her first child with symptoms of faecal urgency and poor perineal sensation, as well as occasional incontinence of flatus and faeces. She sustained a third degree tear during vaginal delivery, having given birth to a baby weighing 3.8 kg after a prolonged second stage of labour requiring the use of forceps for delivery. The referring letter also indicated that endoanal ultrasound showed scarring to the external anal sphincter; however, the internal anal sphincter was found to be normal. Faecal urgency and urge incontinence are generally related to dysfunction of the striated muscle tissue of the external anal sphincter.

All of the symptoms described are high risk indicators of subsequent pelvic floor dysfunction and indeed, on assessment, Emma indicated an unawareness of the need to evacuate her bowel until the rectum became very full, at which stage she experienced extreme urgency. Emma was very distressed, isolated and depressed about her symptoms and had curtailed her activities to a considerable degree since she feared embarrassing incontinence in a public place.

Conservative initial management included daily pelvic muscle and anal sphincter exercise together with a course of neuromuscular stimulation using a home unit borrowed from the clinic. Guidance on lifestyle, optimum fluid and fibre intake as well as general exercise was given. Since Emma's mood seemed low she agreed to see her GP again for advice on depression.

A bulking agent such as ispaghula husk was recommended in order to increase the volume of solid faeces in the rectum, thus alerting Emma to respond to the call to stool. However, a gradual increase in dietary fibre was suggested with the aim of avoiding an exacerbation of incontinence of gas. Support with regular review in the clinic was important in order to encourage Emma to persevere with her treatment plan.

On reassessment she reported some improvement. She found that taking ispaghula husk in the evening resulted in a full bowel action after breakfast next day and although faecal urgency was still acute in the morning she was free from concern about the risk of faecal incontinence for the remainder of the day. However, incontinence of flatus continued to cause embarrassment. She was prescribed antidepressants by her GP and her mood had lifted somewhat.

Nevertheless, Emma found that progress was slow and she agreed to a course of biofeedback, again using a home unit borrowed from the clinic, which would identify her pelvic muscle strength and show her if she was making any progress. Emma was more positive at her subsequent clinic visit and she was satisfied with the progress she had made. She was advised of other tests such as manometry and pudendal nerve terminal motor latency (PNTML). Emma is now due for a follow-up appointment with her obstetrician, who is likely to advise an elective caesarean section at subsequent births.

opportunity to perform a biopsy or remove polyps. The procedure takes about an hour and the patient requires sedation, whereas flexible sigmoidoscopy is quick and simple, taking less than 15 min and requires no sedation or analgesia. Specialist nurse practitioners trained in the procedure, using a thin flexible probe with a camera attached, are providing effective nurse-led clinics. Air or carbon dioxide is pumped into the bowel during sigmoidoscopy; this inflates the bowel, allowing a clearer picture of the bowel mucosa. The air inflation during sigmoidoscopy may reproduce a patient's abdominal pain, suggesting a diagnosis of irritable bowel disease.

A national bowel screening programme launched in April 2006 and phased across England in 3 years uses a dual approach which includes faecal occult blood (FOB) testing and flexible sigmoidoscopy (FOB testing is discussed later in the chapter). This programme is one of the first organised screening programmes for colorectal cancer in Europe. The government has set up seven regional and three national endoscopy training centres in anticipation of the extra demand that the screening programme will create (CancerHelp UK 2006).

Colonic transit time studies

Radiopaque markers are used to confirm slow transit time in those patients experiencing infrequent defecation. Three days prior to the procedure, all laxatives are stopped. Three different sets of markers, distinguishable radiologically by their shapes, are swallowed on each of the 3 days leading up to the procedure. A plain X-ray is taken 120 h after ingestion of the first set of markers and the number of retained markers of each 'shape' counted. The number of retained markers at each time interval (72, 96 and 120 h) is recorded. This simple test provides transit studies with the minimum of radiation exposure.

Manometry

As well as investigating the structure of the colon, its function may also need to be assessed. Manometric tests measure the effectiveness and strength of the anal sphincters, together with the degree of

sensation felt within the rectum. The test usually takes approximately 30 min and involves passing a soft plastic tube, which resembles a urinary catheter, into the rectum. When the balloon is distended, it will demonstrate the effectiveness of rectal contraction and expansion, relaxation of the internal anal sphincter and contraction of the external anal sphincter (the inhibitory and inflation reflexes). The individual will then be asked to pass the balloon out as if it were a stool, and the pressures are measured as the catheter is gradually pulled out.

Balloon capacity and compliance

This test evaluates how well the rectum expands and contracts in response to the entry of faeces. It usually takes approximately 45 min and involves the passing of a deflated balloon into the rectum, which is then inflated with air or water. The patient is asked to indicate when they first feel the balloon in the rectum, when the urge to defecate is felt and when further rectal distension can no longer be tolerated.

Balloon expulsion

This test evaluates the degree of puborectalis muscle relaxation during defecation. Relaxation of this muscle results in an increase in the anorectal angle (see Fig. 8.5), thereby allowing the easy passage of faecal contents from the rectum into the anal canal.

Electromyography

An electromyogram (EMG) records electrical activity within muscles. This test is used to identify and measure any pelvic floor muscle damage. Surface needle electrodes or an intra-anal plug are placed in selected areas of the external anal sphincter and puborectalis muscle. Electrical activity is measured when the muscle contracts. It can be an extremely uncomfortable test, but gives a good indication of whether or not pelvic floor damage is causing or contributing to a constipation problem.

Alternative ways of measuring the electrical activity which are less uncomfortable are by using surface adhesive electrodes or an anal probe. Some centres measure electrical activity continuously over a 24-h period, which gives an extremely reliable and detailed picture.

Faecal occult blood testing

Sudden changes in bowel habit or rectal bleeding may be possible indicators of colorectal cancer. In the UK colorectal cancer is the most common malignant cause of death after lung and breast cancer (NHS Executive 1997) and is a significant health problem throughout all the industrialised nations. It affects both women and men equally, with the prevalence increasing with age. There are 34 500 new cases of colorectal cancer in the UK each year. The incidence of colorectal cancer is escalating, with Scotland having one of the highest incidences in the world (Information and Statistical Division 2000).

What is clear is that early detection of colorectal cancer can be achieved through accurate FOB testing. The National Screening Committee has reviewed the evidence through the meta-analysis of FOB testing studies and found that if FOB testing was available for those aged 50 years or over a 15% reduction in mortality could be achieved (Hardcastle et al 1996, Kronborg et al 1996, Towler et al 1998).

April 2006 should have seen the roll-out of the government's promised national bowel screening programme using FOB tests for all those over 60 years of age. Unfortunately, this deadline was not achieved due to inadequate funding, reflecting the current financial crisis in the NHS. The future of the national screening programme was finally secured in May 2006 with the government agreeing to the financial commitment. However, there is a huge issue around capacity: in order to meet the demand for colonoscopies generated by positive FOB test screening, current waiting times in colonoscopy clinics will need to be reduced. The programme is costing £10 million to set up and aims for national coverage by 2009, by which time 2 million people a year will be receiving the results of their FOB tests through the post. The screening programme will prevent 15% of bowel cancer deaths per year. Currently the money has been agreed for the FOB tests but with little funding going into the upgrading of colonoscopy services. On a positive note, however, the first screening centre opened in Wolverhampton in July 2006 with another in Cambridgeshire to follow shortly.

COMPLEMENTARY THERAPIES

Complementary therapy is a term that covers a broad range of therapies which patients may choose to pursue as an alternative to, or alongside, conventional medical/health care. Amongst the most commonly used complementary therapies are herbalism, acupuncture, aromatherapy and reflexology. In recent years there has been a significant increase in the use of complementary therapies in the UK, with some services (e.g. acupuncture and aromatherapy) now available through the NHS. A number of complementary therapies can be used when caring for patients with bowel problems, but there is little or no research evidence to demonstrate their effectiveness or explain the mechanism through which they may work. The more popular of the complementary therapies employed in management of bowel disorders are discussed below.

Massage and aromatherapy

Massage and aromatherapy have a long and ancient history within medicine, reaching a peak in the late nineteenth and early twentieth century, yet by 1950 the therapies had all but disappeared. Massage and aromatherapy have undergone a revival in clinical practice, particularly within the palliative care, oncology and hospice environments. Abdominal massage, also referred to as bowel or colonic massage, is acknowledged by practitioners to be an effective management option for constipation with the added advantage that it is perceived by most patients as relaxing and giving relief from 'trapped wind' – yet it remains an unproven intervention.

A systematic review of clinical trials into the efficacy of abdominal massage suggests that there are methodological flaws in the existing research, giving rise to calls for more rigorous studies (Ernst 1999). Patients and carers can easily be taught the technique of abdominal massage so that it can be carried out at home. All abdominal massages follow the line of the bowel and the flow of faecal matter in a clockwise circular movement starting at the ascending colon and finishing at the sigmoid colon, avoiding any pressure over the bladder. However, the published data are insufficient to give clear recommendations on the type, intensity and timing of the massage that is most efficacious to the patient. To make an abdominal massage more comfortable, a non-perfumed base oil is used.

Aromatherapy with massage combines the use of essential oils with the massage. Recommended essential oils for abdominal massage are, at a dilution of 1%, Black Pepper (*Piper nigrum*), Roman Chamomile (*Anthemis nobilis*) and Peppermint (*Mentha piperita*) (Preece 2002). Only a qualified aromatherapist should use these oils.

Acupuncture

Acupuncture is an ancient Chinese healing art developed some four to six thousand years ago. It is based on the principle that a 'balance of energy' maintains health. Fine adjustments may be made to the energy potential of bodily organs in order to improve and maintain the body's equilibrium. Acupuncture treatment consists of inserting small sterile needles into certain points, located along identified meridians or energy pathways. The needle acts as a central point through which energy may enter and leave the body, resulting in a subtle adjustment to the energy potential of such a point.

Acupuncture of points both close to the organ requiring treatment, and of points further away, forms the basis of treatment. Points located in the hand and arm are used to treat conditions of the large intestine. Klauser et al (1993) found that acupuncture performed on patients did not significantly affect either stool frequency or bowel transit time when compared with the control group and further research is needed.

Reflexology

Reflexology has been practised for thousands of years in India, China and Egypt, but was only introduced into the West early in the twentieth century. In reflexology the body is divided vertically into 10 different sectors or zones, which extend into the feet and hands. Pressure applied to these zones on the feet or hands is said to stimulate the vital organs in the appropriate sector, by improving the blood and nerve supply and removing uric acid and calcium deposits from nerve endings.

Although pressure zones differ in individuals, it is generally agreed that pressure applied to the outer, fleshy area at the very base of the thumb corresponds to the large colon in hand reflexology. In foot reflexology the arch of the foot corresponds to the large colon, and pressure applied to the heel of the foot is used to treat haemorrhoids. A single-blind study by Tovey (2002) used a reflexology foot massage as the intervention and a non-reflexology foot massage for the control group. The study measured the efficacy of reflexology on the symptoms of abdominal pain, constipation/diarrhoea and abdominal distension in patients suffering with IBS. The results failed to identify any specific benefit for patients with IBS who received reflexology.

On a more positive note, an observational study using reflexology to treat encopresis and constipation in children aged between 3 and 14 years concluded that bowel motions increased and the incidence of soiling decreased (Bishop et al 2003). However, these results should be viewed with some caution as the parents completed the questionnaires and it may be that their involvement in the project made them more aware of their child's needs.

Further research is required to determine the effectiveness of reflexology in the management of bowel disorders.

Herbalism

Herbalism is an ancient form of treatment which seems to be returning to popularity in the Western world, at least partially as a result of increasing interest in 'ecofriendly' ideals. The use of plant extracts and plant-derived medications is generally promoted to help support the body to stimulate its own natural defences, and help in the recovery process, rather than to attack a disease process directly. Linseed is a product of the flax plant and available in most health food shops. A tablespoon of linseeds, soaked overnight, may be sprinkled over food and added to soups and stews; it then acts as a gentle, bulk-forming laxative. As with other complementary approaches to bowel management, the research on linseed is very much in its infancy and further research is needed.

Probiotics

Probiotics are now available in most supermarkets and regularly advertised in the media. A probiotic is a live microbial food supplement, which benefits the body by improving the microbial balance and may help in the treatment of bowel disorders that present with disturbed intestinal bacteria and increased gut permeability. Successful probiotic bacteria are able to survive gastric conditions and colonise in the bowel, at least temporarily, by adhering to the bowel wall. Research into the efficacy of probiotics is still at a relatively early stage but it is thought that probiotics have an anti-inflammatory effect. Potential mechanisms for this anti-inflammatory action are through the production of antimicrobial metabolites, or possibly through their DNA interacting with the bowel epithelium. It is suggested that probiotics may offer a simple adjunct to conventional treatments of inflammatory bowel disease (Shanahan 2000).

CONCLUSIONS

There are multiple factors that may contribute to bowel dysfunction and since conditions such as faecal incontinence have a profound effect on individuals, their families and carers, every opportunity should be taken to prevent problems developing in the first place. Preservation of the pelvic floor musculature and pudendal nerve supply at parturition is extremely important, together with competent and thorough assessment and early intervention should damage present or be suspected. Health professionals need to be proactive in spreading information to patients and the general population about healthy lifestyles, healthy eating and exercise.

A predominant theme emerging from the literature reviewed in this chapter is the importance of assessing patients to identify those who might be at risk of developing constipation (Campbell et al 2001, Richmond 2003, Richmond & Wright 2004). This is further endorsed by Potter et al (2002) who state that the identification of risk factors for constipation in elderly patients is critical to achieving effective management of constipation. Currently there is no effective way of measuring or calculating the risk factors to give an accurate prediction of the risk a patient has of developing constipation. There is certainly scope for the development of such a risk assessment tool but nurses will need to continue to develop a proactive and evidence-based approach to the management of this distressing symptom.

The National Institute for Health and Clinical Excellence (NICE) is preparing a Guideline on the management of faecal incontinence which is due to be published in the summer of 2007.

KEY POINTS FOR PRACTICE

The old aviators' expression 'chocks away!' refers to the removal of small wooden wedges from the wheels of an aeroplane so that it is able to take off. Using this as a basis, here is a final reminder of some of the points made in the chapter.

- Constipation is a symptom identified as the passing of fewer than three stools per week, or excessive straining when having the bowel open.
- Hormonal changes may cause constipation.
- Other causes of constipation may be related to diet, mobility, environment, medication and neurological conditions.
- Constipation in the elderly may be controlled by diet, exercise, toileting after meals, and the administration of suppositories or microenemas if necessary.
- Keep a record of dietary fibre intake as care should be taken when recommending such diets for the elderly and/or the immobile patient.
- Successful treatment depends on accurate diagnosis, as constipation is a symptom not a disease.

- **A**re you sitting comfortably? Correct posture can help to make defecation less strenuous.
- **W**hen administering a laxative, consider the diagnosis and ensure the laxative is appropriate.
- **A**lternatives? Complementary therapies such as acupuncture, herbalism, homeopathy and reflexology have been with us for centuries.

- **Y**es! You can help your patient as 'The size of a deed is measured not so much by its effort, as by its impact' (Lenzkes 1987).

The call of the old aviator to remove a simple obstacle may well be all that is required to set the wheels (or bowels!) in motion.

References

Abd-El-Maeboud K H, El-Naggar T, El-Hawi E M M et al 1991 Rectal suppository: commonsense and mode of insertion. Lancet 338(8770):798–803

Abrams P, Cardozo L, Khoury, Wein A (eds) 2002 Incontinence, 2nd edn. Health Publication, Plymouth, p 985–1044

Abrams W B, Beers M H, Berkow M D 1995 Organ systems: gastrointestinal disorders. The Merck Manual of Geriatrics. Merck Research Laboratories, New Jersey

Addison R 1996 The last resort. Journal of Community Nursing 10(8):18–20

Addison R, Davies C, Haslam D et al 2003 A national audit of chronic constipation in the community. Nursing Times 99(11):34–35

Ahrens T, Prentice D 1998 Critical care certification: preparation, review and practice exams, 4th edn. Appleton & Lange, Stamford, CT

Alessi C A, Henderson C T 1988 Constipation and faecal impaction in the long term care patient. Clinics in Geriatric Medicine 4(3):571–588

American College of Gastroenterology Chronic Constipation Task Force 2005 An evidence-based approach to the management of chronic constipation in North America. American Journal of Gastroenterology 100(supplement 1):1–4

Attar A, Lemann M, Ferguson A et al 1999 Comparison of a low dose polyethylene glycol electrolyte solution with lactulose for treatment of chronic constipation. Gut 44:226–230

Bayliss V, Cherry M, Locke R et al 2000 Pathways for continence care: background and audit. British Journal of Nursing 9(9):590–596

Bennett N, Dodd T, Flatley J et al 1995 Health survey for England. HMSO, London

Bishop E, McKinnon E, Weir E et al 2003 Reflexology in the management of encopresis and chronic constipation. Paediatric Nursing 15(3):20–21

Bradley M 1996 Caring for older people: elder abuse. British Medical Journal 313:548–550

Bradshaw A, Price L 2007 Rectal suppository insertion: the reliability of the evidence as a basis for nursing practice. Journal of Clinical Nursing 16(1):98–103

British National Formulary 2005 British Medical Association, London

Brown S R, Cann P A, Read N W 1990 Effect of coffee on distal colonic function. Gut 31:450–453

Bulmer F 2000 Bowel preparation for rectal and colonic investigation. Nursing Standard 14(20):32–35

Burkitt D P, Walker A R P, Painter N S 1972 Effect of dietary fibre on stools and transit times, and its role in causation of disease. Lancet ii:1408–1411

Campbell A J, Busby W J, Horwath C C 1993 Factors associated with constipation in a community based sample of people aged 70 years and over. Journal of Epidemiology and Community Health 47:23–26

Campbell T, Draper S, Reid J, Robinson L 2001 The management of constipation in people with advanced cancer. International Journal of Palliative Nursing 79(3):110–119

CancerHelp UK 2006 About bowel cancer screening. Cancer Research UK. Online. Available: http://www.cancerhelp.org.uk

Chelvanayagam S, Norton C 1999 Causes and assessment of faecal incontinence. British Journal of Community Nursing 4(1):28–35

Chung B D, Parekd U, Sellin J H 1999 Effect of increased fluid intake on stool output in normal healthy volunteers. Journal of Gastroenterology 28(1):29–32

Cope K 1996 Malnutrition in the elderly: A national crisis. Publication No. 017062-00147-2. Cited in: Sheehy C, Richards-Hall G 1998 Rethinking the obvious: a model for preventing constipation. Journal of Gerontological Nursing 24(3):38–44

Corazziari E, Badiali D, Bazzocchi G et al 2000 Long term efficacy, safety and tolerability of low daily doses of isosmotic polyethylene glycol electrolyte balanced solution (PMF-100) in the treatment of functional chronic constipation. Gut 46(4):522–526

CORE 2005a What is irritable bowel syndrome? CORE, London. Online. Available: www.corecharity.org.uk

CORE 2005b What is coeliac disease? CORE, London. Online. Available: www.corecharity.org.uk

Crotty R 2003 When histories collide. Connolly Publications, London

Cummings J H 1984 Constipation, dietary fibre and the control of large bowel function. Postgraduate Medical Journal 60:811–819

Davies C 2004 The use of phosphate enemas in the treatment of constipation. Nursing Times 100(18):32–34

Department of Health 2000a Good practice in continence services. DH, London

Department of Health 2000b No secrets. DH, London

Department of Health 2001 Reference guide to consent for examination or treatment. DH, London

De Schryver A M, Keulemans Y C, Peters H P et al 2005 Effects of regular physical activity on defecation pattern in middle-aged patients complaining of chronic constipation. Scandinavian Journal of Gastroenterology 40:422–429

Dietz H P, Wilson P D 2005 Childbirth and pelvic floor trauma. Best Practice and Research, Clinical Obstetrics and Gynaecology 19(6):913–924

Dresden K A, Kratzer G L 1959 Sites and frequency of faecal impactions. Journal of the American Medical Association 170:644–647

Eogan M, Daly L, O'Connell P R et al 2006 Does the angle of episiotomy affect the incidence of anal sphincter injury? British Journal of Obstetrics and Gynaecology 113(2):190–194

Ernst E 1999 Abdominal massage therapy for chronic constipation: a systematic review of controlled trials. Forschende Komplementärmedizin 6(3):149–151

Fallon M, O'Neill B 1997 ABC of palliative care. Constipation and diarrhoea. British Medical Journal 315:1293–1296

Fitzpatrick M, O'Herlihy C 2005 Short-term and long-term effects of obstetric anal sphincter injury and their management. Current Opinion in Obstetrics and Gynaecology 17(6):605–610

Fynes M, Marshall K, Cassidy M et al 1999 A prospective randomised study comparing the effect of augmented biofeedback with sensory biofeedback alone on faecal incontinence after obstetric trauma. Diseases of the Colon and Rectum 42(6):753–761

Glia A, Lindberg G 1997 Quality of life in patients with different types of functional constipation. Scandinavian Journal of Gastroenterology 32(11):1083–1089

Grandjean A C, Reimers K J, Buyckx M E 2003 Hydration: issues for the 21st century. Nutrition Reviews 61(8):261–273

Grundy D, Swain A 1996 ABC of spinal injury, 3rd edn. BMJ Publishing, London

Harari D 2004 Bowel care in old age. In: Norton C, Chelvanayagam S (eds) Bowel continence nursing. Beaconsfield Publishers, Beaconsfield

Harari D, Gurwitz J H, Avorn J et al 1996 Bowel habit in relation to age and gender: findings from the National Health Interview Survey and Clinical Implications. Archives of Internal Medicine 156:315–319

Hardcastle J D, Chamberlain J O, Robinson M H et al 1996 Randomised controlled trial of faecal occult blood screening for colorectal cancer. Lancet 348:1472–1477

Heaton K W, Radvan J, Cripps H et al 1992 Defecation frequency and timing, and stoolform in the general population: a prospective study. Gut 33:818–824

Higgins P D, Johanson J F 2004 Epidemiology of constipation in North America. American Journal of Gastroenterology 99(4):750–759

Hoffman N B 1991 Dehydration in the elderly: insidious and manageable. Geriatrics 46(6):33–38

Hojgaard L, Arffmann S, Jorgensen M et al 1981 Tea consumption: A cause of constipation? British Journal of Medicine 282:864

Huether S E, McCane K L 2004 Understanding pathophysiology, 3rd edn. Mosby, St Louis

Information and Statistical Division 2000 Trends in cancer survival in Scotland, 1971–1995. Information and Statistical Division, Edinburgh

Jacobs E J, White E 1998 Constipation, laxative use and colon cancer among middle aged adults. Epidemiology 9(4):385

Kamm M A 1994 Constipation. Medicine International 22(8):305–308

Kenefick N 2004 The epidemiology of faecal incontinence. In: Norton C, Chelvanayagam S (eds) Bowel continence nursing. Beaconsfield Publishers, Beaconsfield

Kinnunen O 1991 Study of constipation in a geriatric hospital, day hospital, old people's home and at home. Ageing 3(2):161–170

Klauser A G, Beck A, Schindlbeck N E et al 1990 Low fluid intake lowers stool output in healthy male volunteers. Zeitschrift für Gastroenterologie 28:606–609

Klauser A G, Rubach A, Bertsche O et al 1993 Body acupuncture: effect on colonic function in chronic constipation. Zeitschrift für Gastroenterologie 31(10):605–608

Kronborg O, Fenger C, Olsen J, Jørgensen O D, Søndergaard O 1996 Randomised study of screening for colorectal cancer with faecal occult blood test. Lancet 348(9040):1467–1471

Kyle G, Prynn P, Oliver H 2005 A procedure for the digital removal of faeces. Nursing Standard 19(20):33–39

Leech K, McDonnell J 1999 Food, fluid and fibre. New Possibilities NHS Trust, Colchester. Cited in: Morrison C 2000 Helping patients to maintain a healthy fluid balance. NTplus Continence Supplement 96(31):3–4

Lenzkes SL 1987 A silver pen for cloudy days. Zonder van Publishing, Michigan, USA

Lukeman D 2003 Mainly children: childhood enuresis and encopresis. In: Getliffe K, Dolman M (eds) Promoting continence: a clinical research resource, 2nd edn. Baillière Tindall, Edinburgh

MacArthur C, Bick D E, Keighley M R 1997 Faecal incontinence after childbirth. British Journal of Obstetrics and Gynaecology 104:46–50

Madden J A J, Hunter J O 2002 A review of the role of the gut microflora in irritable bowel syndrome and the effects of probiotics. British Journal of Nutrition 88(1):67–76

Madoff R D, Parker S C, Varma M G et al 2004 Faecal incontinence in adults. Lancet 364:621–632

Maestri-Banks M, Burns D 1996 Assessing constipation. Nursing Times 92:28–31

Mallet J, Dougherty L 2005 Bowel care. In: Royal Marsden Hospital manual of clinical nursing procedures, 6th edn. Blackwell Scientific, London, p 296

Menter R, Weitzenkamp D, Cooper D et al 1997 Bowel management outcomes in individuals with long-term spinal cord injuries. Spinal Cord 35:608–612

Moriarty K J, Irving M H 1992 Constipation. British Medical Journal 304:1237–1240

Morrison C 2000 Helping patients to maintain a healthy fluid balance. NTplus Continence Supplement 96(31):3–4

Nair P, Mayberry J F 1994 Vegetarianism, dietary fibre and gastro-intestinal disease. Digestive Diseases 12:177–185

National Health Service Centre for Reviews and Dissemination 2001 Effectiveness of laxatives in adults. Effective Health Care 7:1

National Health Service Executive 1997 Improving outcomes in colorectal cancer. The manual. DH, London

National Patient Safety Agency 2004 Patient briefing: ensuring the appropriate provision of manual bowel evacuation for patients with an established spinal cord lesion. DH, London

National Prescribing Centre 2004 The management of constipation. MeReC Bulletin 14(6). Online. Available: http://www.npc.co.uk/MeReC_Bulletins/2003Volumes/Vol14no6.pdf

Norton C 1996a Nursing for continence. Beaconsfield Publishers, Beaconsfield

Norton C 1996b Faecal incontinence in adults. 1: Prevalence and causes. British Journal of Nursing 5(22):1367–1374

Norton C, Christiansen J, Butler U et al 2002 Anal incontinence. In: Abrams P, Cardozo L, Khoury S, Wein A (eds) Incontinence. 2nd International Consultation on Incontinence. Health Publication, London

Norton C, Chelvanayagam S (eds) 2004 Bowel continence nursing. Beaconsfield Publishers, Beaconsfield

Norton C, Whitehead W E, Bliss D Z et al 2005 Conservative and pharmacological management of faecal incontinence in adults. In: Abrams P, Cardozo L, Khoury S, Wein A (eds) Incontinence, vol 2. 3rd International Consultation on Incontinence. Health Publication, Paris

Nursing and Midwifery Council 2002 Code of professional conduct. NMC, London

Patrick J, Culligan J A, Myers R P et al 2005 Elective caesarean section to prevent anal incontinence and brachial plexus injuries associated with macrosomia – a decision analysis. International Urogynaecology Journal 16:19–28

Perry S, Shaw C, McGrother C 2002 Prevalence of faecal incontinence in adults aged 40 or more living in the community. The Leicestershire MRC Incontinence Study Team. Gut 50:480–484

Petticrew M, Watt I, Sheldon T 1997 Systematic review of the effectiveness of laxatives in the elderly. Health Technology Assessment 1:13

Petticrew M, Rodgers M, Booth A 2001 Effectiveness of laxatives in adults. Quality in Health Care 10(4):268–273

Pollack J, Nordenstam J, Brismar S et al 2004 Anal incontinence after vaginal delivery: a five year prospective cohort study. Obstetrics and Gynaecology 104:1397–1402

Popovich J M, Stewart-Amidei C 1991 Alterations in elimination. In: Bronstein K S (ed) Promoting stroke recovery. Mosby-Year Book, St Louis

Potter J M, Norton C, Cottenden A (eds) 2002 Bowel care in older people: research and practice. Royal College of Physicians, London

Powell M, Rigby D 2000 Management of bowel dysfunction: evacuation difficulties. Nursing Standard 14(4):47–51

Preece J 2002 Introducing abdominal massage in palliative care for the relief of constipation. Complementary Therapies in Nursing and Midwifery 5:101–105

Prodigy Guidance 2004 Practical support for clinical governance – constipation. Online. Available: http://www.prodigy.nhs.uk/constipation

Read N W, Celik A F, Katsinelos P 1995 Constipation and incontinence in the elderly. Journal of Clinical Gastroenterology 20(1):61–69

Reedy D F 1988 How can you prevent dehydration? Geriatric Nursing 9(4):224–226

Richards-Hall G, Rakel B, Karstens M et al 1995 Managing constipation using a research protocol. MEDSURG Nursing 4(1):11–21

Richmond J P 2003 Prevention of constipation through risk management. Nursing Standard 17(16):39–46

Richmond J P, Wright M E 2004 Review of the literature on constipation to enable development of a constipation risk assessment tool. Clinical Effectiveness in Nursing 8:11–25

Rodriguez L A G, Ruigomez A 1999 Increased risk of irritable bowel syndrome after bacterial gastroenteritis: cohort study. British Medical Journal 315:565–566

Romero Y, Evans J M, Fleming K C et al 1996 Constipation and faecal incontinence in the elderly population. Mayo Clinic Proceedings 71:81–92

Ross D G 1995 Altered bowel elimination patterns among hospitalised elderly and middle-aged persons: quantitative results. Orthopaedic Nursing 14(1):25–31

Ross H 1998 Constipation: cause and control in an acute hospital setting. British Journal of Nursing 7(15):907–913

Royal College of Nursing 2000 Digital rectal examination and manual removal of faeces: guidance for nurses. RCN, London

Royal College of Physicians 1995 Report of a working party. Incontinence – causes, management and provision of services. RCP, London

Sartor R B 1997 Enteric microflora in IBD: pathogens or commensals? Inflammatory Bowel Disorders 3:230–235

Shafik A 1993 Constipation. Pathogenesis and management. Drugs 45(4):528–540

Shanahan F 2000 Probiotics and inflammatory bowel disease: is there a scientific rationale? Inflammatory Bowel Disorders 6:107–115

Sheehy C, Richards-Hall G 1998 Rethinking the obvious: a model for preventing constipation. Journal of Gerontological Nursing 24(3):38–44

Signorello L B, Repke J 2000 Midline episiotomy and anal incontinence: retrospective cohort study. British Medical Journal 320:86–90

Smith R G, Lewis S 1990 The relationship between digital rectal examination and abdominal radiographs in elderly patients. Age and Ageing 19:142–143

Spiller R 1990 Management of constipation, when fibre fails. British Medical Journal 300:1064–1065

Sullivan A 1999 Hydration for nurses. Nursing Standard 14(8):44–46

Sultan A H, Stanton S L 1996 Preserving the pelvic floor and perineum during childbirth – elective caesarean section. American Journal of Obstetrics and Gynecology 174:192–198

Swidsinski A, Ladhoff A, Pernthaler A et al 2002 Mucosal flora in inflammatory bowel disease. Gastroenterology 22(1):44–54

Talley N J, Fleming K C, Evans J M et al 1996 Constipation in an elderly community: a study of prevalence and potential risk factors. American Journal of Gastroenterology 91(1):19–25

Taskin O, Wheeler J M, Yalcinoglu A I 1996 The effects of episiotomy and Kegal exercises on postpartum pelvic relaxation: a prospective controlled study. Journal of Gynaecological Surgery 12:123–127

Taylor R 1990 Management of constipation. British Medical Journal 300:1063–1064

Thibodeau G A, Patton K T 1993 Anatomy and physiology, 2nd edn. Mosby, St Louis

Thomas G A, Rhodes J, Green J T et al 2000 Role of smoking in inflammatory bowel disease: implications for therapy. Postgraduate Medical Journal 76(895):273–279

Thomas P D, Forbes A, Green J 2003 Guidelines for the investigation of chronic diarrhoea, 2nd edn. BMJ Publishing Group and British Society of Gastroenterology. Gut Supplement V:1–5

Thompson W G, Longstreth G F, Drossman D A et al 1999 Functional bowel disorders and functional abdominal pain. Gut 45:1143–1147

Tovey P 2002 A single-blind trial of reflexology for irritable bowel syndrome. British Journal of General Practice 52(474):19–25

Towers A L, Burgio K L, Locher J L et al 1994 Constipation in the elderly: influence of dietary, psychological and physiological factors. Journal of the American Geriatric Society 42:701–706

Towler B P, Irwig L, Glasziou P et al 1998 A systematic review of the effects of screening for colorectal cancer using faecal occult blood test, hemoccult. British Medical Journal 317(7158):559–565

Tramonte S M, Brand M B, Mulrow C D et al 1997 The treatment of chronic constipation in adults. Journal of General Internal Medicine 12:15–24

Walker J A 2002 Spinal cord injury – autonomic dysreflexia. Professional Nurse 17(9):519–520

Walton J C, Miller J M 1998 Evaluating physical and behavioural changes in older adults. MEDSURG Nursing 7(2):85–89

Weeks S K, Hubbard E, Michaels T K 2000 Key to bowel success. Rehabilitation Nursing 25(2):66–99

Willis J 2000 Bowel management and consent. Nursing Times Plus 96(6):7–8

Zetterstrom J, Lopez A, Anzen B 1999 Anal sphincter tears at vaginal delivery: risk factors and clinical outcome of primary repair. Obstetrics and Gynaecology 94:21–28

Chapter 9

Medication for continence

Deborah Rigby

CHAPTER CONTENTS

Principiis obsta: sero medicina paratur cum mala per longas convaluere mortas. Stop it at the start: it's late for medicine to be prepared when disease has grown strong through long delays.

Ovid, 43 BC to AD 17

INTRODUCTION

It is estimated that over 50 million people in the developed world are affected by urinary and faecal incontinence (Andersson et al 2005) but the development of pharmacological treatment for the different forms of incontinence has been considered slow (Wein & Rovner 2002). There is a wide choice of drugs used to treat bladder and bowel problems but the research is often difficult to compare due to the nature and methodology of the studies. Andersson et al (2005) state that while there is an abundance of drugs, for many of them clinical use is based on the results of preliminary open studies rather than randomised controlled clinical trials. In many studies there have been such high levels of placebo effect that meaningful differences between placebo and active drug are difficult to determine. Nevertheless, drug therapy can be effective, although in some cases patients choose to discontinue their prescribed medication because of unacceptable side effects. It is suggested that drug therapy may be best used as adjunctive therapy to other conservative treatments (discussed in preceding chapters).

Box 9.1   Medication for continence –
summary of common bladder and bowel
problems

- Overactive bladder
- Stress urinary incontinence
- Nocturia
- Nocturnal enuresis
- Underactive bladder
- Bowel management
- Faecal incontinence

This chapter examines the medication options which may be appropriate for the range of bladder and bowel problems indicated in Box 9.1. It then goes on to look at medications which may cause bladder and bowel symptoms and finally discusses the introduction and practical aspects of nurse prescribing. The focus in this chapter is on medications for urinary incontinence (UI) and retention. Medications for bowel care are considered here briefly but are addressed in greater detail in Chapter 8.

MEDICATION TO TREAT THE OVERACTIVE BLADDER

Contraction of the detrusor and relaxation of the outflow region of the bladder and lower urinary tract result from the release of acetylcholine during activation of parasympathetic nerves (see Ch. 2). Anticholinergic agents are the most widely prescribed medications for treatment for overactive bladder and UI (Chapple et al 2002). They work by depressing both voluntary and involuntary detrusor contractions by blocking the muscarinic receptors for acetylcholine on bladder smooth muscle (Fig. 9.1) and therefore reducing feelings of urgency and frequency. Because their action is at receptor level they exert their effect regardless of how the efferent (motor) part of the micturition reflex is activated (Keane & O'Sullivan 2000). Antimuscarinic drugs will also lower intravesical pressure, increase bladder capacity and reduce the frequency of bladder contraction.

Normal bladder contraction is mediated mainly through stimulation of the muscarinic receptors in the detrusor muscle. Five subtypes of muscarinic receptors (M_1–M_5) have been identified using gene cloning techniques. Like most other smooth muscles the bladder contains a mixed population of M_2 (80%) and M_3 (20%) muscarinic receptors. There is general agreement that M_3 receptors are mainly responsible for the contractile response in normal micturition but there is some evidence that M_2 receptors and beta$_3$ adrenergic receptors may also have a role in active relaxation of the detrusor. Muscarinic receptor function may change in different urological disorders such as outflow obstruction, neurogenic bladder dysfunction and diabetes but it is not always clear what this means in terms of detrusor function (Andersson et al 2005). Generally, antimuscarinics can be divided into tertiary and quaternary amines; are well absorbed from the gastrointestinal system; and should be able to pass into the central nervous system, depending on their specific physicochemical properties (Andersson et al 2005).

Although antimuscarinics are commonly used, they lack selectivity for the bladder and their side effects on other organs limit their usefulness. The side effect profile includes dry mouth due to the inhibition of salivary secretion, blurring of near vision (cycloplegia), tachycardia and inhibition of gut motility leading to constipation. All antimuscarinic drugs are contraindicated in narrow-angle glaucoma. Since bladder contractility is decreased and the bladder sphincter smooth muscle tone increased, urinary retention may be a further unwanted side effect. One way to avoid many of the side effects is to administer the drug intravesically (instilled directly into the bladder) although this is only practical for a small number of patients.

The detrusor cell membrane also has a very high density of calcium (Ca^{2+}) channels and detrusor contraction seems to require an influx of extracellular Ca^{2+} through these channels. The significance of this is that there is a potential role for the regulation of entry of Ca^{2+} via the Ca^{2+} channels to manipulate detrusor contractility. Similarly, potassium (K^+) channels have been shown in early research studies to calm detrusor activity because opening the K^+ channels leads to a decrease in Ca^{2+} by reducing the opening probability of the Ca^{2+} channels. This leads to a

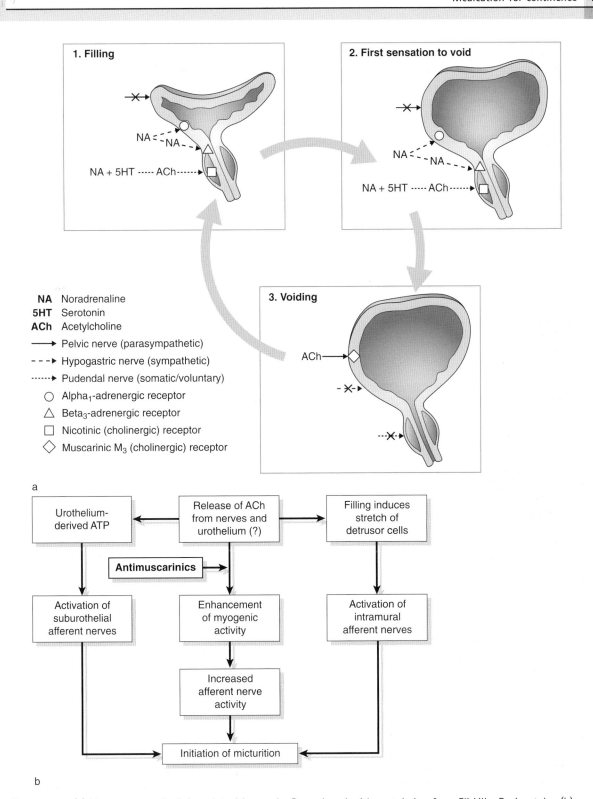

Figure 9.1   (a) Nervous control of the micturition cycle. Reproduced with permission from Eli Lilly, Basingstoke. (b) Effects of antimuscarinic drugs on bladder function. 5HT, serotonin, ACh, acetylcholine; ATP, adenosine triphosphate; NA, noradrenaline.

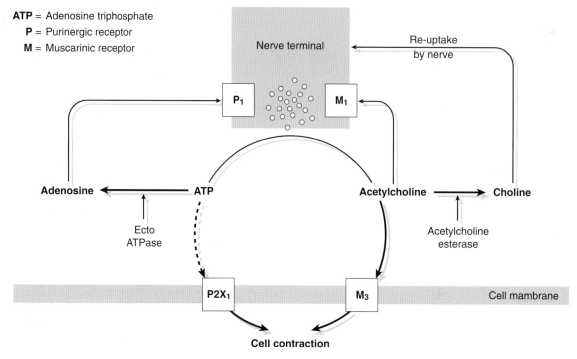

ATP = Adenosine triphosphate
P = Purinergic receptor
M = Muscarinic receptor

Nerve terminal

Re-uptake
by nerve

P_1 M_1

Adenosine ← ATP   Acetylcholine → Choline

Ecto
ATPase

Acetylcholine
esterase

$P2X_1$ M_3 Cell mambrane

Cell contraction

Figure 9.2   Contraction of detrusor muscle cell. ATP, adenosine triphosphate; M, muscarinic receptor; P_1, purinergic receptor.

relaxation of the contraction (Fig. 9.2). However, at this point in time, systemic therapy with Ca^{2+} antagonists or K^+ channel openers does not seem to represent an effective treatment for overactive bladder.

Antimuscarinic drugs with bladder specificity

Tolterodine   (Detrusitol, Detrusitol XL) is a non-selective, antimuscarinic, competitive antagonist with some functional selectivity for the bladder over the salivary glands. This may explain why there is a lower incidence of dry mouth and reduction in withdrawal rate. Tolterodine is available as immediate release (IR; 1 or 2 mg, twice daily) and extended release forms (ER; 2 or 4 mg, once daily). The ER form seems to have some advantages over the IR form in terms of both efficacy and tolerability (Van Kerrebroeck et al 2001).

Trospium   (Regurin) is an antimuscarinic derived from atropine (quaternary ammonium compound). It has no selectivity for muscarinic receptor subtypes and has a very low bioavailability of 5%. It

can achieve therapeutic levels within one week and has been shown to cause reduced cognitive problems compared with other antimuscarinics. It is a well-documented alternative for treatment of overactive bladder (OAB) and seems to be well tolerated. Usual dose is 20 mg twice daily.

Solifenacin   (Vesicare) is the latest in this group of drugs to come onto the UK market. It is a long-acting muscarinic receptor antagonist developed for the treatment of OAB. There is good evidence of effectiveness of 5 mg and 10 mg single doses per day.

Darafenacin   (Emselex) is a selective muscarinic M_3 receptor antagonist and has no detectable effects on cognitive or cardiovascular function. It has been developed as a controlled-release formulation, which means it can be taken once daily. Recommended doses are 7.5 or 15 mg once daily.

Atropine
is rarely used for treatment of OAB because of its systemic side effects which preclude its use. However, it may have a role in intravesical use in patients with neurological detrusor overactivity

for increasing bladder capacity (Enskat et al 2001).

Drugs with 'mixed' action

Some drugs block bladder overactivity by more than one mechanism. They all have some antimuscarinic activity but in addition often have some less specific action on the detrusor muscle which may mean they are effective at lower doses.

Oxybutynin (Ditropan, Cystrin) is the most commonly prescribed treatment in the UK for OAB. It is both antimuscarinic and a direct muscle relaxant. It also has some anaesthetic effect which may be useful when administered intravesically although this is unlikely to play a role when given orally. As a tertiary amine it is well absorbed but undergoes extensive upper gastrointestinal and first-pass hepatic metabolism via the cytochrome P450 system into multiple metabolites. The chief metabolite of oxybutynin (N-desethyloxybutynin; DEO) is also pharmacologically active and is thought to be responsible for the main adverse effect of this drug – troublesome dry mouth. The IR form is recognised for its efficacy and newer antimuscarinic agents are all compared to it. The standard recommended dose is 5 mg three or four times a day; however, a starting dose of 2.5 mg twice daily followed by dose titration is often advised to reduce the side effects.

Oxybutynin extended release (Lyrinel XL) was developed to decrease metabolite formation on the assumption that this would reduce the side effects and improve patient compliance. Dose is 10 mg once daily.

Oxybutynin transdermal patch (Kentera) is a transdermal treatment, used with a twice-weekly dosing schedule. The patch releases a dose of 3.9 mg of oxybutynin in 24 h, bypassing the gut wall metabolism (and release of DEO) with potentially increased therapeutic levels and reduced side effects. Application site pruritus and erythema have been reported in less than 15% of users but this can be a reason for lack of compliance.

Propiverine (Detrunorm) has combined antimuscarinic and calcium channel blocking activity. Twenty per cent of patients on propiverine report adverse side effects, which are mainly anticholinergic in nature. Propiverine is rapidly absorbed but has a high first-pass metabolism. A dose of 15 mg three times a day has been shown to have some beneficial effects for OAB with an acceptable side effect profile.

Flavoxate (Urispas) is an antimuscarinic in which the main mode of action on smooth muscle has not been established. Flavoxate has been found to have moderate calcium antagonist activity but no anticholinergic activity. Although few side effects have been reported, efficacy is not well established compared with placebo or other therapeutic alternatives.

Summary of guidance on medication for OAB

- Antimuscarinic therapy should be tried for a period of 6 weeks to enable an assessment of benefits and side effects. Treatment should be reviewed after 6 months to ascertain continuing need (SIGN 2004).
- Treatment with non-proprietary oxybutynin should be offered as first-line antimuscarinic drug treatment to women with OAB or mixed UI.
- If oxybutynin is not well tolerated, solifenacin, tolterodine or trospium may be considered as alternatives. Women should be counselled regarding the side effects of antimuscarinic drugs.
- Flavoxate, propantheline and imipramine should not be used for the treatment of OAB or UI in women.
- Propiverine may be used to treat frequency in women with OAB, but cannot be recommended for the treatment of UI (NICE 2006).

Drugs acting on membrane channels

Although membrane channels offer a theoretical target for pharmacological intervention, available evidence does not support systemic therapy with calcium agonists or potassium channel openers as effective treatment for OAB.

Other agents

Chilli derivatives

Studies are ongoing to investigate the role of capsaicin and resiniferatoxin in the unstable bladder (see also Ch. 6). Published research on the outcomes of bladder instillations with capsaicin by De Ridder et al (1997) showed that repeated instillations were effective in the treatment of OAB: a single treatment was shown to last 3–6 months with 80% of patients reporting a benefit. The treatment has not become widely available because it does not have a recognised licence for bladder instillation.

Botulinum A toxin (Botox) is a potent neurotoxin which can be injected directly into the detrusor muscle (see Ch. 6). The toxin acts by inhibiting acetylcholine release at the presynaptic cholinergic junction, causing muscle weakness and decreased contractility at the site of the injection. The chemical denervation that occurs is a reversible process as the axons resprout in approximately 3–6 months. Intravesical instillations of botulinum A toxin should only be used in patients with idiopathic detrusor overactivity in the research environment or when they have not responded to conservative treatments such as lifestyle modifications, behavioural techniques and drug therapy. Patients should be informed about the lack of long-term data, and that the use of botulinum A toxin for this indication is outside the UK marketing authorisation for the product. Informed consent to treatment should be obtained and documented (NICE 2006).

Baclofen This skeletal muscle relaxant is used in multiple sclerosis for the relief of chronic muscle spasm. It inhibits motor nerve transmission at spinal level and also depresses the central nervous system. One disadvantage of baclofen is the reduction in muscle tone, therefore affecting the pelvic floor muscle tone.

Imipramine (Tofranil) is a tricyclic antidepressant which has complex pharmacological effects including marked systemic anticholinergic actions and inhibition of reuptake of serotonin and noradrenaline, but its mode of action in detrusor overactivity is unclear. No good quality randomised controlled trials have documented that the drug is effective in the treatment of OAB or stress urinary incontinence (SUI) although it has been used clinically to treat SUI. Imipramine has been shown to have favourable effects in

Table 9.1 Summary level of evidence – drugs used to treat overactive bladder

	Level of evidence	Grade of recommendation
Antimuscarinic drugs		
Tolterodine	1	A
Trospium	1	A
Solifenacin	1	A
Darafenacin	1	A
Atropine	3	D
Mixed action drugs		
Oxybutynin	1	A
Propiverine	1	A
Flavoxate	2	D
Antidepressants		
Imipramine	3	C
Others		
Chilli derivatives (capsaicin)[a]	2	C
Botulinum A toxin[b]	2	B
Baclofen	3	C
Oestrogen	2	C
Desmopressin[c]	1	A

[a] Intravesical
[b] Bladder wall
[c] Nocturia.
Adapted from Andersson et al (2005).

the treatment of nocturnal enuresis in children (Glazener et al 2003) but side effects include dry mouth, reflux oesophagitis, dry skin and the potential to cause cardiac arrhythmias. Imipramine is not licensed in the UK for treatment of OAB or SUI.

Table 9.1 provides a summary of levels of evidence and grades of recommendation relating to drug treatments for OAB. For descriptors of levels of evidence and grades of recommendation, see Box 1.13.

MEDICATION FOR STRESS URINARY INCONTINENCE

The drug treatment of SUI aims to increase the tone of the striated muscle in the urethra and pelvic floor (Fig. 9.3). Whilst it is well recognised

Figure 9.3 The nerve supply to the bladder.

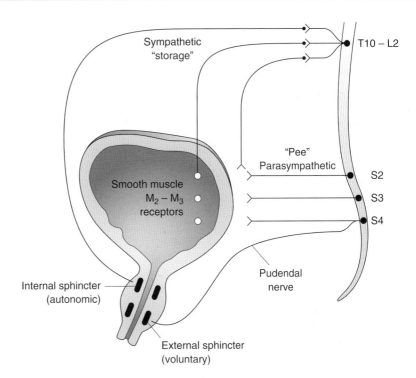

that pelvic floor re-education is first-line management, medication is showing significant potential. The role of serotonin (5HT) receptors is interesting; 5HT receptors are present in the bladder and in the central pathways controlling micturition (Fig. 9.4). There are numerous 5HT subtypes but $5HT_2$ subtypes have been shown to inhibit bladder activity and facilitate reflexes to the striated sphincter muscle (Danuser & Thor 1996).

Adrenoreceptor agonists Drugs with an alpha$_1$-adrenoreceptor agonist effect (e.g. ephedrine, pseudoephedrine and norephedrine) have been used to treat SUI because they increase outflow resistance. However, they are not selective for urethral receptors and side effects include sleep disturbance, headache, tremor and palpitation. Rare, although potentially serious, side effects include cardiac arrhythmias and hypertension and these limit the use of these drugs. None is licensed in the UK for treatment of SUI.

Oestrogens The oestrogen-sensitive tissues of the bladder, urethra and pelvic floor all play a role in the maintenance of continence (see Ch. 2). The urethra has four oestrogen-sensitive functional

layers which contribute to the urethral closure pressure: epithelium, vasculature, connective tissue and muscle. Although oestrogen therapy has been used to treat postmenopausal urgency and urge incontinence for many years, there have been few controlled trials to confirm its benefit. There is ongoing debate about its use for SUI and recent research has suggested that it has little effect in the management of SUI (Castro-Diaz & Amoros 2005). However, it does seem to be of benefit for the irritative symptoms of urgency, frequency and urge incontinence through improvement of urogenital atrophy and atrophic vaginitis (Castelo-Branco et al 2005) rather than a direct effect on urinary incontinence.

Duloxetine (Yentreve) was granted a UK licence in 2004 for the treatment of moderate to severe SUI in women. It is a selective serotonin and noradrenaline reuptake inhibitor (SNRI) and works by improving urethral closure and reducing urinary leakage. In preclinical studies, increased levels of serotonin and noradrenaline in the sacral spinal cord were shown to lead to increased urethral contraction via enhanced pudendal nerve stimulation to the urethral striated sphincter muscle. The ace-

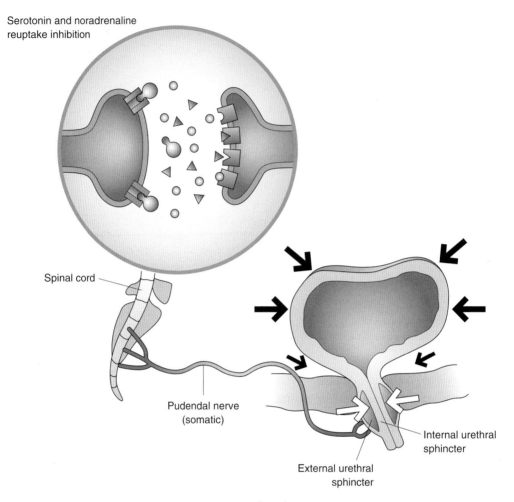

Figure 9.4   Serotonin and noradrenaline reuptake inhibitor (SNRI) mechanism. Reproduced with permission from Eli Lilly, Basingstoke.

tylcholine released by the pudendal nerve stimulates the receptors in the urethral sphincter to increase urethral sphincter contractility during the storage phase of the micturition cycle.

The drug must be used with caution in patients with a history of mania, bipolar disorder or seizures, patients with increased intraocular pressure or those at risk of acute narrow-angle glaucoma, patients taking anticoagulants or products known to affect platelet function and those with bleeding tendencies. Side effects are indicated in Box 9.2. They typically occur in the first week and resolve within a month, but patients should avoid abrupt withdrawal. The recommended dose is 40 mg twice daily. Patients should be reassessed after 2–4 weeks to evaluate benefit and tolerability of the therapy.

Summary of guidance on medication for SUI

- Duloxetine is not recommended as a first-line treatment for women with predominant SUI. Women should be counselled regarding the side effects of duloxetine (NICE 2006).
- Duloxetine should only be used as part of an overall management strategy for SUI in addition to pelvic floor exercises. A 4-week trial is recommended for women with moderate to severe SUI. Patients should be reviewed again after 12 weeks

Box 9.2   Side effects of duloxetine (after Ghoniem et al 2005)

Very common (>10%)	Nausea, dry mouth, fatigue, insomnia, constipation
Common (1–10%)	Anorexia, decreased appetite, thirst, sleep disorder, anxiety, decreased libido, anorgasmia, headache, dizziness (except vertigo), dizziness on discontinuation, somnolence, tremor, blurred vision, nervousness, diarrhoea, vomiting, dyspepsia, increased sweating, lethargy, pruritus, weakness
Uncommon (0.1–1%)	Loss of libido

Table 9.2   Summary level of evidence – drugs used to treat stress urinary incontinence

	Level of evidence	Grade of recommendation
Alpha adrenoreceptor agonist		
Ephedrine	3	D
Norephedrine	3	D
Hormones		
Oestrogen	2	D
Other drugs		
Duloxetine	1	A
Imipramine	3	D

Adapted from Andersson et al (2005).

to assess progress and appropriateness of continued medication (SIGN 2004).

- Intravaginal oestrogen preparations and systemic hormone replacement therapy are not recommended for the treatment of SUI.

Table 9.2 provides a summary of levels of evidence and grades of recommendation relating to drug treatments for SUI.

MEDICATION FOR NOCTURIA

First-line treatment is always correction of any underlying conditions and requires a thorough review of general health and current medication regimen. In patients with peripheral oedema and/or congestive cardiac failure, it is common for fluid to pool in the lower limbs in the daytime and return to the circulation at night when the patient is at rest, with their legs raised. Appropriate management can prevent excessive variation in nocturnal intravascular volume (Fonda et al 2005) but there is limited evidence on the effectiveness of conservative strategies, such as:

- fluid restriction in the early evening
- compression bandages
- restriction of caffeine and alcohol
- late afternoon elevation of legs.

Diuretic treatment   Encouraging urine excretion before bedtime can be a treatment option for nocturnal polyuria. Reynard et al (1998), in a double-blind, placebo-controlled trial, used furosemide (frusemide) 6 h before bedtime to produce diuresis and reduce nocturia. Nocturnal voiding frequency and urine production were significantly reduced.

MEDICATION FOR NOCTURNAL ENURESIS

Desmopressin   Nocturnal polyuria may be due to loss of renal concentrating ability and decreased production of antidiuretic hormone. Desmopressin (DDAVP) is a synthetic analogue of vasopressin which increases urine concentration and reduces total urine output by promoting reabsorption of water in the kidney tubules. It is widely used as a treatment for primary nocturnal enuresis (Glazener et al 2003) (see Ch. 6). It has also been shown to be effective in adult nocturia of polyuric origin (Hilton & Stanton 1982). Adverse side effects of DDAVP are uncommon but there is a risk of water retention and hyponatraemia, which could lead to oedema and heart failure. It is recommended that serum sodium levels should be measured before and a few days after starting treatment or changing the dose. The use of desmopressin for nocturia in adults with non-neurogenic UI is outside the UK marketing authorisation for the product. Informed consent to treatment should be obtained and documented (NICE 2006).

Table 9.3 Summary level of evidence – drugs used to treat nocturia/nocturnal enuresis

	Level of evidence	Grade of recommendation
Vasopressin analogues		
Desmopressin	1	A
Antiprostaglandins		
Aspirin	4	D
Other drugs		
Diuretic	4	D
Imipramine	4	C

Adapted from Andersson et al (2005).

Imipramine In young adults imipramine has been shown to decrease urine output. The effects of imipramine are thought to come from its alpha-adrenergic action on the proximal renal tubules with increased urea and water reabsorption (Hunsballe et al 1997). Further work is required to explore if it has a similar effect on older adults.

Antiprostaglandin (aspirin). There have been some reports indicating that non-steroidal anti-inflammatory drugs (NSAIDs) are effective in reducing symptoms of nocturia. The mechanisms are not well understood but are thought to be mediated by antiprostaglandin (PG) activity. PGs have various effects on kidney, bladder, urethra and sympathetic and parasympathetic nervous systems. Many NSAIDs have serious side effects and careful observation is needed but anecdotal evidence suggests that aspirin may be helpful in reducing nocturia (Le Fanu 2001).

Table 9.3 provides a summary of levels of evidence and grades of recommendation relating to drug treatments for nocturia/nocturnal enuresis.

MEDICATION FOR UNDERACTIVE BLADDER

The aim of treatment is to prevent damage to the upper urinary tract due to failure of the bladder to empty effectively. Cholinergic agonists such as carbachol and bethanechol can enhance detrusor contractions during micturition, provided the problem is not too severe. Their use is limited due to lack of evidence of efficacy but combining a cholinergic drug with an α-blocker has been shown to be effective (Yamanishi et al 2004).

MEDICATION FOR CONSTIPATION

There are over 14 million prescriptions written each year for laxatives, and the annual expenditure on laxatives in England is estimated at £43 billion (including over-the-counter drugs) (Petticrew et al 1999). The management of constipation is based on a combined approach, which includes identifying the cause, reviewing current management strategies (including lifestyle changes), efficacy and concordance. Acute constipation with a full rectum should be treated with either suppositories or microenemas; in severe cases digital removal may be required (see Chs 5, 8). It is important to refer to local policy, including guidance/requirement about digital rectal examination and manual evacuation.

Prolonged treatment with laxatives is not usually necessary but may be required where constipation or faecal impaction recurs when treatment is stopped (Emmanuel 2002). The National Prescribing Centre (2004) recommends that diet and lifestyle changes be implemented where possible and maintained even when laxatives are required. These treatments can help retrain a chronically sluggish bowel. For children, short-term treatment with laxatives, along with retraining to establish regular bowel habits, also helps prevent constipation (see Ch. 8). Laxatives taken by mouth are available in liquid, tablet, gum, powder and granule forms. They work in various ways and as constipation may be drug related, it is also important for the prescriber to be aware of the range of drugs that may cause constipation.

Bulk-forming laxatives are generally considered the safest but can interfere with absorption of some medicines. These laxatives, also known as fibre supplements, are taken with water. They absorb water in the intestine and make the stool softer. Brand names include ispaghula husk (Fybogel, Regulan, Konsyl and Isogel), methylcellulose (Celevac) and sterculia (Normacol). **NB**: Care should be taken in patients with advanced cancer as they require a high fluid intake for such laxatives to be effective (Perdue 2005).

Stimulants cause rhythmic muscle contractions in the intestines. Brand names include senna, bisacodyl, docusate sodium, glycerol and picosulphate, also combined with ispaghula (Manevac).

Stool softeners are also known as emollient laxatives. They cause moisture and fat to penetrate stool to prevent dry hard stool masses. The lubricant effect makes the stools easier to pass. Because this type of laxative changes the quality of the stool mass, it allows for the passage of the softened stool without straining (which may be important following surgery or injury). Products include oral liquid paraffin, docusate sodium and arachis oil enema.

Osmotic laxatives act like a sponge to draw water into the colon for easier passage of stool. Laxatives in this group include lactulose, lactitol, macrogols (Idrolax and Movicol), magnesium hydroxide, magnesium sulphate (Epsom Salts), Carbalax suppositories (also a phosphate salt), microenemas and phosphate enemas.

Phosphate enemas should be used with caution as a review of the literature (Davies 2004) found no conclusive evidence to support the use of these enemas. However, a number of articles reported risks, contraindications and complications.

MEDICATION FOR FAECAL INCONTINENCE

Medications can be very effective in the management of faecal incontinence (FI) because they can be used to either speed up or slow down bowel transit time.

Constipating agents such as loperamide (Imodium) and codeine phosphate are helpful for FI. Loperamide can be titrated from a minimal liquid dose of 0.5 mg/2.5 ml (if small doses once daily or even less are found to be effective) up to 16 mg daily if required. Loperamide is most effective taken in the morning 20 min before food to dampen the gastrocolic reflex, which usually makes the bowel most active. A patient information sheet is available to support treatment regimens, available from http://www.bowelcontrol.org.uk.

Stool-bulking agents include ispaghula husk, bran and methylcellulose, particularly useful in 'mopping up' mucus. A good regimen is often to slow the gut down first with loperamide– reducing the frequency – then aim to bulk the stools to give a more formed stool with better emptying. If bulking agents are added too quickly, stools will become looser. Many people have self-medicated with over-the-counter drugs for years but revisiting a previous regimen with proper support may help improve their condition.

Overflow faecal incontinence due to impaction is best treated with an osmotic laxative – for example, polyethylene glycol (Idrolax or Movicol) or magnesium sulphate. Glycerin suppositories, senna and bisacodyl also aid evacuation and a Carbalax suppository can be helpful to regulate the neurogenic bowel (this includes stroke, multiple sclerosis, Parkinson's disease and spinal cord injury/disease). Over half the cases of diarrhoea in the elderly admitted to hospital with non-malignant disease are due to faecal impaction with overflow (Fallon & O'Neill 1997).

Alpha agonist (phenylephedrine) has been found to increase anal resting tone in healthy volunteers and improve incontinence in patients after formation of an ileal anal pouch (Carapeti et al 2000). A study by Badvie and Andreyev (2005), using phenylephedrine gel, suggested that it may help most patients and in some the improvement may be substantial. Larger, placebo-controlled prospective studies are needed to provide a stronger evidence base.

Glyceryl trinitrate and diltiazem ointment act as a reversible chemical 'sphincterotomy' to treat anal fissures (Malouf et al 2002). Diltiazem seems as efficacious in healing fissures without the undesirable side effect of headaches (Knight et al 2001, Scholefield et al 2003). The National Institute for Health and Clinical Excellence (NICE) is preparing a Guideline on the management of faecal incontinence which is due to be published in the summer of 2007.

MEDICATION CAN CONTRIBUTE TO INCONTINENCE

When UI and FI are identified, medication may in fact be a cause or a contributing factor (Table 9.4).

Table 9.4 Medication likely to cause or exacerbate incontinence

Drug	Use	Possible effects on continence
Diuretics		
Loop diuretics	Management of hypertension, pulmonary	Urinary urgency
Furosemide	oedema, heart failure, oedema	Urge incontinence
Bumetanide		
Thiazides	To relieve oedema due to chronic heart failure	Urinary urgency
Bendroflumethiazide		Frequency
Cyclopenthiazide		Urge incontinence
Metazolone		
Potassium sparing		
Triamterene		
Spironolactone		
Antipsychotic drugs		
Chlorpromazine	Schizophrenia and related psychotic illness	Voiding difficulties
Flupentixol		Decreased awareness
Haloperidol		
Clozapine		
Olanzapine		
Lithium		
Benzodiazepines	Sedation	Decreased awareness
Nitrazepam		Impaired mobility
Temazepam		
Lorazepam		
Barbiturates	Sedation	As above
Amobarbital		
Phenobarbital		
Chloral derivatives	Sedation	As above
Opiate analgesics		
Diamorphine	Pain control	Bladder sphincter spasm causing difficulty
Morphine	Drug abuse	in micturition
		Urge incontinence
		Constipation
Xanthines		
Theophylline (in tea)	Asthma	Increased diuresis aggravates detrusor
Caffeine		instability causing urge incontinence
Alpha agonists		
Pseudoephedrine	Nasal decongestant	Urinary retention in men
Alpha-blockers		
Indoramin	Relax smooth muscle at the bladder neck	Increased urinary flow
		Increased stress leakage
Drugs with antimuscarinic side effects		
Antihistamines	Allergies (e.g. hay fever, rashes)	Voiding difficulties
Pizotifen	Migraine	Reduced awareness of desire to void
Promethazine	Travel sickness	
Tricyclic antidepressants	Depressive illness	Voiding difficulties
Amitriptyline		
Lofepramine		
Imipramine		

Table 9.4 *Continued*

Drug	Use	Possible effects on continence
Calcium channel blockers		
Nifedipine	Angina	Nocturia
	Arrhythmia	Increased frequency
	Hypertension	
Cytotoxics	Malignancies	Haemorrhagic cystitis
Cyclophosphamide		
Ifosfamide		
Alcohol	Social	Impairs mobility
		Reduces sensation
		Increases urinary frequency and urgency
		Induces diuresis
Anticholinesterase	Myasthenia gravis	Bladder sphincter muscle relaxation
Neostigmine	Irritable bowel spasm	causing involuntary micturition
		Control of smooth muscle
		Increased peristalsis
Antimuscarinic drugs, also known as anticholinergics		
Trihexyphenidyl	Parkinson's disease	Voiding difficulties
Procylidine	Drug-induced parkinsonism	Constipation
Hyoscine		
Propantheline		
Homeopathic treatment		
St John's wort	Mild to moderate depression	Voiding difficulty

It is fundamental to the assessment process to establish:

- current prescribed medication
- over-the-counter (OTC) self-medication
- alternative homeopathic medication.

It is well recognised that some drugs can prevent the bladder contracting, thus causing urinary retention; diuretics – by the nature of their pharmacological properties – cause a brisk diuresis. Other medication can cause sedation, reducing the awareness of the need to go to the toilet or the ability to respond in time.

MEDICATION WHICH CHANGES THE COLOUR OF THE URINE

Urine is a natural waste product of the body. It is typically clear, and pale to deep yellow in colour. The colour of urine is due to the pigment urochrome which is derived from the body's destruction of haemoglobin. The more concentrated the urine, the deeper yellow it becomes; changes in colour may reflect diet or medication, or may be due to blood or bile in the urine. Colour as well as taste and smell can be an indication of the patient's condition; equally, drugs and diet can cause the urine to change colour. Ford (1992) linked changes to all the colours of the rainbow (Box 9.3).

THE ROLE OF NURSE PRESCRIBING

Nurse prescribing is a rapidly evolving area of practice with potential to advance nursing roles and improve care delivery. Prescribing also offers nurses greater opportunity for collaborative working to drive national directives forward (Lanyon 2004). Increasing awareness of integrated care and defining specific contributions to meet care delivery mean that nurses from all specialties are redefining their roles in terms of non-medical prescribing (Medicines Control Agency 2002).

> **Box 9.3 Causes of urine colour changes** (after Ford 1992)
>
> - Red   Phenytoin, senna, haematuria, nephritis, beetroot, blackberries
> - Orange   Warfarin or rifampicin, paprika, rhubarb, dehydration
> - Yellow   Nitrofurantoin or sulphonamides, vitamins, asparagus
> - Green   Amitriptyline or indomethacin, jaundice, urine infection
> - Blue   Amitriptyline or triamterene, typhus
> - Purple   Phenolphthalein or senna, high protein diet, porphyrinuria
> - Brown   Iron preparations or metronidazole, liver and gallbladder disease
> - Black   Methyldopa or quinine, malignant melanoma

Alongside these opportunities, nurses must raise their awareness of their ethical and legal responsibilities (Warner 2005). As we develop our knowledge of drugs and interactions to prescribe safely, prescribing offers development opportunities for services, with enhanced case management and greater responsibility in care planning.

Background

Nurse prescribing in the UK has been a long time coming, and the nursing profession has spent more than 20 years lobbying for prescribing rights (Jones 1999). Now nurses can prescribe as independent, extended and supplementary prescribers, and research has shown that nurse prescribing in the community has found a high level of patient satisfaction, an increase in the quality of the relationship between nurses and patients, and better use of nurses' and doctors' time (Brooks et al 2001). The responsibilities of prescribing bring with them additional demands relating to decision making and competency required to practise, but the reality of nurse prescribing is that instead of having to wait for a GP to sign a prescription for a particular catheter, leg bag, appliance, anticholinergic or laxative, patients can receive the prescription they need straight away.

Legal framework for prescribing

The 1968 Medicines Act set out the groups of professionals who could prescribe and the manner in which prescription-only medicines (POMs) could be supplied and administered; this did not include nurses. The Cumberledge Report in 1986 was the first official report to call for nurse prescribing and to recommend that community nurses should be able to prescribe from a limited list of items. In 1992 the Medicines Act was amended to include nurses, midwives and health visitors who were 'of such a description and complied with such conditions as may be specific to order' (i.e. those practitioners who had received training and had appropriate qualifications) and a nurse prescribing formulary was developed.

In 1997 the government established a review of prescribing, supply and administration chaired by Dr June Crown. The first Crown report in 1998 led to the implementation of protocols, later to become patient group directions; the second Crown report in 1999 dealt principally with the question of non-medical prescribing.

In 2000 *The NHS Plan* (DH 2000) endorsed these recommendations and in 2001 the Health and Social Care Act, Section 63, allowed ministers to designate a new category of prescribers and to set conditions for their prescribing. Amendments to NHS regulations enabled the introduction of supplementary and extended prescribing for nurses. It is suggested that by 2008 there will be more non-medical prescribers than medical prescribers, reflecting the changing environment in health care.

Types of nurse prescribing

1. Patient group directions
2. Independent community practitioners
3. Extended formulary prescribing
4. Supplementary prescribing

Patient group directions

Patient group directions (PGDs) are not strictly a form of nurse prescribing but address the supply or administration of a medicine. Many registered allied health professionals (AHPs) and optometrists can also supply or administer a medicine or appliance under a PGD. Under the old name of local prescribing protocols, PGDs are a nationally recognised system for prescribing by nurses. Changes in the Medicines Act, made to enable supply and administration of prescription-only and pharmacy-only medicines by healthcare professionals under PGDs, came into force in August 2000. The implications for nurses are that it provides a framework for the legal supply of medications.

A PGD is a written instruction for the supply or administration of medicines to groups of patients who may not be individually identified before presentation for treatment. Because it is not a form of prescribing, there is no specific training that health professionals must undertake before they are able to work under a PGD. However, certain requirements apply to the use of PGDs and these are outlined below. Guidance on the use of PGDs was issued to the NHS in Health Service Circular 2000/026. The National Prescribing Centre published a guide in 2004.

PGDs can currently be used for the supply or administration of medicines by chiropodists, orthoptists, physiotherapists, radiographers, ambulance paramedics and optometrists, as well as nurses, midwives, health visitors and pharmacists. These health professionals may only do so as named individuals. The Department of Health has made it clear that the majority of clinical care should still be provided on an individual, patient-specific basis. PGDs should be reserved for those limited situations where there is an advantage for patient care, without compromising patient safety.

It its intended that PGDs complement nurse prescribing by providing nurses in acute units, community hospitals and minor injury units with a structured approach to dispense medication for individual patients. The structure is to outline clear and documented lines of professional responsibility and accountability. The PGD also needs to be descriptive of circumstances, criteria for inclusion and exclusion, caution and advice for further action and referral. PGDs should be drawn up by a multidisciplinary group and must be signed by a senior doctor and senior pharmacist, both of whom should have been involved in the group.

The multidisciplinary group should include a representative of any professional group expected to supply or administer medicines under the PGD. A senior person in each professional group should be designated, with the responsibility of ensuring that only fully competent, qualified and trained professionals operate within PGDs. In addition, the PGD must be authorised by the NHS Trust or primary care trust. Some examples of PGDs are available at http://www.druginfozone.nhs.uk and http://www.groupprotocols.org.uk.

Box 9.4   Case study 1: Patient group directions

HISTORY
Kay (54 years old) was seen in the nurse-led continence clinic with symptoms of urinary frequency, urgency and nocturia. Prior to the appointment she had kept a diary of her voiding pattern which showed a daytime frequency ×14 and nocturia ×3, with a maximum voided volume of 200 ml and an average of 100 ml. Kay had a 3-month history of symptoms and when her GP had tested her urine it was NAD. She was well and taking no other medication.

EXAMINATION
On examination a routine urinalysis tested positive to leucocytes, nitrites, protein and blood. A postvoid bladder scan showed a slight residual of 150 ml. An MSU was sent for culture and sensitivity. Kay also admitted to problems with vulval dryness and constipation.

MANAGEMENT PLAN
As part of the management plan Kay was given a 3-day course of trimethoprim 200 mg twice daily using the PGD framework. Fluid intake, bowel management and voiding technique were discussed. She was given a follow-up appointment for 6 weeks to repeat the urine test and to check postvoid residual.

Independent community practitioners

As an independent community practitioner prescriber the nurse is responsible for assessment, diagnosis and prescribing for patients from the *Nurse Prescribers' Formulary* (NPF). The prescriber takes responsibility for the clinical assessment of the patient, establishing a diagnosis and the clinical management required. Following training, nurses may prescribe from a limited formulary of products designed to meet the needs of patients. The NPF consists of appliances, dressings and some medicines, including a small list of prescription-only medicines. The majority of medication is on a general sales list. Community practitioners can also prescribe appliance and wound care management products from a limited list of over 200 items.

Box 9.5   Case study 2: Independent community practitioners

Jane has an indwelling urinary catheter because she has multiple sclerosis and her bladder is now unable to empty without mechanical support. She has recently had a suprapubic catheter inserted but is struggling with the catheter pulling around the site and she is not able to operate the drainage system tap. She has been given night bags to link in but they also have a different tap, which Jane cannot operate.

On inspecting the catheter it was immediately apparent that Jane has a male length suprapubic catheter attached below her knee with a short tube leg bag. As the first change of the catheter is due in 14 days' time, a change to a female length catheter with a catheter valve or belly bag would be more conformable. To relieve her immediate difficulties she was advised to try a catheter valve and a barrel-type bag which she could operate herself. As all catheter and drainage systems are prescribable under the *Nurse Prescribers' Formulary for Community Practitioners*, she was given a prescription there and then, and follow-up via the community nurse was arranged. A letter was sent to the GP for updating records.

Extended formulary prescribing

Prior to 1 May 2006, all first level nurses and registered midwives could train to prescribe from the *Nurse Prescribers' Extended Formulary*. The extended formulary included all general sales list and pharmacy medication prescribable by GPs, together with specific prescription-only medicines. In addition, all items in the NPF could be prescribed. There was, however, a limit to the conditions for which nurses could prescribe. (See also Progressing nurse prescribing below.)

Box 9.6   Case study 3: Extended prescribing

Susan, aged 44, came to the clinic for a routine change of her suprapubic catheter. She has multiple sclerosis and uses an electric wheelchair. It was 2 weeks before her wedding to her long-term partner. She had seen her GP 5 days earlier because of a bothersome vaginal discharge, diagnosed as bacterial vaginosis, and had been given treatment with metronidazole 400 mg twice a day for 7 days. She described the vaginal discharge as worse and offensive.

A vaginal swab was taken and she was given a probable diagnosis of vaginal thrush and a prescription for fluconazole 150 mg single dose orally. At follow-up 3 weeks later she had had some initial symptom relief but felt the discharge and irritation were back. The swab had come back with confirmation of Candida infection.

Supplementary prescribing

Supplementary prescribing is defined as a voluntary partnership between an independent prescriber (doctor or dentist) and a supplementary prescriber. There is an agreed clinical management plan that is patient specific and agreed with the patient and prescriber. For some AHP groups, who work closely with doctors in a team setting, supplementary prescribing might be a sensible solution to improve NHS provision to patients.

Amendments to the Prescription-Only Medicines Order and NHS Regulations to permit supplementary prescribing by nurses and pharmacists came into effect on 4 April 2003. There are no legal restrictions on the medical conditions that may be treated under supplementary prescribing. It is a mechanism that will normally be most useful for the management of chronic medical conditions and health needs. There is no specific formulary or list of medicines for supplementary prescribing. Provided medicines are prescribable by a doctor (or dentist) at NHS expense, and that they are referred to in the patient's clinical management plan, supplementary prescribers will be able to prescribe:

- all general sales list (GSL) medicines and all pharmacy (P) medicines
- appliances and devices prescribable by GPs

- foods and other borderline substances approved by the Advisory Committee on Borderline Substances
- all prescription-only medicines
- medicines for use outside their licensed indications, i.e. off-label prescribing, all black triangle drugs and drugs marked less suitable for prescribing in the *British National Formulary*, unlicensed drugs that are part of a clinical trial that has a clinical trial certificate or exemption
- within their scope of practice.

Supplementary prescribing training for nurses began in January 2003 and the first nurses qualified as supplementary prescribers in April 2003. In May 2004, the Department of Health proposed that more health professionals, including physiotherapists, radiographers, chiropodists and optometrists, should be able to prescribe medicines as supplementary prescribers in partnership with a doctor.

Box 9.7   Case study 4: Supplementary prescribing

Alan, aged 56, is a bus driver and his problem with urinary frequency started 2 years ago. He eventually plucked up courage to see his GP who referred him to a urologist. Following a barrage of tests, including urinalysis, cystoscopy and prostate specific antigen, it was suggested to him that he should try bladder retraining. Life was getting very difficult at work because he was often rostered to a long route with no toilets at the terminus.

Alan was seen in the nurse-led clinic to review his bladder management. The focus of the consultation was on self-help regimes and discussion of medication options. A letter from the urologist confirmed a diagnosis of overactive bladder with a suggestion of treatment with an anticholinergic. This gave a framework within which to work. Alan drank very little for fear of needing to go to the toilet and in an average day only consumed three drinks. He was beginning to reconsider his ability to work because of the inaccessibility of toilets.

Initially it was suggested that he increase his fluid intake, a brave step but essential to allow bladder expansion and reduce the irritation of concentrated urine. A trial period with an anticholinergic was also suggested but Alan was very reluctant because he drives for a living and could not cope with side effects which include blurred vision. Adjuncts to bladder training were explored, following which he tried acupuncture and a TENS unit.

Two months later there had been some improvement but Alan asked if he could give the tablets a try. Using the clinical management plan agreed with the urologist and Alan, he was given a prescription for oxybutynin 5 mg twice a day, a low dose. He understood the possible side effects and the need to continue with his bladder retraining. A letter was sent to his GP to update records and a follow-up appointment in 4 weeks was made to review progress.

Realities and advantages of nurse prescribing

The introduction of nurse prescribing has been generally welcomed within the profession (Allsop et al 2005). Service users benefit the most because nursing services are more responsive (e.g. when clients are discharged home with an indwelling catheter). Although some critics have argued that political motivation to introduce nurse prescribing was driven by a need to save money in the NHS and to free up doctors' time by transferring routine tasks to nurses (Sheppard 2002, McHale 2003), the principle of utilitarianism – the greatest good to the greatest number – is applicable to nurse prescribing in that more clients will benefit from seamless nursing care. A major advantage is the time saved by not having to wait outside a GP's consultation room for a prescription to be signed, although the counter to this is the additional nursing time required to maintain communication with GP surgeries because medical records need updating.

As nurse prescribers, it is imperative to be clinically safe and responsible. This can be developed through careful assessment of patients' needs and an evidence-based approach to prescribing. Mentoring and reflection provide a guided framework to start practice. There are numerous databases available both on the Internet and in other forms to aid prescribing decisions (Box 9.8) and nurses must take care not to feel coerced by users to prescribe if there is not a clinical need. Prescribers also need to ensure they have personal indemnity cover, usually via a trade union, as they take on new responsibilities. Job descriptions and job profiles should also be amended appropriately to obtain vicarious liability cover from employers.

Legal responsibilities

Prescribing comes with legal responsibilities and accountability. This includes dealing with patients'

demands and expectations and recognising that effective prescribing is time-consuming (Timbs 2003). The legal framework applicable to nurse prescribing is Bolam's Law (1957); this states that a level of competence equalling that which can be reasonably expected of a similarly experienced nurse must be attained. By becoming a prescriber, a nurse is regarded both by law and the Nursing and Midwifery Council (NMC) as a specialist and must therefore demonstrate the knowledge and skill appropriate (Warner 2005) (Box 9.9).

Consultation skills

The consultation process is a critical interaction between practitioner and patient so it is important for practitioners to consider their own style of consultation and learn to adapt as appropriate to different clinical situations. The seven step model of consultation discussed by Byrne and Long (1976) provides a useful framework:

- Step 1: Establish a relationship
- Step 2: Establish the reason for consultation
- Step 3: Verbal and physical examination, as appropriate

Box 9.8 Useful sources of information to aid prescribers

- NICE guidelines
- National Service Framework (NSF) publications
- Electronic resources (e.g. Prodigy)
- Local formulary
- Nurse Prescribers' Formulary
- Cochrane Reviews

Box 9.9 Specific competencies for nurse prescribing (National Prescribing Centre 2001)

Knowledge	Skills
Establishing options	Makes a diagnosis and generates treatment options for the patient. Always follows up treatment
Clinical and pharmaceutical knowledge	Has up-to-date clinical and pharmaceutical knowledge relevant to own area of practice
Communicating with patients	Establishes a relationship based on trust and mutual respect Sees patients as partners in the consultation and applies the principles of concordance
Prescribing safely	Is aware of own limitations Does not compromise patient safety
Prescribing professionally	Works within professional and organisational standards Takes personal responsibility for prescribing decisions
Improving prescribing practice	Actively participates in the review and development of prescribing practice
Information in context	Knows how to access relevant information Can critically appraise and apply information in practice
The NHS context	Understands and works with local and national policies that impact on prescribing practice
The team and individual context	Works in partnership with colleagues to benefit patients Is self-aware and confident in own ability as a prescriber

- Step 4: Consideration of diagnosis
- Step 5: Discuss treatment options
- Step 6: Termination of consultation
- Step 7: A parting shot.

In reality, consultations rarely unfold in such a logical way, though all phases are likely to be considered. Much of the available research comparing nurses' and doctors' consultations focuses on the outcomes rather than the process. Most studies have also found that consultations with nurses are slightly longer, that nurses give more information and that they offer more advice and self-care management.

Progressing nurse prescribing

A Department of Health guide to the implementation of nurse independent prescribing was published on the DH non-medical prescribing webpage in April 2006. The *Nurse Prescribers' Extended Formulary* has been discontinued and, from 1 May 2006, qualified nurse independent prescribers (formerly known as extended formulary nurse prescribers) are able to prescribe any licensed medicine for any medical condition within their competence, including some controlled drugs. The non-medical prescribing programme gives patients quicker access to medicines, improves access to services and makes better use of nurses' and other health professionals' skills.

Developing a new cadre of prescribers is undoubtedly resource intensive in the early years. Work Force Development funding in England was, in principle, effective in supporting the implementation of nurse prescribing and training in prescribing skills but the future of funding remains uncertain. In Wales, each individual Trust pays £800 per nurse to access supplementary training modules via local universities. Other practical difficulties include lack of back fill expertise to cover for staff on training programmes and difficulty in finding a committed medical mentor. Clearly it is important to consider enhancing the preparation of preregistration students, through a comprehensive scientific foundation in applied pharmacology, to equip them for postgraduate training in medication management.

Although nurse prescribing has been established in the UK for over 10 years, relatively little is known about the effects this additional role is having on those who are involved in the process. However, it is clear that the introduction of prescribing along with many other centrally driven initiatives is altering the face of nursing practice and continence care (Fisher 2004).

References

Allsop A, Brooks L, Bufton L et al 2005 Supplementary prescribing in mental health and learning disabilities. Nursing Standard 19(30):54–58

Andersson K-E, Appell R, Cardozo L et al 2005 Pharmacological treatment of urinary incontinence. In: Abrams P, Cardozo L, Khoury S, and Wein A (eds) Incontinence, vol 2. 3rd International Consultation on Incontinence. Health Publication, Paris, p 811–854

Badvie S, Andreyev H J 2005 Topical phenylephedrine in the treatment of radiation- induced faecal incontinence. Clinical Oncology 17(2):122–126

Brooks N, Otway C, Rashid C, Kilty L, Maggs C 2001 Nurse prescribing: what do patients think? Nursing Standard 15(17):33–38

Byrne P, Long B 1976 Doctors talking to patients. HMSO, London

Carapeti E A, Kamm M A, Evans B K et al 2000 Topical phenylephedrine increases anal sphincter resting pressure. British Journal of Surgery 86:267–270

Castelo-Branco C, Cancelo M J, Villero J et al 2005 Management of post-menopausal vaginal atrophy and atrophic vaginitis. Maturitas 52(supplement 1):S46–52

Castro-Diaz D, Amoros M P 2005 Pharmacotherapy for stress urinary incontinence. Current Opinion in Urology 15(4):227–230

Chapple C R, Yamanishi T, Chess-Williams R 2002 Muscarinic receptor sub-types and management of overactive bladder. Urology 60(supplement 5A):82–89

Danuser H, Thor K B 1996 Spinal 5HT2 receptor mediated facilitation of pudendal nerve reflexes in the anaesthetised cat. British Journal of Pharmacology 118:150–154

Davies C 2004 The use of phosphate enemas in the treatment of constipation. Nursing Times 100(18):32–35

Department of Health 2000 The NHS plan. DH, London

De Ridder D, Chandiramini V, Dasgupta P et al 1997 Intravesical capsaicin as a treatment for refractory detrusor hyperreflexia. Journal of Urology 158(6):2087–2092

Emmanuel A 2002 Bowel care in older people. Research and practice. Royal College of Physicians Clinical Effectiveness and Evaluation Unit, London

Enskat R, Deaney C N, Glickman S 2001 Systemic effects of intravesical atropine sulphate. BJU International 87(7):613–616

Fallon M, O'Neill B 1997 ABC of palliative care. Constipation and diarrhoea. British Medical Journal 315(7118):1293–1296

Fisher R 2004 District nurses: relationships in nurse prescribing. British Journal of Community Nursing 9(10):416–419

Fonda D, DuBeau C E, Harari D et al 2005 Incontinence in the frail elderly. In: Abrams P, Cardozo L, Khoury S, Wein A (eds) Incontinence, vol 2. 3rd International Consultation on Incontinence. Health Publication, Paris, p 1165–1214

Ford H 1992 Feeling off colour: colour of urine and faeces indicate disease. Nursing Times 89(5):64, 66, 68

Ghoniem G M, Van Leeuwen J S, Elser D M et al 2005 A randomized controlled trial of duloxetine alone, pelvic floor muscle training alone, combined treatment and no active treatment in women with stress urinary incontinence. Journal of Urology 173(5):1647–1653

Glazener C M, Evans J H, Peto R E 2003 Tricyclics and related drugs for nocturnal enuresis in children. Cochrane Database of Systematic Reviews (3) CD002117

Hilton P, Stanton S 1982 The use of desmopressin (DDAVP) in nocturnal frequency in the female. British Journal of Urology 54:252

Hunsballe J, Ritting S, Pedersen E et al 1997 Single dose imipramine reduces nocturia. Journal of Urology 158:830–836

Jones M 1999 Nurse prescribing, now we know what's cooking. Nursing Standard 95(23):4–5

Keane D, O'Sullivan S 2000 Urinary incontinence: anatomy, physiology and pathophysiology. In: Cardozo L (ed) Clinical obstetrics and gynaecology. Baillière Tindall, London

Knight J, Birks M, Farouk R 2001 Topical diltiazem ointment in the treatment of chronic anal fissure. British Journal of Surgery 88(4):553–556

Lanyon M 2004 Nurse prescribing: current status and future developments. Nursing Times 100(17):28–29

Le Fanu J 2001 The value of aspirin in controlling the symptoms of nocturnal polyuria. British Journal of Urology 88:126

McHale J 2003 A review of the legal framework for accountable nurse prescribing. Nurse Prescribing 1(3):107–112

Malouf A J, Buchanan G N, Carapeti E A et al 2002 A prospective audit of fistula-in-ano at St Mark's Hospital. Colorectal Disease 4(1):13–19

Medicines Control Agency 2002 Proposals for supplementary prescribing by nurses and pharmacists and proposed amendments to prescription only medicines. TSO, London

National Institute for Health and Clinical Effectiveness 2006 Urinary incontinence in women. NICE, London. Online. Available: www.nice.org.uk

National Prescribing Centre 2001 Maintaining competency in prescribing: an outline framework to help nurse prescribers. NPC, Liverpool.

National Prescribing Centre 2004 The management of constipation. MeReC Bulletin 14(6). Online. Available: http://www.npc.co.uk/MeReC_Bulletins/2003Volumes/Vol14no6.pdf

Nurse Prescribers' Extended Formulary 2003–2005 For district nurses and health visitors. British Medical Association, London

Perdue C 2005 Managing constipation in advanced cancer care. Nursing Times 101(21):36–40

Petticrew M, Watt I, Brand M 1999 What's the 'best buy' for treatment of constipation? Results of a systematic review of the efficacy and comparative efficacy of laxatives in the elderly. Review. British Journal of General Practice 49:387–393

Reynard J, Cannon A, Yang Q, Abrams P 1998 A novel therapy for nocturnal polyuria: a double blind randomised trial of frusemide against placebo. British Journal of Urology 81:215–218

Scholefield J H, Bock J U, Marla B et al 2003 A dose finding study with 0.1%, 0.2% and 0.4% glyceryl trinitrate ointment in patients with chronic anal fissure. Gut 52(2):254–259

Sheppard E 2002 An important step forward. Nursing Times 98(49):47

SIGN 2004 Management of urinary incontinence in primary care. Scottish Intercollegiate Guidelines Network, Edinburgh. Online. Available: http://www.sign.ac.uk/pdf/sign79.pdf

Timbs O 2003 What pharmacist prescribers can learn from those who have gone before. Prescribing and Medicines Management 5:5

Van Kerrebroeck P, Kreder K, Jonas U et al 2001 Tolterodine study group. Tolterodine once daily: superior efficacy and tolerability in the treatment of overactive bladder. Urology 57(3):414–421

Warner D 2005 Theory of nurse prescribing. Journal of Community Nursing 19(4):12–16

Wein A J, Rovner E S 2002 Definition and epidemiology of overactive bladder. Urology 60(5 supplement 1):7–12; discussion 12

Yamanishi T, Yasuda K, Kamai T et al 2004 Combination of a cholinergic drug and an alpha-blocker is more effective than monotherapy for the treatment of voiding difficulty in patients with underactive detrusor. International Journal of Urology 11(2):88–96

Further Reading

Drug tariff. TSO, London

National Health Service, England and Wales. Electronic drug tariff. Online. Available: http://www.ppa.org.uk/edt/December_2006/mindex.htm

The NPA guide to the Drug Tariff and NHS dispensing for England and Wales. The National Pharmaceutical Association, St Albans

Medicines, ethics and practice: a guide for pharmacists. Royal Pharmaceutical Society of Great Britain, London

Crown Report – Review of prescribing, supply and administration of medicines. NHS Executive, Leeds. Online. Available: www.dh.gov.uk/assetRoot/04/01/17/26/04011726.pdf

Chapter **10**

Catheters and containment products

Kathryn Getliffe and Mandy Fader

INTRODUCTION

Despite advances in treatments and therapies for incontinence, completely reliable bladder or bowel control is not an attainable goal for everyone. Failure to empty the bladder effectively may require intermittent or indwelling catheterisation, whilst some form of containment product may be needed to manage urine leakage as part of a short- or long-term care strategy. Many people, particularly those with disabilities, need support from continence products to contain their incontinence and to enable them to carry out their everyday lives confidently. Successful management with continence products can help people avoid the stigmatizing consequences of incontinence which can otherwise threaten social and working lives, as well as personal relationships (Paterson 2000). This chapter examines the factors which influence choice of appropriate products and their management. Some of the content is adapted from a comprehensive review carried out by the authors and other members of an international team reporting to the 3rd International Consultation on Incontinence (Cottenden et al 2005). The chapter begins with a focus on catheters and then moves on to a wide-ranging discussion of containment products.

CATHETERS

The operation of introducing the catheter, if it do not require intrepidity and courage, requires at least peculiar delicacy, a perfect knowledge of the parts, and above all, a humane and steady temper . . .

John Bell (1810)

INTRODUCTION

Catheters can provide an effective way of draining the bladder for short- or long-term purposes by intermittent or indwelling catheterisation. Short-term catheterisation is usually considered to be up to 14 days (Brosnahan et al 2004) and long-term catheterisation more than 14 days (Niel-Weise & van den Broek 2005). Box 10.1 indicates the conditions where catheterisation may be appropriate.

Box 10.1   Catheter use

- Short-term catheterisation is most commonly used:
  - during surgical procedures and postoperative care
  - for accurate monitoring of urine output in acute illness
  - for instillation of medication directly into the bladder
  - for relief of acute or chronic urinary retention.
- Long-term indwelling catheterisation may be necessary for patients with:
  - bladder outlet obstruction who are unsuitable for surgery
  - chronic retention, often as a result of neurological disease or injury (where clean intermittent catheterisation (CIC) is not possible)
  - conditions resulting in debilitation, paralysis or coma (with skin breakdown and infection pressure ulcers)
  - intractable incontinence where catheterisation enhances quality of life (only where alternative methods have been found to be inappropriate or unsuccessful).

However, catheters are rarely completely trouble free and common complications include:

- leakage
- tissue trauma and/or inflammatory reactions
- catheter-associated infection (CAUTI)
- recurrent blockage caused by encrustation.

Consequently, decisions about catheterisation should only be made where other options are inappropriate or unsuccessful and the balance between effective bladder drainage, impact on quality of life, well-recognised catheter-associated risks and potential long-term complications has been considered (Box 10.2). The following sections focus on long-term use of catheters (intermittent or indwelling) to manage urinary drainage, including choice of catheter and drainage equipment for individual patients, catheter care and minimisation of problems.

Careful planning and thought can often allow effective management of incontinence without catheters, but where catheterisation is necessary, intermittent catheterisation (IC) is the preferred

Box 10.2   Catheter-associated risks and potential long-term complications

- Catheter-associated infection (potential for bacteraemia, urethritis, epididymitis, prostatitis, pyelonephritis)
- Tissue damage from trauma, pressure or inflammatory reactions (potential for meatal erosion, urethral stricture formation)
- Catheter encrustation leading to recurrent blockage
- Frequent bladder spasm leading to leakage and/or the catheter being expelled
- Bladder calculi
- Potential for long-term inflammatory/neoplastic changes in bladder tissue

option because it is generally associated with fewer catheter-associated problems. IC may be performed by patients themselves or a carer (where this is acceptable to both) and offers the added advantage of freedom from drainage bags. Where an indwelling catheter is required the catheter may be inserted into the bladder via the urethra or a suprapubic cystotomy.

Wherever possible the decision to catheterise should be a joint one between the patient, carer (if at home) and the health professional, and should never be made solely for the convenience of the latter. Urinary catheterisation and catheter care remain primarily a nursing responsibility and promoting 'best practice' based on a sound knowledge base, supported by the best available evidence, is critical to providing effective and supportive patient care.

INDWELLING CATHETERISATION

Catheter design

An effective indwelling catheter should include the following design characteristics (Cottenden et al 2005):

- Retained in the bladder effectively, yet easily removable without trauma to tissue
- Soft 'tip' within the bladder to avoid pressure damage to the mucosa

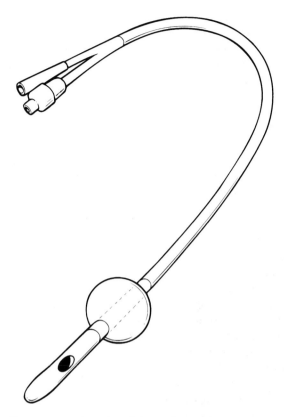

Figure 10.1   A modern Foley catheter.

- Effective drainage while minimising risk of the mucosa being sucked into a drainage channel
- Conforms to the shape of the urethra.

The Foley catheter is the most commonly used of all urethral catheters. In its usual form it has a double lumen shaft (one lumen for urine drainage, the other for inflation and deflation of the retention balloon), a rounded tip and two drainage eyes proximal to the balloon (Fig. 10.1).

Catheter materials

Catheters are made of a variety of materials (Box 10.3) including plastic, latex rubber (with or without a coating), silicone rubber or metal. An effective catheter material should have the following characteristics:

- Soft for comfort, yet sufficiently firm for easy insertion and maintenance of lumen patency in situ

Box 10.3 Selection of appropriate catheter material

Duration of catheterisation		Catheter material
Intermittent		Plastic, with or without hydrophilic coating Metal
Short term	(up to 14 days) (up to 28 days)	Latex or plastic Teflon-coated latex Silver-alloy (may also be selected for longer-term use)
Long term	(more than 14 days) (catheter expected to remain in situ >14 days: recommended time between catheter changes depends on local policy or individualised care plan)	Hydrogel-coated latex Silicone-elastomer-coated latex All silicone

- Elastic recoil, so that an inflated balloon can be deflated again to almost its original size, thus minimising discomfort during catheter removal
- Causing minimal tissue reaction or friction
- Resistant to colonisation by microorganisms and to encrustation by mineral deposits.

Plastic catheters are relatively cheap to manufacture and are commonly chosen for short-term use, up to 14 days. Plastic catheters without a balloon are used for intermittent self-catheterisation (ISC). Some of these are coated with hydrophilic polymers that absorb water, leading to a softer, more flexible catheter with reduced surface friction. Latex catheters are soft and flexible but are restricted to short-term use because of potential irritation due to high surface friction which may cause discomfort during insertion or removal, vulnerability to rapid encrustation by mineral deposits from urine (Cox et al 1989) and the implication of allergic reactions in the development of urethritis and urethral stricture (Cox et al 1989, Pariente et al 2000).

Attempts to minimise catheter complications have led to development of a range of catheter coatings. The most commonly used coatings for long-term use are silicone–elastomer or hydrogel. Hydrogels are hydrophilic polymers which absorb aqueous fluids to produce a soft slippery surface that reduces trauma on insertion or withdrawal of the catheter. They are highly biocompatible, relatively inert and are extensively used in other medical applications such as contact lenses (Nacey & Delahunt 1991). Catheters made of 100%

silicone also minimise tissue irritation and are latex free. These catheters are manufactured by an extrusion process and provide a larger drainage lumen than coated catheters. However, silicone allows the slow diffusion of water, which may occasionally lead to deflation of the balloon and the catheter falling out. The elastic recoil properties also seem more limited and at times this may produce a 'cuff effect' when the balloon is deflated, making catheter removal more difficult and uncomfortable.

Efforts to reduce the risks of CAUTI have included incorporation of antimicrobial surfaces such as silver-alloy. The evidence supporting these catheters is almost exclusively based on short-term catheterisation in acute care settings (Saint et al 2000, Johnson et al 2006). They are licensed for use up to 28 days in the UK but their benefit for long-term catheterised populations is yet to be fully determined (see later discussion on CAUTI).

Catheter size

Catheter size or gauge is measured as the external diameter of the catheter shaft, and is defined in either Charrière units (Ch) or French gauge (Fg). Both scales are identical with one unit equivalent to 0.33 mm (e.g. a 12 Ch or 12 Fg catheter has an external diameter of 4 mm). The diameter of the internal lumen may vary, however, depending on the catheter material and the manufacturing process. For example, catheters formed by the extrusion of a single material, such as silicone,

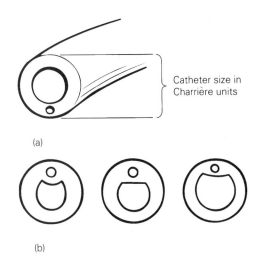

(a)

(b)

Figure 10.2   (a) Catheter size is measured by the external diameter of the catheter. (b) The size of the internal lumen depends on the manufacturing process.

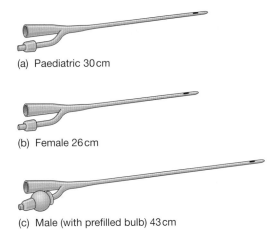

(a) Paediatric 30 cm

(b) Female 26 cm

(c) Male (with prefilled bulb) 43 cm

Figure 10.3   Catheter lengths.

usually have relatively thin walls and large lumens compared with catheters of the same gauge produced by building up layers through dipping and coating on a former.

Urinary flow rate is proportional to the internal diameter of the catheter. The smallest Charrière size (usually 12 for adults) can easily drain normal quantities of urine, including the large volumes produced during diuresis (Ebner et al 1985) (Fig. 10.2). Sizes 12–14 Ch are usually suitable for females and 12–16 Ch for males. Smaller sizes (6–10 Ch) are available for children.

The standard male length catheter (41–45 cm) is available to men and women, but a shorter female length of approximately 25 cm may be more comfortable and discreet for some patients (Fig. 10.3). Whilst the female length should never be used for males as inflation of the balloon within the urethra could result in severe trauma, the longer male length catheter may be more practical for some women, particularly those who are obese, as it provides easier access to the catheter/drainage bag junction. Paediatric catheters are usually approximately 30 cm long.

Catheter balloons

Small balloons are recommended for all patients: 10 ml balloons for adults and 2.5–5 ml balloons for children. Larger catheters and balloon sizes are thought to increase bladder irritability and spasm and present an increased risk of urethral damage if the catheter is expelled (e.g. by bladder spasm). A large balloon also sits higher within the bladder so that a reservoir of urine is retained below the eyes, creating potential for infection. It is important that balloons are inflated with the correct amount of sterile water, as stated on the catheter. Both over- and underinflation can result in balloon distortion so that the tip is angled to one side (Fig. 10.4) which could result in pressure ulceration of the bladder wall.

Drainage equipment

Careful choice of drainage equipment to aid patient independence and self-care is particularly important. A wide range of products is available (Fig. 10.5) and whenever possible patients should have the opportunity to try out:

- different bags, to decide for themselves which type of tap they find easiest to open and close
- different support systems for bodyworn bags, to find the most practical and comfortable – for example, a drainage bag supported by a holster suspended from a belt around the waist, or a leg bag supported by straps around the thigh or calf etc.

Bodyworn bags are preferable for most patients since their attachment to the leg, or suspension

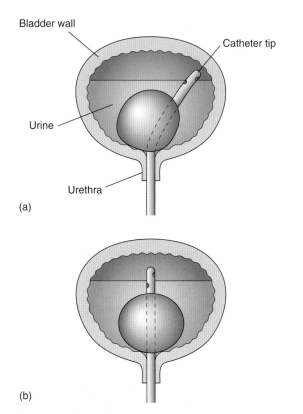

(a)

(b)

Figure 10.4 (a) Underinflated balloons often fail to expand evenly causing the catheter tip to be angled over to one side. (b) A fully inflated balloon allows the catheter tip to be located symmetrically.

from the waist, allows maximum freedom combined with concealment beneath clothing (Fig. 10.6). However, it is extremely important that the bag is emptied frequently to avoid it becoming too heavy and that it is adequately supported so that it cannot suddenly slip, pulling on the catheter and causing urethral trauma. Leg bags are available in a range of capacities (e.g. 350, 500 and 750 ml), with choice being dependent on how frequently the bag is likely to be emptied and the desire for effective concealment. Other features that may affect ease of access and emptying by self-caring patients include the length of the inlet tube, which can vary from around 5 to 40 cm, and the design of the outlet tap. All taps are designed to be opened with one hand but patients commonly find one style more satisfactory than another (Fig. 10.7). This is often related to ease of opening, particularly for those with limited manual strength or dexterity, or to confidence that the tap is securely closed after emptying. To reduce the problem of bulkiness as the bag fills and embarrassing sounds caused by movements of urine, some manufacturers have designed bags which are divided into vertically arranged subcompartments which promote even distribution of urine and greater conformity to the shape of the leg. Plastic surfaces can cause discomfort when

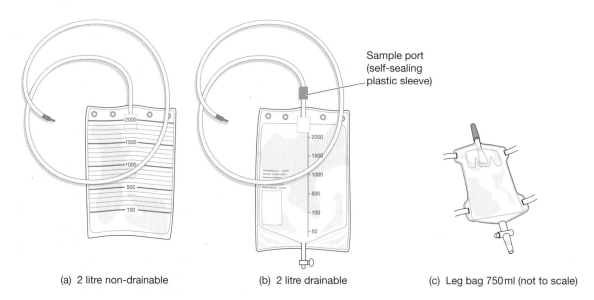

(a) 2 litre non-drainable

(b) 2 litre drainable

(c) Leg bag 750 ml (not to scale)

Figure 10.5 Drainage bag designs.

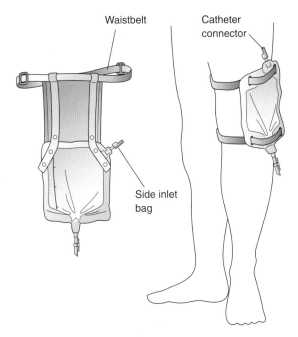

Figure 10.6   Bodyworn urine drainage bags held in place using leg straps (right) and a waist band suspension system (left). Reproduced with permission from Cottenden et al (2005).

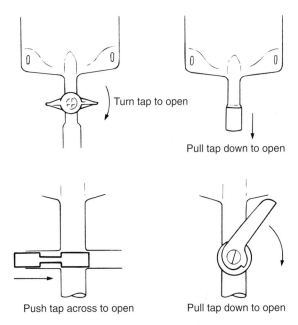

Figure 10.7   Examples of tap designs.

worn next to the skin and some drainage bags have a woven 'coverstock' backing for greater comfort, although this backing can deteriorate with bathing. One solution is to insert the bag into a 'coverstock' sleeve during normal wear, which can be removed for bathing.

At night a larger, freestanding, night drainage bag (capacity 2–4 litres) may replace the smaller leg bag, or be 'linked' to it via an extension to the outlet tap. A simple restraining device is available to minimise the risk of separation of the linked bags during the night since the leg bag tap is left open to allow free drainage. The night drainage bag should be supported on a cardboard or plastic-coated metal stand, which can be obtained on prescription (Fig. 10.8). There is little research evidence to underpin management of drainage bags and guidance on frequency of change is largely based on expert opinion, anecdotal evidence and manufacturer's recommendations. Rooney (1994) found no increase in incidence of CAUTI attributable to reusable urinary drainage bags compared with

sterile bags in 14 patients with neurogenic bladders. Keerasontonpong et al (2003) suggested that bags could be left for more than 3 days in hospitalised patients without increased risk of CAUTI but the authors were reluctant to define how long and recommended further studies.

There are occasional reports in the literature of purple discolouration in urine drainage bags (PUBS – purple urine bag syndrome). This is thought to be related to alkaline urine and high bacterial load (Mantani et al 2003) but the precise cause and significance of the problem remains unclear.

Urine specimens

Most drainage bags provide a sample port for taking urine specimens for analysis. Commonly this is a resealable plastic sleeve located on the inlet tubing, through which a syringe needle can be inserted. It is important that samples are taken from the port and not from the bag, via the tap, since the urine in the bag is likely to contain greater numbers of microorganisms which have had the opportunity to multiply within the reservoir of urine collecting in the bag.

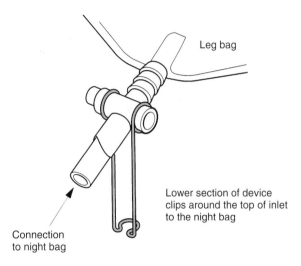

Leg bag

Connection to night bag

Lower section of device clips around the top of inlet to the night bag

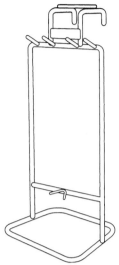

Figure 10.8 Night use: (a) a simple restraining device to secure connection between bags at night; (b) support for a night bag.

Catheter valves

The urine drainage system may be dispensed with altogether if a catheter valve is inserted into the end of the catheter, allowing bladder filling and intermittent drainage (Fig. 10.9). Valves may help to promote maintenance of bladder tone and capacity and are available in several different designs. However, they are unsuitable for patients with poor bladder capacity, detrusor overactivity, ureteric reflux or renal impairment. Patients must be able to manipulate the valve and empty the bladder regularly to avoid overfilling. At night, some valves can be connected to a drainage bag to allow free drainage. A spigot is not a suitable alternative to a catheter valve since it must be removed from the catheter to allow drainage, thereby breaking what is essentially a closed system.

Much of the evidence supporting beneficial effects of catheter valves is anecdotal, but the flushing effect which results from bladder filling and emptying seems likely to contribute to reduced problems with encrustation and blocking. There is stronger evidence of benefits in terms of patient comfort and independence (Fader et al 1997, German et al 1997) and users reported that the most important characteristics for them were: easy to manipulate, leak free, comfortable, inconspicuous and an integral part of the closed system.

'pull open'

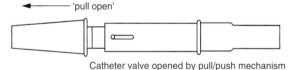

Catheter valve opened by pull/push mechanism

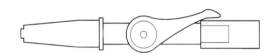

Figure 10.9 Catheter valves.

CATHETER MANAGEMENT

The main aims of catheter management are:

- to relieve and manage urinary dysfunction
- to recognise and minimise risks of secondary complications
- to promote patient dignity and comfort
- to assist patients to reach their own potential in terms of self-care and independence through appropriate education and support
- to provide a cost-effective service.

The skills and knowledge necessary to achieve these aims are complex (Fig. 10.10) and include ongoing assessment of patients and evaluation of both care products and procedures. Local policies

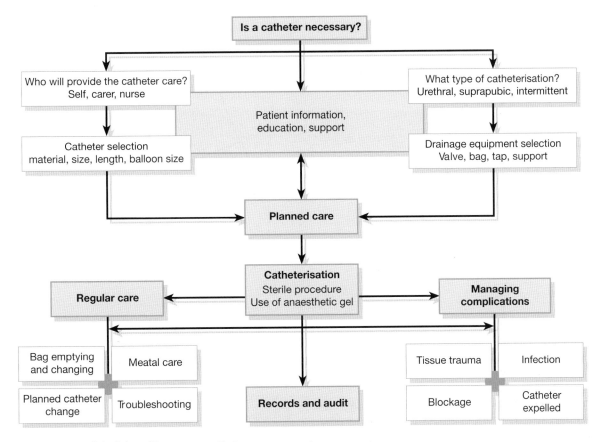

Figure 10.10 Principles of long-term catheter management.

should be referred to for detailed guidance on catheterisation procedure including aseptic technique and use of anaesthetic gel for both males and females.

Catheter-associated risks

There are three main categories of complications which can arise during long-term catheterisation:

- tissue damage and inflammation
- catheter-associated urinary tract infection (CAUTI)
- catheter encrustation leading to recurrent blockage.

TISSUE TRAUMA AND INFLAMMATION

Tissue damage can occur during the catheterisation process or from inflammatory reactions to catheter material. Careful technique and choice of a catheter material that minimises tissue reaction are extremely important. Correct positioning of the drainage bag is also important to minimise risks of hydrostatic suction causing the bladder mucosa to be sucked into the catheter eyes. Positioning the bag no more than 30 cm below the bladder should minimise this risk.

If urethral secretions, or mineral deposits from the urine (see later), have formed hard crusts around the meatus or on the external surface of the catheter and balloon, catheter removal can be painful. Meatal secretions can be removed by gentle washing with soap and water, but catheters should always be observed for signs of encrustation immediately following removal.

Pressure necrosis

Pressure necrosis can be caused in the bladder by the catheter tip pressing continuously on the same

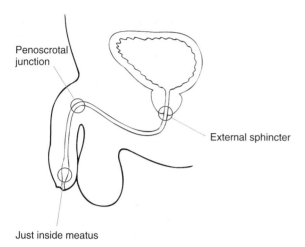

Figure 10.11 Diagram of penoscrotal flexure and potential pressure points.

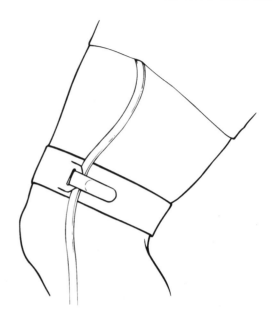

Figure 10.12 Catheter support strap.

location. Regular changing of the catheter and hence the position of the tip will reduce this risk. Severe tissue erosion can occur around the urethral meatus or at other vulnerable points, particularly in the male urethra (Fig. 10.11) if the drainage bag is not effectively supported or there is traction on the catheter or drainage tubing for some other reason (LeBlanc & Christensen 2005). Bags should be emptied when no more than two-thirds full to help reduce risks. Several types of catheter support have been designed to provide a secure support whilst preventing pulling, some of which are available on prescription (Fig. 10.12). If a catheter support is used, it is important that it is not allowed to constrict the catheter or tubing causing a restriction in the urine flow.

CATHETER-ASSOCIATED URINARY TRACT INFECTION

Catheter-associated urinary tract infections (CAUTIs) are widely recognised as a major source of healthcare-associated infections (HAIs) (Plowman et al 1999, Harbath et al 2003) and the frequency of catheter use produces substantial costs to healthcare services, often including unnecessary antibiotic therapy, which may then become a major source of antibiotic-resistant pathogens (Maki & Tambayah 2001). The majority of the existing research on risks of CAUTI has been

Box 10.4 Risk factors for CAUTI

Risk factor	Relative risk (RR)
Prolonged catheterisation >6 days (by 30 days bacteriuria is almost universal)	5.1–6.8
Female	2.5–3.7
Other active sites of infection	2.3–2.4
Diabetes	2.2–2.3
Malnutrition	2.4
Ureteral stent	2.5
Renal insufficiency	2.1–2.6
Improper positioning of drainage tube (above bladder or sagging below drainage bag)	1.9

Adapted from Maki & Tambayah (2001).

conducted in acute care settings where catheters usually remain in place for less than 14 days and many patients' health is already compromised by comorbidities (Brosnahan et al 2004) (Box 10.4). Much less is known about the prevalence of CAUTIs and other HAIs in primary and community care settings (NICE 2003, Niel-Weise & van den Broek 2005). In a recent study of 4010 older people (>65 years) receiving home care in 11

European countries, the prevalence of indwelling catheter use was 5.4% and the risk of a urinary tract infection was 6.5 times greater than for non-catheterised individuals (McNulty et al 2003). Another study of 1004 frail older women living in the community reported a catheter prevalence rate of 38.1%. Prevalence of a urinary tract infection was 21% versus 10% in non-catheterised subjects ($p > 0.001$) and catheterised subjects were more likely to die within a year (Landi et al 2004).

Limitations in the quality and consistency of catheter-related information collected routinely by healthcare services or recorded in patient notes present a major obstacle to robust epidemiological analysis. This is compounded by a lack of clear, standardised criteria used to define CAUTI. Most studies measure the incidence of bacteriuria (presence of bacteria in the urine) and report the number of colony forming units (cfu) detected from culturing 1 ml of urine. The criteria selected to define bacteriuria usually range from $>10^3$ cfu/ml to $>10^5$ cfu/ml but the majority of studies fail to distinguish between asymptomatic bacteriuria and the clinically more important symptomatic bacteriuria.

Entry of microorganisms

The risk of catheter-associated bacteriuria increases by 5–8% per day (Mulhall et al 1988) and despite modern closed drainage systems bacteriuria is virtually inevitable in long-term catheterisation. Microorganisms may gain access to the catheterised bladder in three ways (Fig. 10.13):

- Extraluminal (early) – during the catheterisation procedure

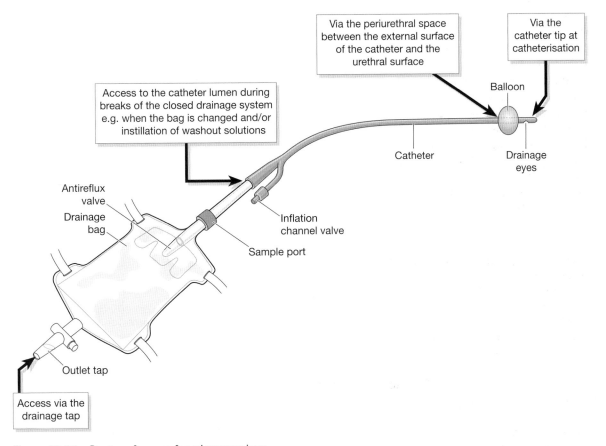

Figure 10.13   Routes of access for microorganisms.

- Intraluminal – by migration within the catheter lumen from the collection bag and/or the catheter drainage tube junction
- Extraluminal (late) – via the mucus film adherent to the external catheter surface.

The comparative importance of these routes is only likely to be of relevance in short-term catheterisation and strategies for prevention of CAUTI, including novel technologies, must address all possible portals of entry. The Department of Health (2001) published guidelines for preventing infections associated with insertion and maintenance of short-term indwelling urethral catheters in acute care. Many of these principles are equally relevant to long-term catheterisation.

Closed drainage systems

The catheter and drainage bag represent a closed system which is not open to the external environment. It is important that the bag is positioned at a level lower than the bladder, such that there is a free flow of urine into the bag, thus preventing collections of stagnant urine within the tubing which can act as a reservoir for growth of microorganisms. The bag should also be positioned such that the tap is not resting on the floor. The non-return valve helps to prevent reflux of urine (and bacteria) into the catheter and bladder if the bag is moved. In order to maintain the effectiveness of the closed system in limiting bacterial access, breaks in the system by disconnecting the bag should be as infrequent as possible. It is generally recommended that bags attached directly to the catheter are changed at weekly intervals unless leakage occurs or the catheter becomes blocked. A high frequency of errors in catheter care, including 'breakages' of the closed system, have been documented in some studies (Mulhall et al 1993) and ongoing, frequent monitoring of adherence to procedures and policies remains important.

Meatal cleansing

There is no evidence that stringent meatal cleansing with or without the use of antiseptic agents will reduce catheter-associated infection. However, it is recommended that urethral secretions are removed on a daily basis using pure or non-perfumed soap and water, with clean wash cloths, to prevent crust formation (Classen et al 1991).

Infecting microorganisms

Complex mixed communities of microorganisms, including a preponderance of Gram-negative bacilli, are commonly found in the urine of catheterised patients. The source of these organisms is often the patient's own bowel flora and microorganisms identified in the urine have also been isolated from the perineum and urethral meatus (Classen et al 1991, Ehrenkranz & Alfonso 1991).

Whilst bacteriuria undoubtedly presents a potential risk of upper urinary tract infection, renal impairment and bacteraemia, the associated risks of morbidity and mortality appear to be related to the underlying health of the patient. Although increased mortality has been associated with urinary catheterisation in one frequently quoted study of acutely ill patients (Platt et al 1982, 1983), this has not been observed to the same extent in other studies (Johnson et al 2006) or for long-term catheterised patients in community care.

Biofilm mode of bacterial growth

Many chronic infections, particularly those involving indwelling devices, such as catheters, implants and prostheses, involve bacterial populations growing as an adherent biofilm (Fig. 10.14). As the biofilm multiplies, it becomes firmly 'cemented' to the catheter surface by secretion of a polysaccharide matrix or 'glycocalyx' (Marrie & Costerton 1983, Getliffe 1992). Biofilm members are generally less susceptible to host defences and antimicrobial agents than free-living organisms (Trautner & Darouiche 2004) and common urinary pathogens such as *Escherichia coli*, although killed in the urine by antimicrobial agents, may persist in the biofilm and restart the cycle of infection. Slow growth rate and nutrient deprivation within the biofilm may be important factors in reducing bacterial pathogenesis and susceptibility to antibiotic agents (Brown et al 1988). The biofilm mode of growth may explain why many patients, with heavily colonised urinary catheters, experience few overt symptoms of infection.

Figure 10.14   Electron micrograph showing thick layer of adherent bacteria on the catheter surface forming a living biofilm.

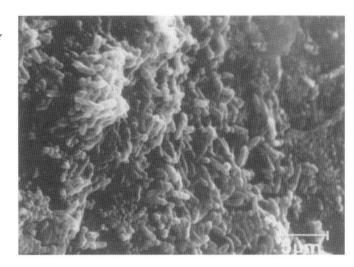

Catheter materials to minimise CAUTI

None of the currently available catheter materials is resistant to biofilm formation. There is increasing evidence of a reduced risk of CAUTI in the short term when silver-alloy coated catheters are used (Saint et al 2000, Johnson et al 2006); however, the potential for longer term protection is unclear. Johnson et al (2006), in their systematic review of antimicrobial catheters, conclude that it is difficult to provide robust analysis of the clinical efficacy and cost–benefit of silver-alloy catheters due to variations in study design, small study sizes and lack of data on clinically meaningful endpoints or long-term catheter use. Most published clinical trials are highly context-dependent, and results are likely to be influenced by a variety of factors including patient groups, antimicrobial usage patterns, background bacteriuria rate, local catheter use, management practices, etc. Consequently, decision-makers need to make careful assessment of appropriateness for their own particular setting.

Antimicrobial agents incorporated into the catheter material or other efforts to disrupt matrix or glycocalyx components offer alternative possibilities (Darouiche et al 1999, Lee et al 2004, Tenke et al 2004). Stickler et al (2003) have attempted to inhibit biofilm development by inflation of the balloon with an antiseptic solution which then diffuses throughout the catheter material, but all of these potential interventions require further testing and consideration of risks of developing resistant strains.

Antibiotics and antiseptic therapies

In the absence of clinical symptoms it is generally accepted that bacteriuria should not be treated with antibiotics (Cravens & Zweig 2000). Similarly, although irrigation of the bladder with antibiotic or antiseptic solutions has been advocated in the past, and continues to be used in some places (Getliffe & Newton 2006), this practice cannot be recommended. Eradication of microorganisms is rarely achieved and the emergence of resistant strains is favoured (Gopal Rao & Elliott 1988). In particular, the benefits of the widespread use of chlorhexidine in bladder washouts (or catheter maintenance solutions), lubricating gels and antiseptic cleaning solutions has been disputed (Davies et al 1987). Chlorhexidine is ineffectual against a number of commonly occurring urinary pathogens, but may remove sensitive bacteria in the normal urethral flora, allowing subsequent colonisation by more resistant organisms.

Certain strains of bacteria may be particularly difficult to eradicate. In a study of nursing home patients, Sabbuba et al (2003) showed that a single genotype of *Proteus mirabilis* can persist in the urinary tract despite many changes of catheter, periods without catheter and antibiotic therapy.

If antibiotic therapy is prescribed, there is evidence from a randomised controlled trial (RCT) involving 54 nursing home residents that changing the catheter immediately prior to the start of antibiotics is significantly associated with better clinical outcomes (Raz et al 2000).

Fluid intake

A high fluid intake of more than 2 litres per day has been traditionally recommended for catheterised patients (Wilson 1997). The rationale behind this is twofold:

- diuresis will assist in voiding microorganisms from the bladder
- a dilute urine will impair bacterial growth and reduce the concentration of encrustation components.

However, biofilms adhere strongly to catheter surfaces and are unlikely to be removed by increased urine flow in a catheter on continuous drainage. Although there is no clear evidence that drinking large quantities of fluid will actually prevent catheter-associated infection, Stickler and Hughes (1999) showed that dilute urine did slow the swarming behaviour of *P. mirabilis* (a common uropathogen) and therefore may also slow biofilm development. It remains sensible to encourage catheterised patients to drink sufficient fluids to avoid constipation or dehydration, especially as many have restricted mobility and may be unable to prepare their own drinks. Urine that is very concentrated may cause irritation of the bladder mucosa and potentiate problems of bladder spasm. In addition, concentrated urine commonly has a strong odour, which patients may find upsetting.

Cranberry juice

Crushed cranberries have been used as a herbal remedy for urinary tract infection for centuries. Cranberry juice is now available as a soft drink or in capsule or tablet form, and has been shown to reduce bacteriuria and pyuria in an RCT conducted with elderly, non-catheterised women (Avorn et al 1994). The mechanism of action against infection may relate to the acidity of the berries and concomitant lowering of the urinary pH, to the bacteriostatic effects of the metabolic by-product, hippuric acid, which is excreted in the urine and/or to an inhibitory effect on the bacterial adherence of some microorganisms, including *E. coli*, to the bladder mucosa (Schmidt & Sobata 1988, Ofek et al 1991). Although antiadherent properties could be particularly advantageous to catheterised patients, the effects are likely to vary with differing organisms and Stickler and Hughes (1999) were unable to detect any inhibitory effect on *P. mirabilis* by oral intake of cranberry juice in their laboratory study.

Cranberry juice or capsules offer a simple and acceptable form of therapy for most patients and may be beneficial, but much of the evidence is anecdotal and further well-controlled investigations on catheterised patients are necessary to confirm or refute its potential benefits to them. Box 10.5 provides a summary of key aspects of care in relation to catheter-associated infection.

CATHETER ENCRUSTATION AND RECURRENT BLOCKAGE

Recurrent catheter blockage caused by encrustation affects around 50% of long-term catheterised patients and presents a problem which is both distressing to patients and carers, and costly to health services in terms of time and resources. Although catheter blockage may result from a number of causes, including twisted drainage tubing, bladder spasm or the pressure of a constipated bowel on the adjacent urethra (see Box 10.8), by far the most common cause of recurrent blockage is the deposit of mineral salts or encrustations on the catheter surface. These deposits may occur both within the lumen of the catheter and on outer surfaces of the tip and balloon where they may cause pain and trauma due to tissue abrasion during catheter removal (Fig. 10.15).

Causes of catheter encrustation

The major components of catheter encrustations are struvite (magnesium ammonium phosphate) and calcium phosphates (Ohkawa et al 1990, Getliffe 1992) which precipitate from the urine under alkaline conditions produced by activity of

- Catheter care should include good personal hygiene around the meatal area during daily hygiene care
- Effective hand washing techniques and wearing of gloves must be employed whenever catheters and bags are handled, and strict attention paid to infection control protocols
- Catheterisation is a sterile procedure and modern drainage equipment provides a sealed system that should not be broken more often than absolutely necessary
- There is no clear evidence that stringent meatal cleansing, addition of antiseptic agents to the drainage bag, bladder washouts with chlorhexidine or similar reagents, drinking large volumes of fluid or regular consumption of cranberry juice will prevent or eradicate catheter-associated infection
- Antibiotic treatment for asymptomatic bacteriuria is not recommended (except in at-risk patients)
- Bacteriuria may be almost inevitable in long-term catheterisation, but it is particularly important to minimise or prevent risks of cross-infection for patients in institutionalised care and for patients at home, who depend on carers and health professionals coming into the home to provide catheter care
- Silver-alloy coated catheters may be effective in the short term but long-term benefits are unknown

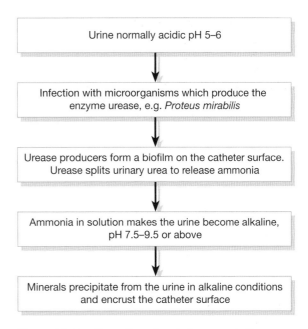

Figure 10.16 Formation of catheter encrustations.

the bacterial enzyme urease. Urease catalyses the breakdown of urinary urea to release ammonia. Ammonia in solution is alkaline, resulting in an increase in urine pH from a normally slightly acidic condition to a pH in the region of 7.5–9.5 (Fig. 10.16). One of the most commonly occurring, potent urease producers is *P. mirabilis*, which is often present in the patient's own normal bowel flora. Figure 10.17 is an electron micrograph of the luminal surface of an encrusted catheter showing the large 'coffin-shaped' crystals of struvite surrounded by the 'rubble-like' calcium phosphate.

Blockers and non-blockers

Despite considerable variation in the tendency of individual patients to develop catheter encrustation, it is generally possible to classify patients into broad categories of 'blockers' or 'non-blockers' (Kunin et al 1987, Getliffe 1992, 1994a, Choong et al 1999) where:

- 'blockers' are defined as those patients who consistently and repeatedly develop extensive encrustation on their urinary catheters within a few days to a few weeks, resulting in shorter

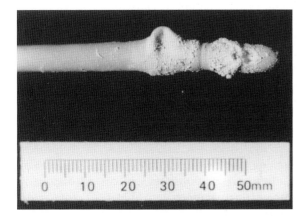

Figure 10.15 An encrusted catheter.

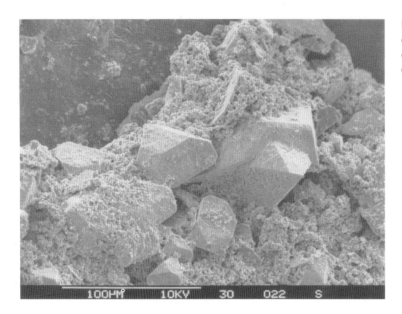

Figure 10.17 Electron micrograph of catheter encrustations showing large crystals of struvite and 'rubble-like' calcium phosphate.

catheter life because of diminished flow and leakage

- 'non-blockers' are those patients who do not form encrustations even when the catheter is left in place for weeks to months (Kunin et al 1987).

Proactive care – planned catheter changes

The recognition of patients as 'blockers' and 'non-blockers' is useful because it allows proactive care to be planned. If a characteristic 'pattern of catheter life' can be identified for an individual patient the catheter can be changed according to a planned schedule to precede the predicted blockage (Getliffe 1994a). It is suggested that the 'life' of at least three to five catheters needs to be recorded in order to identify a clear pattern (Norberg et al 1983). Catheters should be examined carefully for signs of encrustation after removal and not simply assumed to be blocked because of failure to drain well. It may also be helpful to monitor the pH of the urine with an indicator strip since alkaline urine is a strong indicator of potential encrustation. Some patients know their bodies and their catheters extremely well and have a sense of impending blockage. An example of a catheter management chart to aid monitoring of 'catheter life' is shown in the case study in Box 10.6. Another

useful innovation is an indicator inserted into the drainage bag which changes colour as the urine becomes increasingly alkaline.

Using a catheter valve

There is some evidence from laboratory studies that when urine flow is intermittent through use of a catheter valve, the 'flushing' mechanism may increase the time that catheters require to become blocked. The most beneficial effect was recorded when urine was released from the bladder at 4-h intervals during the day and at night by an automatic valve (Sabbuba et al 2005).

Catheter maintenance solutions

Whilst planned catheter changes can limit the occurrence of blockage, frequent recatheterisation can also be a potential source of trauma or distress for patients (Getliffe 1994a). For these patients, instillation of an acidic catheter maintenance solution to reduce encrustation may be helpful to prolong the period of catheter life. Laboratory studies have demonstrated success in dissolving catheter encrustations with Suby G or other acidic solutions but saline is not effective since its pH is neutral (Hesse et al 1989, Getliffe 1994b).

Box 10.6   Case study 1

Mr P was in his mid-70s and had problems of retention of urine due to benign enlargement of his prostate gland. In view of his age and general health he was considered unfit for surgery and his retention was managed by use of an indwelling urethral catheter. Whilst Mr P was happy with the catheter as an effective alternative to surgery, there were times when the catheter suddenly became blocked and the resulting retention of urine caused him considerable pain and distress. Most often the blockage seemed to occur in the early hours of the morning and Mr P would wake feeling an urgent need to void. He was unwilling to call his GP before surgery hours although the longer he waited the more painful his bladder became. Even when the surgery finally opened at 8.30 a.m. he often had to wait several

more hours until the doctor or district nurse was able to visit and change the catheter.

The district nurse was concerned about Mr P's recurrent problem and decided to try to identify the likely cause. She began to keep a chart on which she recorded the characteristics of each 'catheter life' (see Fig. 10.18). Prior to this time Mr P's catheters had been expected to stay in situ for approximately 12 weeks, only to be changed earlier if blockage occurred. After monitoring the 'lives' of three catheters a pattern began to emerge. Mr P's catheters appeared to stay patent for about 3 weeks but tended to block soon after that.

Catheter blockage can sometimes be caused by twisted tubing, bladder spasm or by constipation if the loaded rectum presses on the urethra. However, the

---

Indwelling Catheter Management Chart — CASE STUDY

Name .... MR P

Catheter type ...... BARD BIOCATH (MALE)

Catheter size .... 14 CH

G.P. ....

District Nurse ....

Contact Number ....

Evaluate the current pattern of 'catheter life' after every three catheters and revise care if necessary

Date of catheter change	Previous catheter's 'life' (in days)	Reason for change P – planned B – blocked O – other	Urine pH *pH INDICATOR*	Visible encrustation?	Catheter maintenance solution protocol e.g. 50 ml Suby G 2 x weekly	Next catheter change due	Signature
22/1/01	23	B	ALKALINE RED	YES AROUND EYES	No	12 WEEKS 16/4/01	BS
19/2/01	28	B	ALKALINE RED	No	No	12 WEEKS 19/5/01	BS
15/3/01	25	B	ALKALINE RED	YES	No	3 WEEKS 5/4/01	BS

Evaluate LAST CATHETER CUT OPEN. ENCRUSTATION BLOCKING LUMEN. URINE CONSISTENTLY ALKALINE — SMELLS OF AMMONIA. SAMPLE TO LAB. SEEMS TO BLOCK AFTER ABOUT THREE WEEKS. PLANNED CHANGES AT 3 WEEKS (BEFORE BLOCKAGE!)

5/4/01	21	P	RED	NO	No	3 WEEKS 26/4/01	BS
26/4/01	21	P	RED	YES, ON TIP	No	3 WEEKS 17/5/01	BS
17/5/01	21	P	RED	YES, ON TIP	NO	3 WEEKS 7/6/01	BS

Evaluate 3 WEEK PLAN SEEMS OK. SAMPLE CONTAINS P. MIRABILIS (KNOWN TO CAUSE ALKALINE URINE + CATHETER ENCRUSTATION). LAST CATHETER CUT OPEN. STILL ENCRUSTING BUT STAYS PATENT FOR ABOUT 3 WEEKS. CONTINUE CHANGE AT 3 WEEKS

Figure 10.18   Extract from Mr P's 'catheter life' chart (simplified chart).

Box 10.6 *Continued*

most common cause of recurrent catheter blockage is the build-up of mineral deposits, or encrustation, inside the catheter lumen. By observing each catheter carefully when it was removed it was often possible to see evidence of encrustation on the tip or around the eyes. Two catheters were cut open showing encrusting mineral deposits inside filling the lumen. Mineral salts are precipitated if the urine becomes alkaline due to infection with particular bacteria which release ammonia from urinary urea. By monitoring the pH of the urine, with indicator paper which turns pink or red in alkaline conditions (B. Braun, Sheffield), it was clear that Mr P's urine was alkaline. The most likely cause was infection with an organism that could release ammonia. This was confirmed when a urine sample was sent for microbiological analysis and the organism *Proteus mirabilis*, which is commonly associated with problems of catheter encrustation, was identified.

Antibiotics are not usually very successful at eradicating this type of catheter-associated infection, partly because bacteria stick firmly to the catheter surface forming a biofilm which is unresponsive to antibiotics and partly because the organism is often present in the patient's own bowel providing a continued source of reinfection. The catheter could be replaced with a new 'clean' one whilst a course of antibiotics is tried if it is considered that the organism has been introduced by cross-infection, but since Mr P was living at home this seemed unlikely. The district nurse decided to instigate a regime of planned catheter changes at 3-weekly intervals, i.e. just prior to the likely event of a catheter blockage occurring.

Although Mr P's urine remained alkaline and there were signs of encrustation around the tip of some catheters when they were removed, this regime proved effective and further blockage rarely occurred. Mr P was greatly relieved, especially as he now felt able to go on holiday with his daughter and family without the uncertainty and fear of his previous catheter problems. A few years later, when it became necessary for Mr P to go into residential care, the fact that his catheter was relatively trouble free was an important factor in his acceptance at the centre of his choice.

Potential risks

Potential risks to the bladder can arise from the instillation procedure and/or from the reagent used. Traditional 'bladder washouts' have been performed using a 60 ml bladder syringe fitted to the funnel end of the catheter. Although this method allows active flushing of the catheter and bladder, the physical forces exerted on the bladder mucosa may be considerable (Elliott et al 1989). Despite the 'washout' being performed as an aseptic technique, any breakage of the closed drainage system inevitably increases the risk of introducing infection. The availability of pre-packed, sterile solutions of 50 or 100 ml offers a convenient method for nurses or patients to perform catheter maintenance and to minimise the risks of introducing infection.

Weak citric acid solutions (Box 10.7) such as Suby G are the usual reagent of choice, since all acidic reagents may cause some irritation to mucosal tissues as indicated by Kennedy et al (1992). In a small RCT of Suby G, Solution R and saline in 25 female patients with long-term cathe-

Box 10.7 Catheter maintenance solutions available in the UK

• Suby G	3.23% citric acid solution, pH 4, containing magnesium oxide to minimise tissue irritation, aimed at reducing encrustation
• Solution R	6% citric acid solution, pH 2, containing magnesium carbonate, aimed at dissolving encrustations
• Mandelic acid 1%	An acidic solution, pH 2, aimed at inhibiting the growth of urease producers
• Saline 0.9%	A neutral solution, pH 7, recommended for flushing of debris and small blood clots (not recommended for catheter encrustation)
• Chlorhexidine 0.02%	An antiseptic solution aimed at preventing or reducing bacterial growth, in particular *E. coli* and *Klebsiella* species (not recommended for catheter encrustation or preventing (AUTI)

ters, a high percentage of red blood cells was found in the drainage fluid following use of Suby G, indicating some degree of tissue irritation. Increased shedding of urothelial cells was noted with all three solutions. Although there were limitations in the design of this study, there is clearly a need for further clinical studies to determine if these outcomes are clinically important or if the mucosa recovers rapidly (Donmez et al 1990).

Dissolution of catheter encrustations may also be achieved by Solution R, but the benefits may be outweighed by potential inflammatory tissue reactions to a stronger acid solution, which limits the frequency with which this solution can be used. It is probably of most value used prior to catheter removal if external encrustations on the catheter tip and balloon cause pain and tissue trauma when the catheter is withdrawn. Solution R may also be useful in dissolving encrustations which are blocking the catheter by instilling the solution as far as the blockage and leaving it in place to dissolve the encrustations for up to 15–20 min. The most commonly available range of prepacked solutions is shown in Box 10.7.

How much and how often?

The relative lack of either experimental or clinical research-based evidence makes it extremely difficult to provide clear guidance on the optimum use of catheter maintenance solutions (Getliffe 1996, Getliffe et al 2000). Studies using a laboratory model of catheter encrustation have shown that 50 ml is as effective as 100 ml at reducing encrustations and also that two sequential washes with 50 ml may be more effective at reducing encrustation than a single washout with either 50 or 100 ml (Getliffe et al 2000). One manufacturer markets a delivery device which contains 'twin' washes of 50 ml which can be helpful for patients with severe encrustation problems, but two washes are not necessarily required for every patient. It seems likely that even smaller volumes would still completely fill the catheter lumen and bathe the tip, and could perhaps be used more frequently (e.g. on alternate days) without increasing the risks of tissue irritation. Pomfret (1995) discusses the instillation of 'mini-bladder washouts' in 10 patients experiencing severe problems with catheter

encrustation and blockage. Subjective evidence suggested that, for many of them, there appeared to be a reduced frequency of blockage.

Catheter maintenance solutions are not advocated for all patients and even where they may be appropriate it makes sense to develop an individualised regime based on the smallest volume and lowest frequency that helps extend catheter life to an acceptable duration. It is not expected that this management approach will necessarily prevent encrustation completely but it can help reduce the frequency of catheter blockage.

Oral acidification of urine

Although efforts to acidify urine through dietary means are attractive there is a lack of any robust evidence of effectiveness from cranberry juice (Morris & Stickler 2001) or ascorbic acid (vitamin C) (Nahata et al 1977) although most studies to date have been poorly controlled. Evidence from laboratory-based studies also suggests that attempts to reduce urinary pH in the presence of urease producers are ineffective because lower pH can act as a trigger for more urease production to raise the pH again (Bibby et al 1995).

Individualised patient care

In research studies which focus on a population of patients who are all 'blockers' it may be difficult to demonstrate the efficacy of different management approaches because of wide intragroup variations (e.g. in characteristic patterns of catheter life). Therefore it is always important for practitioners to look carefully, not only at the research evidence available, but also at the way in which it was collected. Strategies which may not appear to be effective for all 'blockers' may nevertheless extend the catheter life of individual patients.

Using a catheter valve to allow the bladder to fill and subsequently empty when the valve is opened has the potential to create a flushing action which could help reduce build-up of encrustation and deserves further study in the clinical setting.

PATIENT SUPPORT

It is important not to underestimate the psychological and social effects of long-term catheterisation. For some patients faced with long-term urinary dysfunction, catheterisation may be viewed depressingly as the 'beginning of the end', marked by the need for an invasive device to control what should be a normal bodily function. However, for others, a catheter can provide an improved sense of freedom and independence in the knowledge that their urine loss is contained. In some cases a catheter can make the difference between coping at home and the alternative of institutional care.

Information and practical advice

Patients may require a great deal of educational help and support, particularly in the early days following catheterisation. An explanation of the purpose of the catheter and its care is important for all patients who are not unconscious or cognitively impaired and should include not only verbal discussion but also provision of written information to which patients and carers can continue to refer. A range of useful booklets and brochures is available from specialist manufacturers and charities. The main educational issues that should be addressed include the following:

- What a catheter is and why it is needed
- Simple anatomy and physiology of the urinary tract, illustrating the position of the catheter
- Personal hygiene, especially handwashing before and after handling the catheter or drainage bag
- Connecting and disconnecting bags
- Disposal of urine and cleaning of bags
- Dietary advice, avoiding constipation, fluid intake
- Dealing with catheter problems, including when and where to call for help
- Obtaining supplies
- Sexual activity.

Quality of life

Quality of life for people with urinary catheters has not been studied adequately. Anecdotal information suggests that many people find a urethral catheter uncomfortable but there is a general lack of published evidence from research studies. In one study at a Veterans Affairs Medical Center in

the USA, 30% of catheterised patients surveyed reported that they found the indwelling catheter embarrassing, 42% reported that it was uncomfortable, 48% complained it was painful and 61% said that it restricted their activities of daily living (Saint et al 1999). Qualitative data from some small scale studies suggest that major QoL issues involve stigma related to exposure and urine accidents, sexuality and acceptance/non-acceptance of living with a catheter (Roe 1990, Wilde 2003). Other concerns include disruptions to daily living because of catheter-related problems (e.g. blocking, leaking, symptomatic CAUTI, catheter change process).

Sexual activity

Sexual activity is not precluded by the presence of a urethral catheter although catheterisation will influence sexuality and may contribute to physical and psychological problems including impaired body image, loss of libido, embarrassment, discomfort and retrograde ejaculation in men (Seymour 1998, Roe & May 1999, Pateman & Johnson 2000, Wilde 2003). In males the catheter can be folded back along the length of the penis and secured in place with a condom. In females it can be helpful to reassure the couple that the catheter is not in the vagina and can be taped across the lower abdomen to keep it out of the way. A 'rear approach' may also be a more comfortable position. KY jelly can be used to aid lubrication. However, patients may prefer to consider the possibility of a suprapubic insertion or the temporary removal and subsequent replacement of the catheter. In some cases the patient or partner may be taught how to remove the catheter prior to sexual activity and recatheterise subsequently. Healthcare professionals need to be alert to these issues, even in the case of elderly patients. They must be prepared to facilitate discussions, which patients may find difficult to initiate, in a sensitive manner and be able to offer guidance or other sources of advice.

Troubleshooting

Some practical hints for dealing with common problems associated with urethral catheterisation are offered in Box 10.8.

Box 10.8 Troubleshooting – urethral catheters

URINE DOES NOT DRAIN

- Check the drainage bag is below the level of the bladder
- Check for kinked tubing
- Empty the bag – urine will not drain if the bag is very full
- If it is suspected that the bladder mucosa may be occluding the catheter eyes, raise the bag above the level of the bladder briefly to release negative hydrostatic pressure and then position the bag no more than around 30 cm below the bladder
- Check for constipation
- Change the catheter and inspect for encrustation

URINARY BYPASSING

- Check for kinked tubing
- Check for constipation
- Change the catheter and inspect for encrustation and blockage
- If there is a possibility of bladder irritation/spasm:
  - consider increasing fluid intake to dilute urine
  - check for systemic symptoms of infection
  - check for bladder calculi by X-ray or ultrasound
  - replace the catheter with a smaller size
  - consider anticholinergic medication

HAEMATURIA

- Small amounts of blood may be caused by trauma or infection
- If severe, seek medical help urgently

THE INFLATION BALLOON DOES NOT DEFLATE

- Check for kinked tubing
- Try a different syringe. Leave in place; the water may seep out over a period of time
- Try to relieve constipation, if present. This may cause pressure on the inflation channel
- Try to remove or dislodge debris blocking the deflation channel by gently 'milking' the catheter along its length or inserting a few drops of sterile water into the inflation channel (no more than 1–2 ml)
- Attach a sterile needle to a 10 ml syringe and insert into the catheter arm just above the inflation valve. If the valve is faulty the water may be withdrawn gently via the syringe
- Never cut the catheter. If it is under traction it may recoil inside the urethra
- Never cut off the inflation valve. If the balloon does not deflate it will no longer be possible to try alternative simple methods
- Never attempt to burst the balloon by overinflating it – a cystoscopy will be required to remove fragments! Remaining fragments may result in formation of calculi
- Consult local nursing policy for further advice

NB: Always have a spare catheter available!

SUPRAPUBIC CATHETERISATION

For some patients the insertion of an indwelling catheter suprapubically, i.e. into the bladder through the abdominal wall, may offer some advantages over the urethral route. This technique may be necessary following urethral or pelvic trauma, and may also be appropriate for urinary retention or voiding problems caused by prostatic obstruction or urethral stricture. The suprapubic route can be particularly useful for women with neuropathy since urethral catheterisation forces them to sit on a urethral catheter. A lack of mobility, which prevents changing the seated position, can cause pressure on the catheter, which in turn could cause erosion of the bladder neck and urethra. Hypercontractility of the neuropathic bladder also increases the risk of the catheter being expelled, with concomitant trauma to urethral tissue. A suprapubic insertion can also be the method of choice for patients with restricted hip mobility (e.g. due to arthritis), those with urethral scarring resulting from trauma or tumours, or those who are sexually active.

Some benefits of the suprapubic route

There is evidence of high levels of satisfaction and an improved quality of life associated with suprapubic catheterisation in patients requiring long-term drainage due to neuropathic bladder dysfunction (Sheriff et al 1998). Some of the advantages of suprapubic compared to urethral insertion include the following:

- No risk of urethral trauma, necrosis or catheter-induced urethritis
- Greater comfort, particularly for patients who are chairbound

- Access to the entry site is easier for cleansing and catheter change
- Greater freedom for expression of sexuality
- Facilitation of trials of voiding after major/urological surgery. The drainage tubing can be clamped and the ability to void urethrally assessed prior to removal of the suprapubic catheter.

The major contraindication to suprapubic catheterisation is in patients with haematuria of unknown origin or with known carcinoma of bladder since there are clear risks associated with inflicting trauma on tumour cells. Suprapubic catheters may also be inappropriate for small contracted or fibrotic bladders (resulting from long-term free drainage by urethral catheter) and in some very obese patients where the catheter will be trapped between folds of skin and adipose tissue.

Catheter insertion

Although suprapubic catheterisation is gaining wide acceptance it is not entirely without risks. Catheter insertion requires a minor surgical procedure through an incision in the abdominal wall (cystotomy), with potential risks to structures adjacent to the bladder, especially large and small intestines with resultant peritonitis. The procedure is normally undertaken by a medical practitioner under local or general anaesthetic, under strict aseptic conditions (Figs 10.19, 10.20) but can be carried out by an appropriately trained and competent nurse, with due adherence to UKCC guidelines (1992). Gujral et al (1999) reported on 164 patients who had their first suprapubic catheter inserted by a continence adviser/urology nurse specialist, with no evidence of serious complications.

Catheter change

Once the abdominal channel has become established (about 4 weeks) a Foley catheter can be changed routinely by experienced nursing staff on the ward or in the community, usually without the use of local anaesthetic. Patients or carers may also be taught to change the catheter for themselves. It

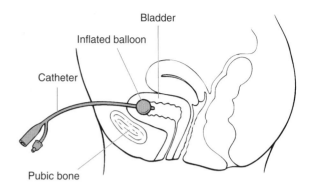

Figure 10.19   Suprapubic catheter in position.

is important to carefully observe the angle of the catheter as it leaves the abdomen and the length of the exposed portion of the catheter as this will help insertion of the new catheter along the established pathway. Insertion of a little anaesthetic gel down the side of the old catheter will help to lubricate it and facilitate its removal after deflation of the balloon. If the balloon has not returned to its original flat position or there is some encrustation on the catheter a gentle pull may be necessary to remove it and can result in a little bleeding. The new catheter should be inserted as quickly as possible whilst the tract is still easy to follow. A delay of only a few minutes can result in partial obliteration of the tract as the detrusor fibres contract (Iacovou 1994).

Suprapubic catheter management

Although the principles of catheter management are similar to the management of urethral catheters, there are differences. The suprapubic catheter emerges at right angles to the abdomen and may require support in this position. Its location may also present some difficulties in dressing and carrying out personal hygiene. Secretions around the cystotomy site can be removed while bathing or with soap and water. If staining of clothing by secretions is a problem, a simple dressing may be applied but is often unnecessary. One relatively minor complication, which can be a great nuisance to patients, is persistent weeping from small patches of granulation tissue which develop

Figure 10.20   Introduction of a suprapubic catheter.

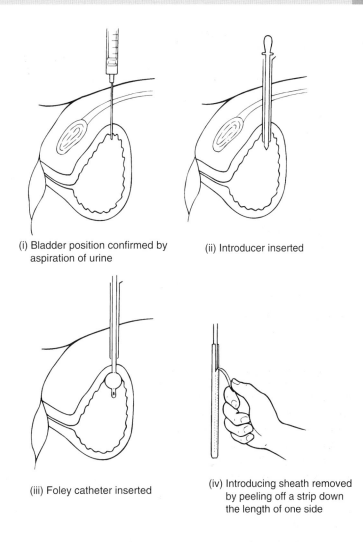

(i) Bladder position confirmed by
aspiration of urine

(ii) Introducer inserted

(iii) Foley catheter inserted

(iv) Introducing sheath removed
by peeling off a strip down
the length of one side

alongside the catheterisation site. Reference should be made to local wound management or catheter care protocols to deal with this problem. Evans and Feneley (2000) report on a study of the nursing management of 113 patients with long-term suprapubic catheters in the community. These authors found that 60% of patients required a dressing around their suprapubic site and 42% of patients regularly received either a bladder washout or catheter maintenance solution instillation. Persistent urethral leakage can sometimes be a difficulty, most commonly in females.

It is suggested that there may be a reduced risk of CAUTI in short-term suprapubic catheterisation due to the greater spatial separation from potential contamination by bowel microorganisms but the evidence is inconclusive. For long-term use, suprapubic catheters are susceptible to catheter-associated infection, biofilm formation and to catheter encrustation and blockage in the same way as urethral catheters (Getliffe 1992, Shah & Shah 1998). Other potential risk factors are also similar to those encountered in urethral catheterisation and include bladder spasm, loss of bladder tone and pressure necrosis (Addison & Mould 2000). There is some evidence to suggest that bladder calculi may be more common in suprapubic catheterisation and Shah and Shah (1998) recommend annual ultrasound and cystoscopy to check for these.

Common problems with suprapubic catheters

- If no urine drains after changing the catheter, ensure the drainage bag is below the level of the bladder. Also encourage the patient to drink beforehand.
- If there is leakage through the urethra, check for kinked tubing. If bladder spasm is a problem, consider anticholinergic medication. Surgical closure of the urethra may be necessary as a last resort.
- Overgranulation of tissue at the insertion site can be ignored if it is not causing concern to the patient. Refer to local wound management or catheter care protocols if further action is required.

INTERMITTENT SELF-CATHETERISATION

Intermittent catheterisation (IC) is the act of passing a catheter into the bladder to drain urine via the urethra or other catheterisable channel such as a Mitrofanoff continent urinary diversion. Clean intermittent self-catheterisation (CISC), originally introduced by Lapides et al (1972), is the preferred option for bladder drainage for patients who can manage this technique as it provides greater independence and personal control over bladder function. Since the catheter is passed intermittently into the bladder and immediately removed when drainage has ceased, ISC avoids many of the problems associated with the retention of a catheter in situ.

Wyndaele (2002) examined complications of IC in a review of 82 trials. Urinary tract infection was the most frequent complication and catheterisation frequency and the avoidance of bladder overfilling were recognised as important preventative measures. The study concluded that the most critical preventative measures were good education of all involved in IC, good patient adherence to protocol, use of an appropriate catheter material and good catheterisation technique. Similar findings were reported by Campbell et al (2004) in a follow-up of children with spina bifida who had used IC for at least 5 years.

Teaching ISC technique

The residual urine volume should not be less than 100 ml to make the technique worth teaching and can be measured postvoiding by ultrasound bladder scan or by draining the residual through an intermittent catheter. Some patients may need to be taught the technique prior to surgery if there is a risk of incomplete bladder emptying post surgery. Provided the importance of regular bladder drainage is understood, ISC can be practised by males and females and can be taught to older people and to children as young as 4 years old with parental supervision (Eckstein 1979, Pilloni et al 2005).

An appropriate level of manual dexterity is essential and as a general rule if people can write and feed themselves they have the dexterity to catheterise (Fowler 1998). Disabilities such as blindness, lack of perineal sensation, tremor, mental disability and paraplegia do not necessarily preclude mastery of the technique (Doherty 2001) and a range of catheter handling aides can be used to enhance manual skills.

Location of the urethra may sometimes be more difficult for females but can usually be accomplished easily with practice once they have a better understanding of their own anatomy and often with the use of a mirror in the first instance. If patients are unable to carry out the procedure for themselves, the technique can be taught to carers but local protocols on 'consent' must be complied with and health professionals are still responsible for ensuring the care provided is both effective and safe.

Advantages of ISC

The main advantages of ISC include:
- greater opportunity for patients to reach their own potential in terms of self-care and independence
- reduced risk of some common catheter-associated problems:
  - urethral trauma . . .   risk reduced
  - urinary tract infection . . . risk reduced
  - encrustation . . .   risk removed
- better protection of the upper urinary tract from reflux

- reduced need for equipment and appliances, e.g. drainage bags
- greater freedom for expression of sexuality and positive body image
- potential for improved continence between catheterisations.

Frequency of catheterisation

Catheterisation should follow a regime designed to suit the needs of the individual patient but it is generally accepted that this should be no more than every 2 h during the day and that sleep should be undisturbed as far as possible. Some patients catheterise far less frequently, and in some cases, where inefficient voiding leads to a gradual collection of a large residual, ISC may be necessary only once a day or even on alternate days. Alternatively, an extra catheterisation may be appropriate prior to an activity that may limit access to a toilet for some time or prior to sexual activity. Anticholinergic drugs may be helpful for patients experiencing symptoms of frequency, urgency or nocturia (see Ch. 9).

Individual care plans help to identify appropriate catheterisation frequency based on discussion of individual voiding dysfunction and impact on quality of life, frequency/volume charts, functional bladder capacity and ultrasound bladder scans for residual urine volume. In an adult, catheterising frequently enough to avoid residual urine greater than 400–500 ml is a general principle but bladder capacity should be guided by urodynamic findings and renal function.

Types of catheter for ISC

Types and characteristics of catheters for ISC vary considerably. Catheters for ISC do not require a retention balloon and are usually more rigid than indwelling catheters to aid self-insertion. They are typically comprised of a clear plastic (PVC) tube with two eyes at the tip and often with a funnel at the other end (Fig. 10.21). The funnel helps patients with poor eyesight to identify the correct end for insertion and also allow patients to observe the colour/concentration of the urine.

Plain uncoated catheters are packed singly in sterile packaging and are frequently reused after

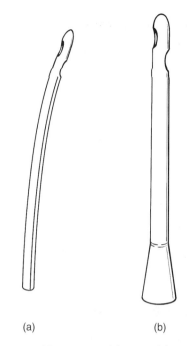

(a)　　　　　　　　　　(b)

Figure 10.21　ISC catheters: (a) Scott; (b) Nelaton.

cleaning with soap and water, boiling, disinfectant soaks or microwave. Cleaned catheters are air-dried and stored in a sealed plastic container. Coated catheters are intended to improve catheter lubrication and ease of insertion. The most common coatings are hydrophilic polymers which absorb water when wetted to form a slippery surface. An alternative is a prelubricated catheter and several of these products have an integral collection bag which allows greater flexibility for the user and are efficient for hospital use. Coated catheters are intended for single use only, though in terms of cumulative use over time they are more expensive than uncoated catheters. A trial reported by De Ridder et al (2005) suggests that UTI is reduced in hydrophilic catheter users compared with uncoated PVC catheter users and further exploration of these findings is needed (Moore et al 2007). One of the difficulties in determining the prevalence of UTI is at least partially due to the variable definitions of UTI used (see earlier discussion of CAUTI).

ISC catheter sizes are in the range 6–20 Ch, most of which are available on prescription. The most common sizes for female use are 10–12, and

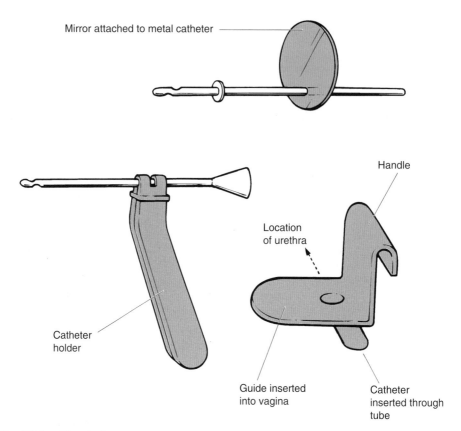

Mirror attached to metal catheter

Handle

Location of urethra

Catheter holder

Guide inserted into vagina

Catheter inserted through tube

Figure 10.22   ISC handling devices.

12–14 for males, although males with a history of urethral strictures may require a larger size. A number of handling devices can be used to assist patients with limited manual dexterity (Fig. 10.22). Patients should have the opportunity to try different catheters and to choose which best suits their needs and lifestyle. Nurses should also ensure they are competent to teach the technique.

A full programme of teaching and follow-up support should be offered after careful assessment and identification of patients who are:

- willing to accept the concept of self-catheterisation
- motivated and have sufficient mental ability to understand the technique
- are sufficiently agile and manually dextrous to perform ISC.

Patient education for ISC

It is important not to assume that all patients are comfortable with the idea of ISC and it is sensible to explore their expectations, goals and motivation before commencing a teaching programme (Box 10.9). Booklets and videos are available from many manufacturers of ISC products and provide useful information for patients, families and carers. If possible it is a good idea to watch the video with the patient or carer who is learning the technique to help answer specific questions and allay fears. The programme of teaching and support should include:

- discussion with patients about their individual bladder dysfunction and the reasons for self-catheterisation
- discussion of personal anatomy and identification of urethral orifice

Box 10.9 Guidelines for intermittent self-catheterisation

Helpline number, in case of problems: ....
1. Wash and dry hands immediately before catheterising, after adjusting clothing.
2. Wash genital area if necessary:
   Females: Part labia and cleanse from front to back.
   Males: Cleanse tip of penis and pull back foreskin to clean around glans, insert anaesthetic gel if required
3. Adopt a suitable position such as one of the following, checking that the other end of the catheter is towards the toilet or the container so that you won't spill any urine:
   Female: Lying with the knees apart, sitting on a toilet or bidet.
            Standing with one leg raised on the toilet or bath.
            Squatting against a wall.
            Sitting in an empty bath.
   Male: Standing over a toilet, sitting on a toilet or chair
4. Gently insert the catheter, with or without a lubricating agent:
   Female: Insert inside the urethra, sloping slightly down from front to back, until urine begins to come out. If you miss and go into the vagina, remove the catheter, wash it and start again.
   Males: Hold the penis at an angle of 60° to horizontal with slight tension applied to straighten urethral curves. Just before the catheter enters the bladder you may notice some resistance as the catheter passes through the external sphincter.
            If the catheter won't go in, stop and try again later. Don't make yourself sore.
            Provided you are gentle you won't do any damage; if you push the catheter in too far, it will simply curl up in the bladder.
5. When urine flows, stop insertion.
6. Observe colour of urine:
   – pale yellow is desirable
   – dark yellow, strong smelling indicates a concentrated urine. Increase your fluid intake.
7. When urine drainage ceases, slowly withdraw the catheter to ensure all the urine is drained. It may help to bend forward slightly to aid drainage, or to press on your tummy just above the pubic bone. If the catheter cannot be withdrawn easily, stop, relax by giving a loud sigh and try to imagine letting go, cough slightly and then gently withdraw.
8. Wash the catheter in running water (with soap if wished) after use, allow to air dry and store in a sealed plastic box or bag. Dispose of after 1 week.

NB: Self-lubricating catheters such as 'Lofric' (AstraTech) and 'Easicath' (Conveen) are designed for single use only.

- performance of ISC, including identification of the most comfortable position, followed by observation of the patient's technique
- discussion of hygiene, including importance of handwashing and cleansing of genitalia
- cleaning, storage and reuse of catheters, and subsequent disposal. Reusable catheters may be washed carefully and stored in an airtight box. They should be disposed of after 5–7 days. Single-use catheters should not be reused according to manufacturers (although some patients do wash and reuse them for a limited time)
- possible difficulties and what to do (see Common problems)

- dietary advice and avoidance of constipation
- obtaining supplies, on prescription
- follow-up visits, usually every 1–2 weeks initially, then as required. Importance of follow-up appointments with consultant as appropriate.

Common problems with ISC

- UTI – the prevalence of reported UTIs varies widely in the literature; however, relatively high proportions of patients have chronic bacteriuria although the prevalence is lower than in patients with indwelling urethral catheters (Maes & Wyndaele 1988, Shekelle et al 1999).

- Sometimes the catheter will not go in at the first attempt. Usually if left for a while the catheter can be inserted at the next try. Dipping the catheter in water may aid lubrication.
- Sometimes the catheter will not come out. The patient should be advised to leave it for a few minutes, try to relax and 'let go' of the catheter, then cough gently and withdraw it.
- If urethral bleeding occurs it may be helpful to prevent the bladder filling above 450 ml. Atonic bladders can become stretched to hold very large volumes and surface capillaries become enlarged. This may result in bleeding when the bladder is artificially emptied (Doherty 2001).

ISC requires a high level of patient commitment and may be abandoned, particularly during times of physical or psychological stress, or during pregnancy. It is important that patients performing ISC have regular follow-ups with their consultant to ensure there is no evidence of damage to the upper urinary tract.

Children

There are a small though not insignificant number of children who require regular catheterisation during the course of the school day per urethra or Mitrofanoff stoma. A care plan should be drawn up by a continence adviser/paediatric community nurse and/or school nurse, together with the child's consultant, the child and the parents. With adequate training and suitable facilities, many children are able to carry out ISC themselves either on a toilet or from a wheelchair. Good interagency working between health, education and social services in partnership with the child and parents is essential for effective care. Further detail is beyond the scope of this book but key sources of further information are included in Chapter 5.

EVALUATION OF CATHETER CARE PRACTICE

Documentation

Thorough documentation is important to ensure patient safety, consistency in delivery of high quality care and effective monitoring. It also protects the nurse. If care has been not been docu-mented, a court of law may assume that it was not done. This could be used to support accusations of unprofessional conduct. The UKCC guidelines for records and record keeping (1998) should be adhered to. Use of a catheter record card is recommended. This can accompany the patient to hospital if needed. At each catheterisation the following data should be recorded in the patient's notes:

- Date of insertion and reason for catheterisation
- Catheter type, size including length, balloon size
- Batch number, manufacturer and date of expiry, so that in the event of a fault it can be reported to the manufacturer and/or Department of Health and easily traced
- Type of lubricant or anaesthetic gel used
- Any difficulty on insertion or removal of previous catheter
- Planned care protocol and expected date of review/catheter removal or next change
- Signature of the person inserting the catheter.

KEY POINTS FOR PRACTICE

- Non-invasive methods for management of urinary dysfunction are preferable to catheterisation where possible
- Clean intermittent catheterisation is a treatment of choice for patients needing to use a catheter and with residual urine >100 ml
- Suprapubic catheterisation can be an appropriate alternative to urethral catheterisation for many patients, following appropriate risk assessment
- Self-caring patients should receive appropriate education and ongoing support and have an opportunity to try different drainage equipment to optimise ease and independence
- Good handwashing practice (before and after handling catheters and drainage equipment) and maintenance of a closed system are important to reduce the risks of cross-infection
- Where recurrent catheter blockage is a problem, aim for 'planned care' not 'crisis care'. Monitoring of 'catheter life' can often establish a pattern of recurrent catheter encrustation in susceptible patients and allow recatheterisation to be planned prior to problem development

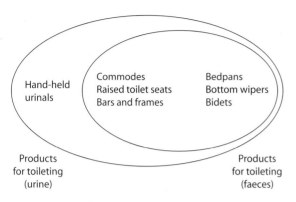

Figure 10.23   Categories of products ⁻prevent incontinence by assisting toileting. Re   ⁻with permission from Cottenden et al (20⁻

Products
for toileting
(urine)

Products
for toileting
(faeces)

Hand-held
urinals

Commodes
Raised toilet seats
Bars and frames

Bedpans
Bottom wipers
Bidets

CONTAINMENT PROD⁻
CONTINENCE CARE

INTRODUCTION

The aim of this section
navigation through t'
continence products
optimum products
needs.

TYPES OF PRO⁻
NEEDS

Continence products may be a⁻
broad categories: products to prevent inc⁻
by assisting toileting (Fig. 10.23) and products⁻
manage urinary retention or to contain/control
urinary and/or faecal incontinence (Fig. 10.24).

Choosing the most appropriate products can be
difficult and the algorithms in Figures 10.25 and
10.26 are intended to help determine which category of product is most likely to benefit an individual. The answers to three questions are
needed:

- Is there urinary incontinence or faecal incontinence, or both?
- Is there urinary retention with or without
  incontinence?
- Are there problems with toilet access (e.g. prox-
  imity or design of the toilet, mobility or urgency
  problems for the patient)?

Selecting appropriate products requires consultation with the patient (and their carers) and is
usually best carried out in the individual's living
environment (rather than in a clinic) to determine
practical and contextual issues as well as individual characteristics and preferences (Gibb & Wong
1994, Paterson et al 2003). Box 10.10 lists factors
which should be considered during assessment
and are known to influence the suitability of products for different patient needs.

PRODUCTS FOR ASSISTING TOILETING

Hand-held urinals

⁻ndividual impairments such as limited mobility
⁻lems with hip abduction can restrict an
⁻bility to access a toilet. Hand-held
⁻ll, portable devices designed
⁻ing when toilet access is
⁻, helpful for people who
⁻r urgency when fast toilet
⁻avoid incontinence.

⁻or 'bottle' is a familiar product to
⁻d has changed little in decades.
⁻s come with a detachable non-spill
⁻aining a flutter valve to impede
⁻urine from the urinal. There are no
⁻trials of such products but it is likely
⁻ain factors in determining suitability for
⁻als are the ease of grasping and holding
⁻ ⁻al in place and the stability of the urinal
when not in use (to avoid spillage). Disposable
hand-held urinals for both men and women are
available which are usually 'flat' packed or pocket-
sized and are designed for travel and 'emergency'
purposes.

Female urinals

Female hand-held urinals come in many different
shapes and sizes (Fig. 10.27). Most are designed
for multiple use and are usually made from
moulded plastic. Some are intended for single use
and are made from flexible plastic or cardboard.
Some have handles to facilitate grip and positioning and are designed to hold bladder-sized

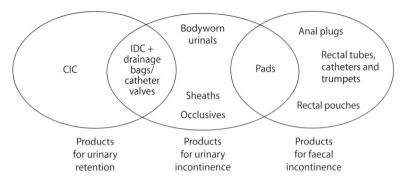

Figure 10.24   Categories of products to manage urinary retention or to contain/control urinary and/or faecal incontinence. CIC, clean intermittent catheterisation; IDC, indwelling catheter. Reproduced with permission from Cottenden et al (2005).

CIS = Clean Intermittent Catheterisation;
IDC = Indwelling Catheterisation

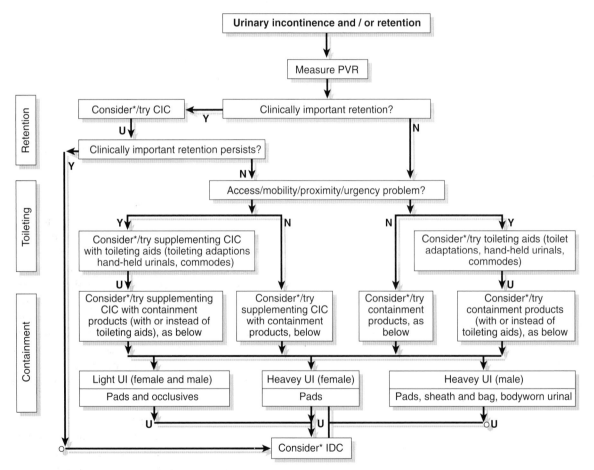

Y = Yes   N = No   U = Unsatisfactory outcome

PVR = Post-void residual urine

* NB physical characteristics; cognitive ability; personal preferences etc.

Figure 10.25   Algorithm for choosing products for urinary incontinence (UI) and/or retention. CIC, clean intermittent catheterisation; IDC, indwelling catheter; N, no; U, unsatisfactory outcome; Y, yes. * Physical characteristics, cognitive ability, personal preferences, etc. Reproduced with permission from Cottenden et al (2005).

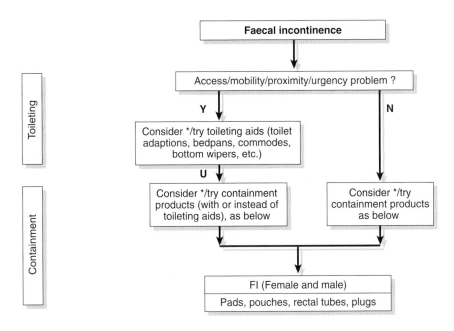

Y = Yes   N = No   U = Unsatisfactory outcome

* NB physical characteristics; cognitive ability; personal preferences etc.

Figure 10.26   Algorithm for choosing products for faecal incontinence (FI). N, no; U, unsatisfactory outcome; Y, yes. * Physical characteristics, cognitive ability, personal preferences, etc. Reproduced with permission from Cottenden et al (2005).

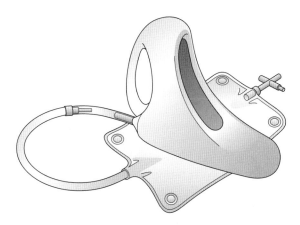

Figure 10.27   A female urinal. Reproduced with permission from the Continence Foundation (http:// www.continence-foundation.org.uk).

volumes of urine (200–500 ml); others have small capacities but are designed for use with drainage bags. Macintosh (1998) provides guidance on assessment to help select appropriate urinals. Female hand-held urinals have only been the subject of one published trial (Fader et al 1999). The findings from this study of 37 community-based women showed that many products were successful when used in the standing/crouching position or when sitting on the edge of a chair/bed/wheelchair. Fewer worked well for users sitting in a chair/wheelchair. Only one worked even reasonably well when users were lying/semi-lying. In general, this study showed that individuals with higher levels of dependency and with limited ability to change position are likely to find fewer urinals suitable for their needs.

Recommendation for practice

- Assessment of the individual's manual dexterity, hip abduction and ability to adopt different postures will help to determine the suitability of different designs.
- If possible, offer users a range of products to experiment with before making a selection. Some continence services provide a library of products for short-term loan for this purpose.

Box 10.10 Key elements of patient assessment for products (adapted from Cottenden et al 2005)

Element	Rationale
Independence/assistance	If a carer is required to apply or change the product then it may be important to involve them in the selection of the product and to establish their willingness and ability to use it
Nature of incontinence	The frequency, volume and flow rate of the incontinence influences product suitability. Generally smaller, more discreet products should be tried before larger bulkier products
Mental acuity	Mental impairment can affect the person's ability to manage the product. Products that resemble usual underwear (e.g. some absorbents) may be easiest to manage. Products that have health implications if used incorrectly (e.g. occlusives or catheter valves) should be avoided if mental impairment is present
Mobility	Impaired mobility may make some product choices impractical or require toilet or clothing modification to allow effective use of the product
Dexterity	Problems with hand or finger movement can make it difficult to use some products, e.g. taps on leg bags, straps with buttons
Eyesight	Impaired eyesight limits effective application and management of some products
Physical characteristics	Anthropometrics (e.g. height, and waist, thigh and penile circumference) will influence the comfort and effectiveness of a product
Leg abduction problems	Difficulty with leg abduction can make the use of some products impractical or ineffective
Lifestyle	Daily activities can influence the choice of product and a mixture of products may provide optimum management. Different products may be most satisfactory for daytime and going out (when discreetness may be a priority) and nighttime or staying in (when comfort may be a priority) or for holidays (when large quantities of disposables may be a problem)
Laundry facilities	Reusable continence products and bed linen may be very heavy when wet and take a long time to dry. It is important to check that the person doing the laundry has the ability and facilities to cope
Disposal facilities	Ability to appropriately, safely and discreetly dispose of the selected products needs to be considered
Personal preferences	Different people like different products and, where possible, patients should be given a choice of products with which to experiment to determine the most satisfactory product
Personal priorities	Everyone wants to avoid leakage but other factors such as discreetness may be more or less important to individuals

Commodes and bedpans

Some people with mobility problems and other disabilities find using a toilet difficult and slow. Toilet adaptations such as raised toilet seats, padded seats and grab rails can be very helpful in enabling individuals to access the toilet easily and comfortably. However, if the toilet is inaccessible or cannot be reached quickly enough to avoid incontinence, commodes and other toileting receptacles (such as female urinals, see above) need to be considered.

Commodes comprise a frame supporting a toilet seat with a pan (disposable or washable) beneath to receive urine and faeces. Commodes have changed little over the last 20–30 years and researchers have generally found that commode design is far from ideal. Problems with poor trunk support, aesthetics, comfort and pressure ulcer prevention have been identified, as well as concerns about risks of falls and commode instability (Medical Devices Agency 1993, Nelson et al 1993, Nazarko 1995). Concerns from patients also include lack of privacy and embarrassment about using the commode, unpleasant smells and the poor physical appearance of the commode (Naylor & Mulley 1993). Using a 'shower chair' over a toilet is an alternative option that can provide the mobility and support advantages of a commode, together with the privacy of a toilet (Nazarko 1995). An adapted shower chair based on users' needs has been developed by both Nazarko (1995) and Malassigne and colleagues (1995).

Simple moist wipes can be helpful for people who have difficulties with bottom wiping; bottom-wiping devices may also be useful, although there is no published research about them.

Recommendations for practice

- If at all possible, access to a toilet should be made available for defecation.
- If direct transfer to a toilet is impossible or unsafe, a sani-chair/shower chair should be offered in preference to a commode wherever possible.
- If a commode is used, care should be taken to ensure good trunk support, that the chair is stable and that methods of reducing noise and odour are available.
- Patients vulnerable to pressure ulcers should not sit on a commode/sani-chair/shower chair for prolonged periods.
- With commodes and sani-chairs/shower chairs, the user's bottom should never be visible to others and transportation to the toilet and use of the toilet or commode should be carried out with due regard to privacy and dignity.
- Bedpans and other portable receptacles should be avoided for defecation purposes.
- The person should be given a direct method of calling for assistance when left on the toilet/commode/sani-chair/shower chair.

PRODUCTS FOR CONTAINING/CONTROLLING INCONTINENCE

Absorbent products

Absorbent products are available in a wide range of sizes and absorbencies encompassing light through to very heavy incontinence. Absorbent products may be classified into two broad categories – disposable (single use) and reusable (washable) – with each category dividing into two subcategories: bodyworn products (worn on the person) or underpads (placed under the person). Within each subcategory are different design groups such as diapers and pull-ups which are subdivided (usually by size) according to the severity of incontinence. Some designs are further subdivided into those intended for men, women or children. This classification is shown in Table 10.1. Although absorbent pads are most commonly used for urinary incontinence, they are also used by individuals for both faecal and urinary/faecal incontinence; however, there have been no published studies which specifically address this issue.

Incidental findings from evaluations of products indicate that absorption capacity alone does not determine whether a user will choose to use a product. Some users may have frequent, low flow rate loss of small amounts of urine, whereas others may be dry for days but then have a high volume, high flow rate incontinence incident. Both may prefer to use pads for light incontinence. Mobile and independent community-dwelling women of all levels of incontinence are reported to generally prefer small pads and are often willing to change them frequently rather than use larger products

Table 10.1 Classification of absorbent continence products

Categories	Disposable (single use)		Reusable (washable)	
Subcategories	Bodyworns	Underpads	Bodyworns	Underpads
Design groups*	Inserts	Bedpads	Inserts	Bedpads
	Diapers	Chairpads	Diapers	Chairpads
	Pull-ups		Pull-ups	
	Pouches		Pouches	
Subgroups	Groups subdivide according to the severity of incontinence (light or moderate/heavy) and the sex of the intended users			

* The products within a given design group may vary considerably in their features and the materials from which they are made.

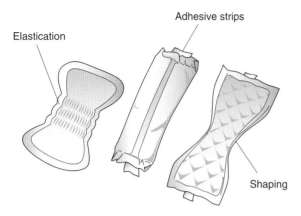

Figure 10.28 Disposable inserts for light incontinence. Reproduced with permission from the Continence Foundation (http:// www.continence-foundation.org.uk).

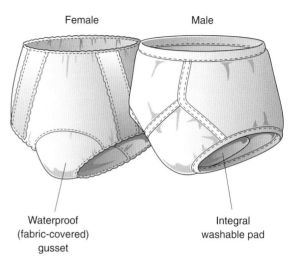

Figure 10.29 Reusable pull-up pants (also known as pants with integral pad for lightly incontinent women (left) and men (right). Reproduced with permission from the Continence Foundation (http:// www.continence-foundation.org.uk).

and change them less often (Fader et al 1987). Conversely, dependent, immobile individuals may prefer the security of larger products despite the loss of relatively low urine volumes due to their dependence on others for pad changing. Hellstrom et al (1993) found that patients were more satisfied with their products once their urine loss had been determined by pad weighing and appropriately absorbent products were provided. However, in practice, it is probably hard to justify the need for pad weighing to determine which absorbents should be provided; if there is doubt about which group a patient falls into, then the patient should be offered small pads for light incontinence in the first instance and the size of pad titrated upwards as necessary. A Cochrane Review (Brazzelli et al 2004) of absorbent products found only six studies that met the review criteria and no firm conclusions could be drawn. However, the literature does provide some guidance regarding product selection and includes a more recent review (Fader et al 2007).

Absorbent products for women with light incontinence

There are three main product designs for women with light incontinence: disposable inserts, reusable pants with integral pad and reusable inserts (Figs 10.28, 10.29). There have been no direct comparisons of the different designs, but studies of single designs have been undertaken. In separate studies, disposable inserts have been found to have good leakage performance and high acceptability (Clarke-O'Neill et al 2004) whilst reusable pants with integral pad have been found to have poorer leakage performance, but with similar overall opinion scores to disposable inserts (Clarke-O'Neill et al 2002). It is likely that reusable pants are cheaper in the long term than disposable inserts, but economic comparisons have not been studied. Reusable pants have a more 'normal' appearance than disposable inserts and may be particularly useful for occasional incontinence when disposable pads might still be dry when discarded.

As an alternative to disposable inserts, menstrual pads may make an acceptable and cheaper alternative (Baker & Norton 1996); however, products have changed in the last 10 years and current comparative performance is not known.

Recommendations for practice

- Most disposable inserts for light incontinence are likely to be satisfactory for patients in terms of leakage, but patients may have individual preferences and should be offered a selection to try where possible.
- Menstrual pads may be sufficient for some patients with very light incontinence.

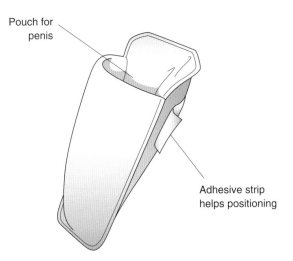

Pouch for penis

Adhesive strip helps positioning

Figure 10.30 Disposable pouch for men. Reproduced with permission from the Continence Foundation (http:// www.continence-foundation.org.uk).

- Reusable pants are an acceptable and probably cost-effective alternative to disposable inserts for women with very light incontinence, but are more likely to leak than disposable inserts and are not recommended for heavier urine loss.

Absorbent products for men with light incontinence

There are two main product designs specifically for men with light incontinence: pouches (Fig. 10.30), which are designed to hold the penis only, and leafs, which are larger, more open pouches, designed to hold the penis and scrotum. Most available pouches and leafs are disposable, although some reusable variants are available. Men may also use insert pads or reusable pants with integral pads (see Figs 10.28 and 10.29).

Macaulay and colleagues (2005) evaluated four designs for men with light incontinence – six pouches and six leafs, a disposable absorbent insert pad, and washable pants with integral pad. Results showed that pouch design performed worse than the leaf or insert design. The most common problems with the pouch were 'staying in place' and difficulties reinserting the penis in the pouch once the pouch was wet. The washable pants with integral pad received both good and bad scores (either loved or hated) and scored well for staying in place but poorly for leakage.

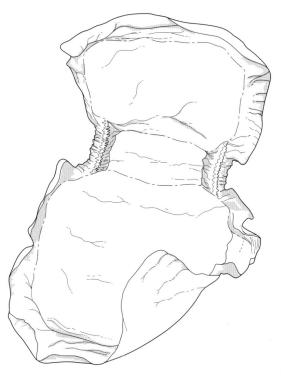

Figure 10.31 Disposable insert for moderate/heavy incontinence. Reproduced with permission from Cottenden et al (2005).

Recommendations for practice
- Disposable leafs appear to be the most acceptable and effective design for men with light incontinence.
- Washable pants with integral pad are likely to be most suitable for men with very light incontinence who have difficulty keeping a product in place.

Absorbent products for men and women with moderate/heavy incontinence

Disposable bodyworn inserts and diapers are the most common designs used for moderate/heavy incontinence (Figs 10.31, 10.32). More recently, modified diapers and pull-ups (Figs 10.33, 10.34) have been introduced which are designed to be easier to apply. Reusable counterparts are available to most disposable bodyworn designs, but they have a much smaller market. Reusable and disposable bedpads are also available and may be used

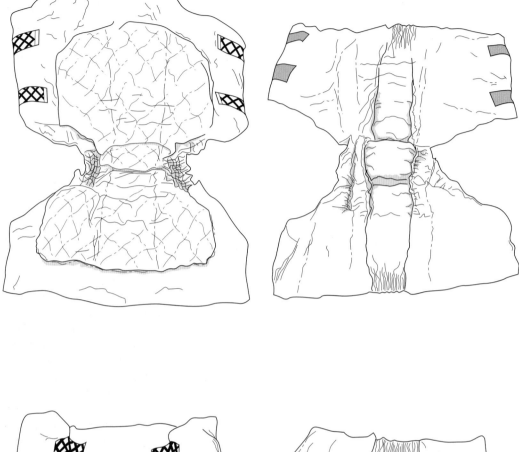

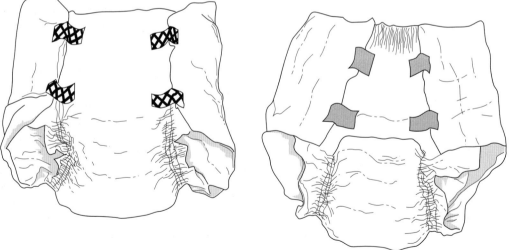

Figure 10.32   Disposable diaper shown open, and with tabs secured. Reproduced with permission from Cottenden et al (2005).

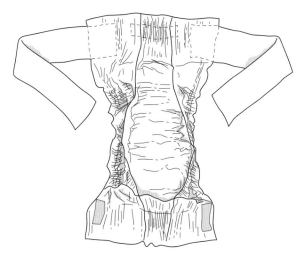

Figure 10.33 Disposable T-shaped diaper. Reproduced with permission from Cottenden et al (2005).

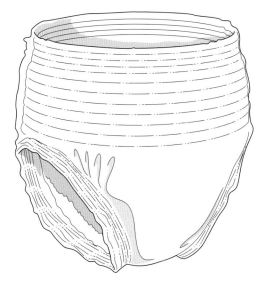

Figure 10.34 Disposable pull-up. Reproduced with permission from Cottenden et al (2005).

on the bed at night with or without the support of a bodyworn product. The use of disposable and reusable chairpads is not recommended because their public display undermines dignity.

Disposable and reusable bodyworn pads

There have been several studies of disposable bodyworn absorbent products. It has been demonstrated that pads are less likely to leak if pants

are worn and that close-fitting mesh pants are better than normal pants (Clancy & Malone-Lee 1991). Studies of single designs of products show that absorbent products that purport to be similar vary widely in performance. For example, the least successful diaper (based on 'overall opinion') was found to be unacceptable to 100% of the test subjects while the most successful was unacceptable to only 6% (Medical Devices Agency 1999).

Trials of reusable versus disposable products for moderate/heavy incontinence have generally been small and products have changed considerably since they were performed (Dolman 1988, Hu et al 1989, Harper et al 1995). The literature indicates that disposable bodyworn products generally perform better than reusables in terms of skin condition and leakage. More recently, Macaulay et al (2004a) carried out a pilot study of 14 reusable products and found that performance varied widely, although generally the products had poor leakage performance and were not liked. However, some terry towelling products showed promise, indicating that reusable bodyworn products may have potential, but more research is needed to test their efficacy and acceptability.

Because clinical evaluations are expensive and time-consuming, laboratory evaluation procedures are in widespread use. Few have been clinically validated but there are some clinically validated International Standards relating to leakage performance. ISO 11948-1 (1996) concerns large pads for heavy incontinence. It describes a simple method for measuring the absorption capacity of pads in the laboratory that was shown to correlate well with leakage performance (Cottenden & Ledger 1993, Cottenden et al 2003). This laboratory test (the Rothwell method) is now in common use in the UK and provides a basis for selecting similar products with which to make direct comparisons (for cost purposes) or to select promising pads for inclusion in clinical trials.

Recommendations for practice

- Individual needs and priorities vary; however, where possible, it is preferable to offer a choice of products for experimentation.
- Disposable diaper designs should be selected over insert pads if leakage is a problem and dis-

posable products with superabsorbers should be selected over those without. The use of close-fitting elasticated pants also helps to reduce leakage.

- Discreetness is a high priority for many users during the daytime and smaller, less bulky designs are preferable, although this must be balanced against the risk of leakage.
- Costs: Cost issues are complex. Cheaper pads do not necessarily save money and expensive pads do not necessarily work better than cheaper ones. Pads that have high leakage may lead to higher laundry costs and higher caregiver burden.

Disposable and reusable underpads

There are few trials comparing different disposable bedpads (Thornburn et al 1992, Brown 1994). However, their role is likely to be limited to providing additional support to bodyworn products when used in the bed; they are not acceptable during the daytime when bodyworn products should be worn under clothing to maintain dignity.

Reusable bedpads have generally been found to be well received when tested in older clinical trials (reviewed by Cottenden 1992) but there have been no recent comparisons with bodyworn products. They are easier to anchor in place (usually with flaps) than disposable bedpads and often have a higher level of absorbency, but the person must be naked below the waist (if the bedpad is not being used to support a bodyworn pad) and this is unacceptable to some people.

In institutional settings reusable bedpads are commonly used by multiple patients and the risk of cross-infection has been examined by Cottenden et al (1999). In this study laundering was shown to destroy all known pathogenic organisms, although some commensal flora were isolated in small numbers. It was concluded that foul wash laundry had left bedpads safe for multiple patient reuse with no demonstrable risk of cross-infection.

Absorbent pads for children

Most children are expected to achieve daytime dryness by around the age of 3, but some children take longer to become dry and some (e.g. children with learning and physical disabilities) may never reach this goal (see Chs 5 and 7). These children usually require absorbent products to contain leakage.

To date there has been only one study of absorbent products for children and this compared the diaper design with the newer pull-up design (Macaulay et al 2004b). Findings indicated that, overall, diapers were preferred for nighttime use by the majority of parents and that less than half of parents preferred pull-ups for daytime. Pull-ups were found to be particularly appropriate for older children and those who were attempting independent toileting, provided they did not have faecal incontinence and did not wear callipers or adapted footwear. The authors recommended that both diapers and pull-ups be supplied for children, with pull-ups (which are 50% more expensive than diapers) being provided for selected children during the daytime.

Recommendations for practice

- Diapers and pull-ups meet different needs of children and both should be made available to children with disabilities, depending on assessment.

Products for men

Sheaths

Penile sheaths are a commonly used device for men. They consist of a tube of thin, impermeable, elastic material such as latex or silicone (similar to a condom) which is applied to the penis and held in place with adhesive. The tip of the sheath is attached to a urine drainage bag. Sheaths are most suitable for men with sufficient penile length on which to attach the sheath (see also Ch. 4).

There are many varieties of sheath (Fig. 10.35); they may be self-adhesive or have a separate adhesive strip to wrap around the penis before applying the sheath. External strips to be used over the top of the sheath are also available. Some sheaths have plastic applicators designed to facilitate application or to enable sheath application with minimal hand contact. Internal flanges may be incorporated to prevent urine draining back from the tubing onto the penis and there may be special features to prevent kinking of tubing.

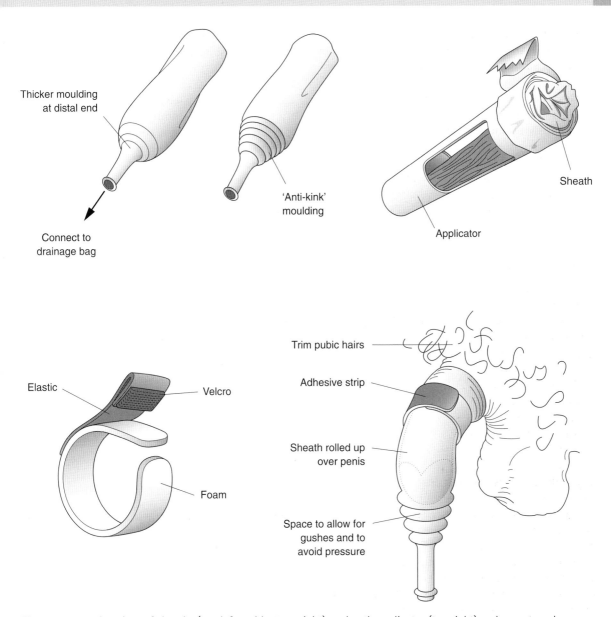

Figure 10.35 A variety of sheaths (top left and bottom right), a sheath applicator (top right) and an external fixation strip (bottom left). Reproduced with permission from the Continence Foundation (http:// www.continence-foundation.org.uk).

Sheath use can be troublesome for skin health. There are reports of skin irritation, allergic responses and compression injury in the literature (Golji 1981, Jayachandran et al 1985), and regular skin observation and good genital hygiene have been recommended. Sheaths have also been associated with urine infections. Ouslander and colleagues (1987) reported that 40% of 30 nursing home sheath users (mean period of use, 35.9 months) developed at least one UTI, but reported rates have been lower than would be expected from an indwelling catheter which might otherwise be an option.

Evaluations of sheaths have found that staying in place and freedom from leakage are important issues for men, followed by comfort and ease of application and removal (Nichols & Balis 2000). A comparison of self-adhesive sheaths with sheaths with a separate adhesive strip showed that self-adhesive sheaths were more successful for overall performance and ease of application (Thelwell et al 1995). A further evaluation of all self-adhesive sheaths on the UK market found that the ease with which a sheath could be put on was found to be the best predictor of overall performance and that, surprisingly, sheaths with an applicator were less successful than those without an applicator (Fader et al 2001).

Recommendations for practice

- Men should be given the opportunity to experiment with different products before making a final selection.
- In general, sheaths with self-adhesive should be selected rather than those in which the adhesive is supplied separately.
- In general, sheaths without applicators should be selected rather than those with an applicator, although a sheath applicator should be considered if a carer is applying the sheath.
- Latex allergy status should be determined.
- Monitoring of skin health should take place.

Male bodyworn urinals

A variety of devices other than sheaths, such as pubic pressure urinals, are available for men. They comprise a ring or cone that is held firmly against the pubis with belt or strap arrangements (similar to a jock-strap), which is connected to a drainage bag which may be disposable or reusable (Fig. 10.36). These devices are not in widespread use and require careful fitting to be successful; however, they can be particularly useful for men with a retracted penis who are unable to use a sheath. There has been no published research evaluating these products.

Occlusive devices for urinary incontinence

Female occlusive devices

Female occlusive devices are designed to prevent urine leakage by occlusion of the urethra and fall into three categories: at the external meatus, in the urethra (intraurethral devices) or via the vagina (intravaginal devices).

Devices that occlude at the external meatus Urethral occlusion devices have been developed to block urinary leakage at the external urethral meatus (Fig. 10.37). Several devices have utilised either adhesive or mild suction to occlude urinary loss at the urethral meatus. In addition to the simple barrier effect, compression of the wall of the distal urethra has been hypothesised to contribute to continence. Although these devices have tended to show favourable results in trials, they have not been popular and none is currently available on the UK market.

Intraurethral devices Urethral inserts are silicone cylinders that are self-inserted or removed at the patient's discretion. These devices comprise external retainers or flanges to prevent intravesical migration and proximal balloons to hold the device in place. They act by causing occlusion either in the urethra itself or at the external urethral meatus (Balmforth & Cardozo 2003). The FemSoft (Rochester Medical Corporation, USA) is the only urethral insert currently distributed in the UK. It has a soft, compressible, mineral oil-filled silicone layer with an insertion probe. Before insertion, the fluid distends the proximal end of the cylinder; as the user pushes the device (guided by the insertion probe) into the urethra, fluid transfers automatically to the distal end, allowing the device to pass through the urethra. Once in place, fluid flows back to the proximal end to hold the device in place. Dunn et al (2002) demonstrated that the FemSoft was effective in preventing leakage from six women during an exercise session. However, use of intraurethral devices has also been shown to be associated with UTI, haematuria and discomfort (Staskin et al 1996).

Intravaginal devices Support of the bladder neck to correct urinary stress incontinence has been achieved, with varying success, utilising (i) traditional tampons, (ii) pessaries and contraceptive diaphragms, and (iii) intravaginal devices specifically designed to support the bladder neck (Fig. 10.38). Simple tampons and pessaries have been found to reduce urinary incontinence in small studies of women with stress urinary incontinence (Suarez et al 1991, Nygaard 1995). Intravaginal devices designed specifically to support the bladder neck are also available and include a

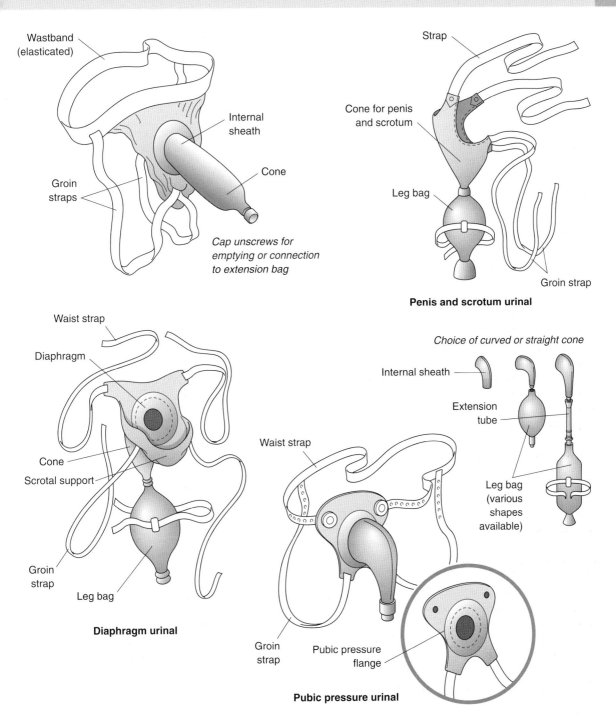

Wastband
(elasticated)

Internal sheath

Cone

Groin straps

Cap unscrews for emptying or connection to extension bag

Strap

Cone for penis and scrotum

Leg bag

Groin strap

Penis and scrotum urinal

Waist strap

Diaphragm

Cone

Scrotal support

Groin strap

Leg bag

Diaphragm urinal

Waist strap

Groin strap

Pubic pressure flange

Pubic pressure urinal

Choice of curved or straight cone

Internal sheath

Extension tube

Leg bag (various shapes available)

Figure 10.36 A variety of pubic pressure bodyworn urinals for men. Reproduced with permission from the Continence Foundation (http:// www.continence-foundation.org.uk).

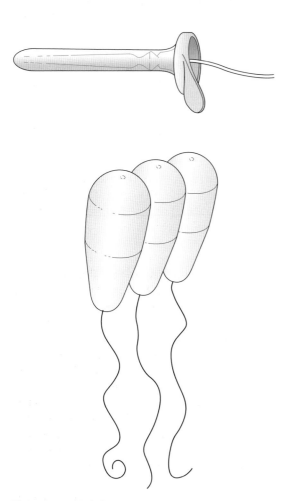

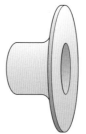

Figure 10.37 A female internal (above) and external (below) occlusive device. Reproduced with permission from Cottenden et al (2005).

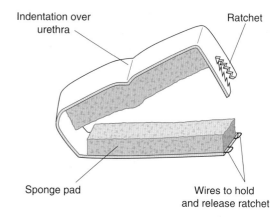

Figure 10.39 Male occlusive device. Reproduced with permission from Cottenden et al (2005).

Figure 10.38 A female intravaginal occlusive device. Reproduced with permission from the Continence Foundation (http:// www.continence-foundation.org.uk).

reusable device (Introl) and disposable single-use devices such as the Conveen Continence Tampon.

Studies of all the devices have mainly been small. Problems with fitting the reusable device were found by Moore et al (1999). Thyssen et al (1999) reported improvements in urinary incontinence on 24-h pad tests for the disposable device, as did Hahn and Milsom (1996), but discomfort was an associated problem for some women. There are few data on long-term use of these products.

Recommendations for practice

- Vaginal support devices may be considered a treatment option for women with stress urinary incontinence but successful long-term use is uncertain.

Male occlusive devices

Male occlusive devices aim to prevent urine leakage by compressing the penis. A variety of designs are available but occlusion is usually achieved with either a clamp or a peri-penile strap (Fig. 10.39). Such devices have the potential advantages of low cost and simplicity compared with a sheath and drainage bag.

There has been only one published study comparing different occlusive devices. Moore et al (2004) evaluated three different devices in a cross-over study involving 12 men. Each of the devices significantly ($p < 0.05$) reduced mean urine loss. The Cunningham clamp was rated most positively; however, cavernosal artery blood flow was significantly reduced. Overall, the authors concluded that, used correctly, the Cunningham clamp can be an effective method of controlling urinary incontinence in men with stress urinary incontinence who are cognitively intact and aware of bladder filling, and have normal genital sensation, intact penile skin and sufficient manual dexterity to open and close the device.

Recommendations for practice

- Male occlusive devices should be considered for selected men with stress urinary incontinence who are cognitively intact and aware of bladder filling, and have normal genital sensation, intact penile skin and sufficient manual dexterity to open and close the device.

SKIN HEALTH AND CONTINENCE PRODUCTS

The skin of an incontinent individual will be regularly exposed to contact with urine and/or faeces and damage to the skin is the main physical health consequence of urinary and faecal incontinence (Ersser et al 2005). The majority of current knowledge about the effects of urine and faeces on skin has been obtained from studies with pads or pad materials on animals, healthy infants and on body areas such as the forearm or back of adults. Where clinical trials have been conducted, they have usually been on infants and rarely on adults using pads. Skin irritation within the pad occlusion area is usually termed diaper dermatitis in infants and perineal dermatitis in adults.

The aetiology of diaper dermatitis has been examined using a hairless mouse model with patches of urine and faeces (Berg et al 1986, Buckingham & Berg 1986) and showed that the irritant potential of urine was evident after continuous exposure (10 days). Faeces were found to be more irritant through the action of proteases and lipases but the combination of urine and faeces caused significantly higher levels of irritation than urine or faeces alone. The authors concluded that the presence of faecal urease results in the breakdown of urinary urea, causing an elevation in pH, which increases the activities of faecal proteases and lipases leading to skin irritation.

Hydration dermatitis (Tsai & Maibach 1999) occurs following prolonged exposure of the skin to water. Such prolonged occlusion (as within a continence product) has been demonstrated to reduce skin barrier function (Fluhr et al 1999) and significantly raise microbial counts and pH (Faergemann et al 1983). Zimmerer et al (1986) demonstrated that overhydrated skin has a higher coefficient of friction and is more susceptible to abrasion damage than normally hydrated skin. The role of microorganisms is less certain. It is thought that bacterial or fungal infection is secondary to alterations in the skin barrier that allow penetration of the microorganisms (Faria et al 1996). A product that simply maintains wet and occluded skin (even without the additional constituents of urine and faeces) is therefore likely to cause skin irritation and increase skin permeability to other irritants.

Berg (1987) analysed the aetiological factors contributing to infant diaper dermatitis and developed a model (Fig. 10.40) to show its development and resolution. However, the applicability of this model to adults with incontinence has not been tested, and other factors such as poor mobility and prolonged pressure – which are common in frail, older adults – are not accounted for in this model. In addition, this model assumes the presence of urinary and faecal incontinence, which is much less common in adult populations than urinary incontinence alone. The prevalence of perineal dermatitis in adults has varied widely in studies (Table 10.2), probably due to difficulties in reliably rating perineal dermatitis and the confounding presence of reactive hyperaemia (blanchable erythema), particularly on the sacrum and buttocks.

Pressure ulcers and incontinence

The role of urinary and faecal incontinence in the development of pressure ulcers is uncertain. Studies aiming to identify risk factors for the development of pressure ulcers have generally found that the presence of both urinary and faecal incontinence was a risk (Brandeis et al 1994, Bergquist & Frantz 1999), but some studies have only found faecal rather than urinary incontinence to be a risk factor (Spector & Fortinsky 1998, Theaker et al 2000). Pressure ulcer risk assessment scales all have a subscale of incontinence or moisture level, and the main mechanism for the development of pressure ulcers has been thought to be

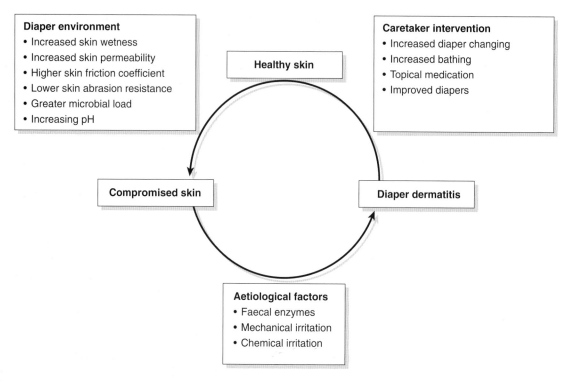

Figure 10.40   Berg's model of diaper dermatitis. Adapted from Berg (1987).

Table 10.2   Studies reporting prevalence of diaper (perineal) dermatitis in adults

Authors	Sample (n)	Prevalence of dermatitis (%)
Keller et al (1990)	Older people: long stay (95)	53
Lyder et al (1992)	Older people: psychogeriatric wards (15)	33
Brown (1994)	Adults: acute medical wards (166)	35
Schnelle et al (1997)	Older people: nursing home residents (100)	94
Gray (2004)	Adults: ambulatory, urodynamics (50)	42

the increased friction and increased vulnerability to abrasion of wet skin.

Recently, Fader et al (2003) examined the effects of absorbent continence pads on mattress interface pressures using an articulated model or 'phantom' as the subject and found that the presence of a pad significantly and substantially increased the peak pressures recorded between the buttocks and the pad by around 20%. Peak pressures were frequently found at the locations of pad creases and it was considered that pad folding and compression may contribute to raised interface pressures. It is therefore possible that continence product use contributes to the formation of pressure ulcers by raising interface pressures.

Clinical studies of the impact of products and product materials on skin health

Product manufacturers introduced diapers with superabsorbent polymers (SAP) in the 1980s, which were designed to reduce skin wetness, buffer pH and reduce urinary/faecal contact in order to help prevent diaper dermatitis. Clinical studies to evaluate the efficacy of diapers with different materials, in particular SAP, have generally shown that the presence of SAP reduces the risk of dermatitis compared to those without, and compared to conventional washable diapers (Lane et al 1990, Brown 1994).

Clinical studies of skin–care products and nursing practices to maintain or improve skin health

Specialised cleansers are commonly used to prevent and treat dermatitis; however, clinical studies have not demonstrated robust differences in skin outcomes when using different cleansing regimes. Some studies have shown indirect benefits, such as savings in nursing time (Whittingham & May 1998, Lewis-Byers & Thayer 2002), and generally cleansers have received favourable staff opinion compared with soap and water. However, no detailed comprehensive economic analyses have been undertaken.

The effects of different pad changing regimes on skin health have also been investigated (Fader et al 2003). Eighty-one subjects from 20 nursing homes were studied using a cross-over design of two pad changing regimes: either changing the pad once during the night or not changing the pads at all during the night. No significant differences were found on measures of skin health, but skin on the less frequent changing regime was found to be significantly wetter (measured by transepidermal water loss). In addition, five subjects developed stage II pressure ulcers in the no-pad changing regime compared with none in the once per night changing regime. The authors stated that it could not be concluded that leaving patients all night in pads without changing was safe for skin health.

Recommendations for practice

- Absorbent pads with SAP should be selected in preference to those without.

- Absorbent pads should be changed regularly to minimise wet skin.
- Patients with faecal or double incontinence should be changed as soon as possible after incontinence has occurred to prevent the development of dermatitis from protease and lipase activity.
- Patients should be washed gently at times of pad change with either soap and water or cleansers. Cleanser may be less time-consuming than soap and water.
- Barrier creams may be applied to skin within the pad area to reduce water penetration of the skin.
- Buttock and sacral areas should be protected using topical skin barrier products, containment products or diversion devices in patients vulnerable to perineal dermatitis or pressure ulcers.

CONCLUSIONS

Selecting effective products for continence management can be challenging for nurses, particularly as there are so many product designs and varieties to choose from. This chapter has examined the range of products available and summarised the evidence to inform their selection, but there is nevertheless insufficient evidence to make informed choices in many product areas. Innovation and product development can mean that research in this area can quickly become outdated and lose clinical currency. Evidence-based product selection and evidence-based purchasing of products require a consistent programme of research to ensure that optimum continence management with products is delivered by nurses.

References

Addison R, Mould C 2000 Risk assessment in suprapubic catheterisation. Nursing Standard 14(36): 43–46

Avorn J, Monane M, Gurwitz J H et al 1994 Reduction in bacteriuria and pyuria after ingestion of cranberry juice. Journal of the American Medical Association 271(10):751–754

Baker J, Norton P 1996 Evaluation of absorbent products for women with mild to moderate urinary incontinence. Applied Nursing Research 9(1):29–33

Balmforth J, Cardozo L D 2003 Trends toward less invasive treatment of female stress urinary incontinence. Urology 62(4 supplement 1):52–60

Bell J (1810) cited in Bloom et al 1994

Berg R W 1987 Etiologic factors in diaper dermatitis: a model for development of improved diapers. Pediatrician 14 (supplement 1):27–33

Berg R W, Buckingham K W, Stewart R L 1986 Etiologic factors in diaper dermatitis: the role of urine. Pediatric Dermatology 3(2):102–106

Bergquist S, Frantz R 1999 Pressure ulcers in community-based older adults receiving home health care. Prevalence, incidence, and associated risk factors. Advances in Wound Care 12(7):339–351

Bibby J M, Cox A J, Hukins D W L 1995 Feasibility of preventing encrustation of urinary catheters. Cells and Materials 2:183–195

Bloom D A, McGuire E J, Lapides J 1994 A brief history of urethral catheterisation. Journal of Urology 151:317–325

Brandeis G H, Ooi W L, Hossain M et al 1994 A longitudinal study of risk factors associated with the formation of pressure ulcers in nursing homes. Journal of the American Geriatrics Society 42(4):388–393

Brazzelli M, Shirra E, Vale L 2004 Absorbent products for containing urinary and/or faecal incontinence in adults. Cochrane Database of Systematic Reviews (2):CD001406

Brosnahan J, Jull A, Tracy C 2004 Types of urethral catheters for management of short-term voiding problems in hospitalised adults. Cochrane Database of Systematic Reviews (1):CD004013

Brown D 1994 Diapers and underpads, Part 1: Skin integrity outcomes. Ostomy and Wound Management 40(9): 20–26, 28

Brown M R W, Allison D G, Gilbert P 1988 Resistance of bacterial biofilms to antibiotics: a growth related effect. Journal of Antimicrobial Chemotherapy 22:777–783

Buckingham K W, Berg R W 1986 Etiologic factors in diaper dermatitis: the role of feces. Pediatric Dermatology 3(2):107–112

Campbell J, Moore K, Voaklander D et al 2004 Complications associated with clean intermittent self-catheterisation in children with spina bifida. Journal of Urology 171(6):2420–2422

Choong S K, Hallson P, Whitehead H N et al 1999 The physicochemical basis of urinary catheter encrustation. BJU International 83:770–775

Clancy B, Malone-Lee J 1991 Reducing the leakage of body-worn incontinence pads. Journal of Advanced Nursing 16(2):187–193

Clarke-O'Neill S, Pettersson L, Fader M et al 2002 A multicentre comparative evaluation: washable pants with an integral pad for light incontinence. Journal of Clinical Nursing 11(1):79–89

Clarke-O'Neill S, Pettersson L, Fader M et al 2004 A multicenter comparative evaluation: disposable pads for women with light incontinence. Journal of Wound, Ostomy and Continence Nursing 3(1):32–42

Classen D C, Larsen R A, Burke J P et al 1991 Prevention of catheter-associated bacteriuria: clinical trials of methods to block three known pathways of infection. American Journal of Infection Control 19:136–142

Cottenden A M 1992 Aids and appliances for incontinence. In: Roe B (ed) The promotion and management of continence. Prentice Hall, Englewood Cliffs, NJ

Cottenden A M, Ledger D J 1993 Predicting the leakage performance of bodyworn disposable incontinence pads using laboratory tests. Journal of Biomedical Engineering 15(3):212–220

Cottenden A, Moore K N, Fader M et al 1999 Is there a risk of cross-infection from laundered reusable bedpads? British Journal of Nursing 8(17):1161–1163

Cottenden A M, Fader M J, Pettersson L et al 2003 How well does ISO 11948-1 (the Rothwell method) for measuring the absorption capacity of incontinence pads in the laboratory correlate with clinical pad performance? Medical Engineering and Physics 25(7):603–613

Cottenden A, Bliss D, Fader M et al 2005 Management with continence products. In: Abrams P, Cardozo L, Khoury S, Wein A (eds) Incontinence. Health Publications, Paris, p 149–253

Cox A J, Millington R S, Hukins D W L et al 1989 Resistance of catheters coated with a modified hydrogel to encrustation during an in vitro test. Urology Research 17: 353–356

Cravens D D, Zweig S 2000 Urinary catheter management. American Family Physician 61(2):369–376

Darouiche R O, Smith J A, Hanna H et al 1999 Efficacy of antimicrobial impregnated bladder catheters in reducing catheter associated bacteriuria: a prospective randomized, multi-centre clinical trial. Urology 54(6):976–981

Davies A J, Desai H N, Turton S et al 1987 Does instillation of chlorhexidine into the bladder of catheterised geriatric patients help reduce bacteriuria? Journal of Hospital Infection 9:72–75

De Ridder D, Everaert K, Fernandez L et al 2005 Intermittent catheterisation with hydrophilic-coated catheters (Speedicath) reduces the risk of clinical urinary tract infection in spinal cord injured patients: a prospective randomised parallel comparative trial. European Urology 48(6):991–995

Department of Health 2001 Guidelines for preventing infections associated with the insertion and maintenance of short-term indwelling urethral catheters in acute care. Journal of Hospital Infection 47(supplement):S39–S46

Doherty W 2001 Indications for and principles of intermittent self catheterisation. In: Pope Cruikshank J, Woodward S (eds) Management of continence and urinary catheter care. British Journal of Nursing Monograph. Mark Allen, Dinton

Dolman M 1988 Continence: the cost of incontinence. Nursing Times 84(31):67–69

Donmez T, Erol K, Baycu C et al 1990 Effects of various acidic and alkaline solutions used to dissolve urinary calculi on the rabbit urothelium. Urology International 45: 293–297

Dunn M, Brandt D, Nygaard I 2002 Treatment of exercise incontinence with a urethral insert: a pilot study. Physician and Sports Medicine 30(1):53–55

Ebner A, Madersbacher H, Schober F et al 1985 Hydrodynamic properties of Foley catheters and its clinical relevance. In: Proceedings of the International Continence Society 15th Meeting, London

Eckstein H B 1979 Intermittent catheterisation of the bladder in patients with neuropathic incontinence of urine. Zeitschrift fur Kinderchirurgie und Grenzgebiete 28(4): 408–412

Ehrenkranz N J, Alfonso B C 1991 Failure of bland soap handwash to prevent hand transfer of patient bacteria to urethral catheters. Infection Control and Hospital Epidemiology 12:654–662

Elliott T S J, Reid L, Gopal Rao G et al 1989 Bladder irrigation or irritation. British Journal of Urology 64:391–394

Ersser S J, Getliffe K A, Voegeli D et al 2005 A critical review of the inter-relationship between skin vulnerability and urinary incontinence and related nursing intervention. International Journal of Nursing Studies 42:823–835

Evans A, Feneley R 2000 A study of current nursing management of long-term suprapubic catheters. British Journal of Community Nursing 5(5):240–245

Fader M, Barnes E, Malone-Lee J, Cottenden A 1987 Choosing the right garment. Nursing Times 83:78–85

Fader M, Pettersson L, Brooks R 1997 A multi-centre comparative evaluation of catheter valves. British Journal of Nursing 6(7):359–367

Fader M, Pettersson L, Dean G et al 1999 The selection of female urinals: results of a multicentre evaluation. British Journal of Nursing 8(14):918–925

Fader M, Pettersson L, Dean G et al 2001 Sheaths for urinary incontinence: a randomized crossover trial. BJU International 88(4):367–372

Fader M, Clarke-O'Neill S, Cook D et al 2003 Management of night-time urinary incontinence in residential settings for older people: an investigation into the effects of different pad changing regimes on skin health. Journal of Clinical Nursing 12(3):374–386

Fader M, Cottenden AM, Getliffe K 2007 Absorbent products for light urinary incontinence in women. Cochrane Database of Systematic Reviews (in press)

Faergemann J, Aly R, Wilson D R et al 1983 Skin occlusion: effect on Pityrosporum orbiculare, skin PCO_2, pH, transepidermal water loss, and water content. Archives of Dermatological Research 275(6):383–387

Faria D T, Shwayder T, Krull E A 1996 Perineal skin injury: extrinsic environmental risk factors. Ostomy and Wound Management 42(7):28–34, 36

Fluhr J W, Lazzerini S, Distante F et al 1999 Effects of prolonged occlusion on stratum corneum barrier function and water holding capacity. Skin Pharmacology and Applied Skin Physiology 12(4):193–198

Fowler C 1998 Bladder problems. In: Multiple sclerosis: information for nurses and health professionals. Information Pack. MS Research Trust, Letchworth

German K, Rowley P, Stone D et al 1997 A randomised crossover study comparing the use of a catheter valve and a leg bag in urethrally catheterised male patients. British Journal of Urology 79:96–98

Getliffe K A 1992 Encrustation of urinary catheters in community patients. PhD Thesis, University of Surrey

Getliffe K A 1994a The characteristics and management of patients with recurrent blockage of long-term urinary catheters. Journal of Advanced Nursing 20:140–149

Getliffe K A 1994b The use of bladder washouts to reduce urinary catheter encrustation. British Journal of Urology 73(6):696–700

Getliffe K A 1996 Bladder instillations and bladder washouts in the management of catheterised patients. Journal of Advanced Nursing 23:548–554

Getliffe K A, Newton T 2006 Catheter-associated urinary tract infection (CAUTI) in primary and community health care. Age and Ageing 35(5):477–481

Getliffe K A, Hughes S C, Le Claire M 2000 The dissolution of urinary catheter encrustation. BJU International 85:60–64

Gibb H, Wong G 1994 How to choose: nurses' judgements of the effectiveness of a range of currently marketed continence aids. Journal of Clinical Nursing 3(2):77–86

Golji H 1981 Complications of external condom drainage. Paraplegia 19(3):189–197

Gopal Rao G, Elliott T S J 1988 Bladder irrigation. Age and Ageing 17:373–378

Gray M 2004 Preventing and managing perineal dermatitis: a shared goal for wound and continence care. Journal of Wound, Ostomy and Continence Nursing 31(supplement 1):S2–S9

Gujral S, Kirkwood L, Hinchcliffe A 1999 Suprapubic catheterisation: suitable procedure for clinical nurse specialists in selected patients. British Journal of Urology 83(9): 954–956

Hahn I, Milsom I 1996 Treatment of female stress urinary incontinence with a new anatomically shaped vaginal device (Conveen Continence Guard). British Journal of Urology 77(5):711–715

Harbath S, Sax H, Gastmeier P 2003 The preventable proportion of nosocomial infections: an overview of published reports. Journal of Hospital Infection 54:258–266

Harper D W, O'Hara P A, Lareau J et al 1995 Reusable versus disposable incontinent briefs: a multiperspective crossover clinical trial. Journal of Applied Gerontology 14(4): 391–407

Hellstrom L, Ekelund P, Larsson M et al 1993 Adapting incontinent patients' incontinence aids to their leakage volumes. Scandinavian Journal of Caring Sciences 7(2): 67–71

Hesse A, Schreyger F, Tuschewitzki G J et al 1989 Experimental investigations on dissolution of encrustations on the surface of catheters. Urology International 44:364–369

Hu T W, Kaltreider D L, Igou J 1989 Incontinence products: which is best? Geriatric Nursing 10(4):184–186

Iacovou J W 1994 Supra-pubic catheterisation of the urinary bladder. Hospital Update 20(3):159–162

Jayachandran M D, Moopan U M M, Kim H 1985 Complications from external (condom) urinary drainage devices. Urology 25(1):31–34

Johnson J J, Kuskowskil M A, Wilt T J 2006 Systematic review: antimicrobial urinary catheters to prevent catheter-associated infection in hospitalized patients. Annals of Internal Medicine 144(2):116–126

Keerasontonpong A, Thearawiboon W, Panthawanan A et al 2003 Incidence of urinary tract infection in patients with short-term indwelling urethral catheters: a comparison between a 3-day urine drainage bag change and no change regime. American Journal of Infection Control 31(1):9–12

Keller P A, Sinkovic S P, Miles S J 1990 Skin dryness: a major factor in reducing incontinence dermatitis. Ostomy/Wound Management 30:60–64

Kennedy A P, Brocklehurst J C, Robinson J et al 1992 Assessment and use of bladder washout/instillations in patients with long-term indwelling catheters. British Journal of Urology 70:610–615

Kunin C M, Chin Q F, Chambers S 1987 Formation of encrustations on indwelling urinary catheters in the elderly: a comparison of different types of catheter materials in 'blockers' and 'non-blockers'. Journal of Urology 138:899–902

Landi F, Cesari M, Onder G et al 2004 Indwelling urethral catheter and mortality in frail elderly women living in the community. Neurourology and Urodynamics 23(7):697–701

Lane A T, Rehder P A, Helm K 1990 Evaluations of diapers containing absorbent gelling material with conventional disposable diapers in newborn infants. American Journal of Diseases of Children 144(3):315–318

Lapides J, Ananias C D, Silber S J et al 1972 Clean intermittent self-catheterisation in the treatment of urinary tract disease. Journal of Urology 107:458–461

LeBlanc K, Christensen D 2005 Addressing the challenge of providing nursing care for elderly men suffering from urethral erosion. Journal of Wound, Ostomy and Continence Nursing 32(2):131–134

Lee S J, Kim S W, Cho Y H et al 2004 A comparative multicentre study on the incidence of catheter-associated urinary tract infection between nitrofurazone-coated and silicone catheters. International Journal of Antimicrobial Agents 24(supplement 1):S65–69

Lewis-Byers K, Thayer D 2002 An evaluation of two incontinence skin care protocols in a long-term care setting. Ostomy/Wound Management 48(12):44–51

Lyder C H, Clemes-Lowrance C, Davis A et al 1992 Structured skin care regimen to prevent perineal dermatitis in the elderly. Journal of ET Nursing 19(1):12–16

Macaulay M, Clarke-O'Neill S, Fader M et al 2004a A pilot study to evaluate reusable absorbent body-worn products for adults with moderate/heavy urinary incontinence. Journal of Wound, Ostomy and Continence Nursing 31(6):357–366

Macaulay M, Fader M, Pettersson L et al 2004b A multicenter evaluation of absorbent products for children with incontinence and disabilities. Journal of Wound, Ostomy and Continence Nursing 31(4):235–244

Macaulay M, Pettersson L, Fader M et al 2005 Absorbent products for men with light incontinence: an evaluation. Report 05020. Medical Devices Agency, London

Macintosh J 1998 Realising the potential of urinals for women. Journal of Community Nursing 12(44):1739–1741

McNulty C, Freeman E, Smith G et al 2003 Prevalence of urinary catheterization in UK nursing homes. Journal of Hospital Infection 55:119–123

Maes D, Wyndaele J 1988 Long-term experience with intermittent self-catheterisation. Neurology and Urodynamics 73:273–274

Maki D G, Tambayah P 2001 Engineering out the risk for infection with urinary catheters. Emerging Infectious Diseases 7(2):342–347

Malassigne P, Nelson A L, Cors M W et al 1995 Design of the advanced commode-shower chair for spinal cord injured individuals. Journal of Rehabilitation, Research and Development 37:373–382

Mantani N, Ochiai H, Imanishi N 2003 A case control study of purple urine bag syndrome in geriatric wards. Journal of Infection and Chemotherapy 9(1):53–57

Marrie T, Costerton J W 1983 A scanning electron microscopic study of urine droppers and urine collecting systems. Archives of Internal Medicine 142:1135–1141

Medical Devices Agency 1993 Basic commodes: a comparative evaluation. Disability Equipment Assessment Report A5. MDA, London

Medical Devices Agency 1999 All-in-one disposable body-worn pads for heavy incontinence. Disability Equipment Assessment Report IN4. MDA, London

Moore K H, Foote A, Burton G et al 1999 An open study of the bladder neck support prosthesis in genuine stress incontinence. British Journal of Obstetrics and Gynaecology 106(1):42–49

Moore K N, Schieman S, Ackerman T et al 2004 Assessing comfort, safety, and patient satisfaction with three commonly used penile compression devices. Urology 63(1):150–154

Moore K N, Getliffe K A, Fader M 2007 Techniques and strategies for long-term bladder management by intermittent catheterisation in adults and children. Cochrane Database of Systematic Reviews (in press)

Morris N S, Stickler D J 2001 Does drinking cranberry juice produce urine that is inhibitory to the development of crystalline, catheter-blocking Proteus mirabilis biofilms? British Journal of Urology 88(3):192–197

Mulhall A B, Chapman R G, Crow R A 1988 Bacteriuria during indwelling urethral catheterisation. Journal of Hospital Infection 11:253–262

Mulhall A B, King S, Lee K et al 1993 Maintenance of closed urinary drainage systems: are practitioners more aware of the dangers? Journal of Clinical Nursing 2:135–140

Nacey J N, Delahunt B 1991 Toxicity of first and second generation hydrogel-coated latex urinary catheters. British Journal of Urology 67:314–316

Nahata M C, Shrimp L, Lampman L et al 1977 Effect of ascorbic acid on urine pH in man. American Journal of Hospital Pharmacology 34:1234–1237

National Institute for Clinical Excellence 2003 Prevention of healthcare associated infection in primary and community care. NICE, London. Online. Available: http://www.nice.org.uk/pdf/CG2fullguidelineinfectioncontrol.pdf

Naylor J R, Mulley G P 1993 Commodes: inconvenient conveniences. British Medical Journal 307(6914):1258–1260

Nazarko L 1995 Commode design for frail and disabled people. Professional Nurse 11(2):95–97

Nelson A, Malassigne P, Amerson T et al 1993 Descriptive study of bowel care practices and equipment in spinal cord injury. Spinal Cord Injury Nursing 10(2):65–67

Nichols T, Balis N 2000 Male external urinary catheter design survey. In: Proceedings of the 32nd Annual Wound, Ostomy, Continence Conference, Toronto, Ontario

Niel-Weise B S, van den Broek P J 2005 Urinary catheter policies for long-term bladder drainage. Cochrane Database of Systematic Reviews (1):CD004201

Norberg B, Norberg A, Parkhede U 1983 The spontaneous variation in catheter life in long stay geriatric patients with indwelling catheters. Gerontology 29:332–335

Nygaard I 1995 Prevention of exercise incontinence with mechanical devices. Journal of Reproductive Medicine 40(2):89–94

Ofek I, Coldhar J, Zafriri D et al 1991 Anti-Escherichia coli adhesin activity of cranberry and blueberry juices [letter]. New England Journal of Medicine 324(22):1599

Ohkawa M, Sugata T, Sawaki M et al 1990 Bacterial and crystal adherence to the surfaces of indwelling urethral catheters. Journal of Urology 143:717–721

Ouslander J G, Greengold B, Chen S 1987 External catheter use and urinary tract infections among incontinent male nursing home patients. Journal of the American Geriatrics Society 35(12):1063–1070

Pariente J L, Bordenave L, Jacob F et al 2000 Cytotoxicity assessment of latex urinary catheters on cultured human urothelial cells. European Urology 38(5):640–643

Pateman B, Johnson M 2000 Men's lived experiences following transurethral prostatectomy for benign prostate hypertrophy. Journal of Advanced Nursing 31(1):51–58

Paterson J 2000 Stigma associated with post-prostatectomy urinary incontinence. Journal of Wound, Ostomy and Continence Nursing 27(3):168–173

Paterson J, Dunn S, Kowanko I et al 2003 Selection of continence products: perspectives of people who have incontinence and their carers. Disability and Rehabilitation 25(17):955–963

Pilloni S, Krhut J, Mair D et al 2005 Intermittent catheterisation in older people; a valuable alternative to an indwelling catheter. Age and Ageing 34(1):57–60

Platt R, Polk B F, Murdock B et al 1982 Mortality associated with nosocomial urinary-tract infection. New England Journal of Medicine 307:637–642

Platt R, Polk B F, Murdock B et al 1983 Reduction of mortality associated with nosocomial urinary tract infection. Lancet 1:893–897

Plowman R, Graves N, Griffin M et al 1999 The socio-economic burden of hospital-acquired infection. Public Health Laboratory Service, London

Pomfret I 1995 Bladder irrigation. Journal of Community Nursing Dec:24–29

Raz R, Schiller D, Nicolle L 2000 Chronic indwelling catheter replacement before antimicrobial therapy for symptomatic urinary tract infection. Journal of Urology 164(4):1254–1258

Roe B H 1990 Study of the effects of education on the management of urine drainage systems by patients and carers. Journal of Advanced Nursing 15(5):517–524

Roe B H, May C 1999 Incontinence and sexuality: findings from a qualitative perspective. Journal of Advanced Nursing 30(3):573–579

Rooney M 1994 Impacting health care: study of a reusable urinary drainage system. Spinal Cord Injury Nursing 11(1):16–18

Sabbuba N, Mahenthiralingam E, Stickler D J 2003 Molecular epidemiology of Proteus mirabilis infections of the catheterized urinary tract. Journal of Clinical Microbiology 41(11):4961–4965

Sabbuba N, Stickler D J, Long M J et al 2005 Does valve regulated release of urine from the bladder decrease encrustation and blockage of indwelling catheters by crystalline Proteus mirabilis biofilms? Journal of Urology 173(1):262–266

Saint S, Lipsky B, Baker P 1999 Urinary catheters: what type do men and their nurses prefer? Journal of the American Geriatrics Society 47(120):1453–1457

Saint S, Veenstra D L, Sullivan S D et al 2000 The potential clinical and economic benefits of silver alloy urinary catheters in preventing urinary tract infection. Archives of Internal Medicine 160:2670–2675

Schmidt R D, Sobata A E 1988 An examination of the anti-adherence activity of cranberry juice on urinary and non-urinary bacterial isolates. Microbios 55:173–181

Schnelle J F, Adamson G M, Cruise P A et al 1997 Skin disorders and moisture in incontinent nursing home residents: intervention implications. Journal of the American Geriatrics Society 45(10):1182–1188

Seymour W 1998 Coping with embarrassment: bodily continence. In: Remaking the body: rehabilitation and change. Routledge, London

Shah J, Shah N 1998 Percutaneous suprapubic catheterisation. Urology News 2(5):11–12

Shekelle O G, Morton S C, Clark K A et al 1999 Systematic review of risk factors for urinary tract infection in adults with spinal cord dysfunction. Journal of Spinal Cord Medicine 22(4):258–272

Sheriff M K M, Foley S, McFarlane J, Nauth-Misir R, Craggs M 1998 Long-term supra-pubic catheterisation: clinical outcome and satisfaction survey. Spinal Cord 36(3):171–176

Spector W D, Fortinsky R H 1998 Pressure ulcer prevalence in Ohio nursing homes: clinical and facility correlates. Journal of Aging and Health 10(1):62–80

Staskin D, Bavendam T, Miller J et al 1996 Effectiveness of a urinary control insert in the management of stress urinary incontinence: early results of a multicenter study. Urology 47(5):629–636

Stickler D J, Hughes G 1999 Ability of Proteus mirabilis to swarm over urethral catheters. European Journal of Clinical Microbiology and Infectious Diseases 18(3):206–208

Stickler D J, Jones G L, Russell A D 2003 Control of encrustation and blockage of Foley catheters. Lancet 361(9367):1435–1437

Suarez G M, Baum N H, Jacobs J 1991 Use of standard contraceptive diaphragm in management of stress urinary incontinence. Urology 37(2):119–122

Tenke P, Reidl C, Jones G et al 2004 Bacterial biofilm formation on urological devices and heparin coating as preventative strategy. International Journal of Antimicrobial Agents 23(supplement 1):67–74

Theaker C, Mannan M, Ives N et al 2000 Risk factors for pressure sores in the critically ill. Anaesthesia 55(3):221–224

Thelwell S, Symon C, Gay S et al 1995 Penile sheaths: a comparative evaluation. Disability Equipment Assessment Report A15. Medical Devices Agency, London

Thornburn P, Cottenden A, Ledger D 1992 Continence. Undercover trials. Nursing Times 88(13):72–78

Thyssen H, Sander P, Lose G 1999 A vaginal device (continence guard) in the management of urge incontinence in women. International Urogynecology Journal and Pelvic Floor Dysfunction 10(4):219–222

Trautner B W, Darouiche R O 2004 Role of biofilm in catheter-associated urinary tract infection. American Journal of Infection Control 32(3):177–183

Tsai T F, Maibach H I 1999 How irritant is water? An overview. Contact Dermatitis 41(6):311–314

UKCC 1992 The scope of professional practice. UKCC, London

UKCC 1998 Records and record keeping. UKCC, London

Whittingham K, May S 1998 Cleansing regimens for continence care. Professional Nurse 14(3):167–172

Wilde M H 2003 Life with an indwelling catheter: the didactic of stigma and acceptance. Qualitative Health Research 13(9):1189–1124

Wilson J 1997 Control and prevention of infection in catheter care. Nurse Prescriber/Community Nurse 3(5):39–40

Wyndaele J J 2002 Complications of intermittent catheterisation: their prevention and treatment. Spinal Cord 40(10):536–541

Zimmerer R E, Lawson K D, Calvert C J 1986 The effects of wearing diapers on skin. Pediatric Dermatology 3: 95–101

Chapter **11**

Service organisation and delivery

Karen Logan and Kathryn Getliffe

Coming together is a beginning
Keeping together is progress
Working together is success

Henry Ford

INTRODUCTION

This chapter focuses on the development of continence services and clinics, with a particular emphasis on integration of services across traditional boundaries of primary and secondary care, outlining the benefits of multidisciplinary working across a range of specialties. Although the service context is largely the UK National Health Service (NHS) and local health economies (NHS Trusts), many of the issues addressed are common to those experienced in other countries (Box 11.1) and therefore much of the chapter content has potential for wider application.

Moving towards integrated continence services – background and context

Integrated care has been described by Hands (1999) as the explicit basis for improvement in both efficiency and effectiveness – in other words, improved treatment outcomes for individual patients, promotion of population health and cost-effective services. Despite the existence of a comprehensive NHS in the UK for over 50 years, many services can still be remarkably disintegrated and

Box 11.1   Key objectives for service development

- Access to early assessment in community care settings
- Accurate and timely diagnosis
- Appropriate level of specialist service provision by multidisciplinary teams
- Appropriate referral for investigations and surgery or a specialist consultant opinion
- Efficiency and effectiveness (from patient, professional and service perspectives)

most would agree that this has been true for continence services until recently. However, there is growing recognition of the importance of integrated continence services (ICS) in order to promote best practice in continence care – see *Good Practice in Continence Service* (DH 2000a) and the National Service Frameworks (NSFs) (see also Ch. 1).

Although there is an increasing evidence base which demonstrates the benefits of integration of services (Speakman 1999, Pomfret 2001, Logan & Proctor 2003), many organisations struggle with the problems of operationalising recommendations for best practice in this area. A survey of continence services in England, evaluating the measures taken by NHS Trusts to implement an integrated service as recommended in the Department of Health (2000a) guidance, showed that only 8% were planning to appoint a Director of Continence Services, despite this being a key recommendation (Thomas et al 2004). This was disappointing since a lack of strong leadership from an agreed clinical champion is likely to impede progress towards successful integration of services.

Other common barriers to service development include funding, skill mix, professional autonomy and multiprofessional working. It must also be recognised that territorialism (geographical and interprofessional) can and does hinder progress and effective teamworking; in many organisations it appears that this is the main barrier to integration. Despite the above concerns and the somewhat daunting prospect of attempting to integrate

and modernise continence services in the face of financial barriers, much can be achieved with minimum financial investment by capitalising on NHS reorganisation, utilisation of existing resources and creative use of staff vacancies (Logan & Proctor 2003).

DEVELOPING THE SERVICE

The aim to integrate continence services reflects a broader recognition of the benefits of multiagency, multiprofessional working, designed to enable patients to access services appropriate to their needs in primary care, and to reduce inappropriate referral and length of waiting lists in secondary care (DH 2000b, Wanless 2003). Separation of primary and secondary care in continence services is inappropriate and leads to delays in treatment, unnecessary diagnostic pathways such as urodynamic investigations for many patients, and time wasted on unplanned, duplicated and repeated activities (Hands 1999). Artificial boundaries which have grown around different NHS roles or institutions (e.g. tertiary referral units) tend to impede patient-centred integration and interdisciplinary contributions to treatment and care. The strengths of both primary and secondary services need to be brought together within a context of shared care.

Making a business case

Incontinence places huge burdens on individuals, carers and services, yet because it is not life threatening and is generally a symptom of an underlying cause, rather than being perceived as a disease in its own right, it can be difficult to achieve appropriate recognition at high levels within organisations. This creates challenges in acquiring additional resources in the face of more pressing priorities such as cancer and heart disease. Incontinence must be considered and presented to managers as a chronic condition, profoundly affecting the health and well-being of individuals. There is strong evidence that incontinence is very common – indeed more common than other chronic conditions such as asthma, diabetes and depression (see Ch. 1) – and has a negative impact on quality of life (Milsom et al 2001) (see also Ch. 1). Incontinence is also associated with increased risk of falls and hospitalisation (Brown et al 2000) and generates a huge burden on NHS resources and costs.

This important information and evidence should be used as strong ammunition when developing a business case to lobby for resources. Continence advisers/clinical leads need to be familiar with, and ready to quote from, relevant health service strategy documents (published at local, national and international levels) if they are to be successful in influencing managers and service commissioners. By learning to 'speak' their language and understand their priorities, it becomes easier to command attention and make an attractive case which also fits in with their local targets.

Political awareness

Political awareness is a vital skill which must be utilised continuously to get continence on the commissioning agenda and keep it there. The ability to influence decisions at a strategic level is critical at a time when competition for resources is high. Although influencing change and capitalising on opportunities is never easy, it is always necessary to think ahead and be able to demonstrate a good understanding of current policy and government targets. Developing skills in business case and report writing is essential to facilitate development of new services or redesign/improve existing ones and being well prepared to submit bids for money, often at short notice, is highly advantageous. 'Buddying' up with a respected manager within the organisation can be a beneficial strategy to produce a template business case that is transferable, adaptable and retained in readiness for when an opportunity presents itself.

Working towards integration

Good Practice in Continence Services (DH 2000a) outlined a set of principles for improving health and tackling health inequalities in service provision for people with bladder and bowel dysfunction. The document called for new ways of working and new partnerships, whilst recognising that successful models might be different in different localities

(see Ch. 1). One example, reported by Pomfret (2001), incorporates an innovative, multidisciplinary, line management structure that includes physiotherapists and occupational therapists in continence advisory roles as well as continence nurses. This was successfully introduced in a community NHS Trust in response to opportunities arising from local restructuring, professional interests and opportunistic use of vacancies. However, a model of this kind may be less practical where the context for service delivery spans primary and secondary care interfaces across several different Trusts.

Incontinence impinges on all specialties and consequently there is a need for specialists in all fields to be stakeholders in a comprehensive service, employing a shared vision that encourages and fosters joined-up thinking and joined-up working across the boundaries. The model described by Logan and Proctor (2003) is an example of joint working across all directorates involved in continence management (Box 11.2). It is, in essence, 'a virtual continence service', held together by a designated clinical leader who has the authority and ability to lead the relevant stakeholders. Integration is about shared interdisciplinary care and a useful description is provided by Pritchard and Hughes (1995):

> The responsibility for the healthcare of the patient is shared between individuals or teams who are part of separate organisations or where substantial organisational boundaries exist.

In the absence of this approach health professionals are commonly working in relative isolation, often 'reinventing the wheel' or, worse still, working to different standards with little or no continuity.

Integrated continence care pathways

Historically, continence services have been viewed as low status services frequently associated with the stigma of incontinence (Goldstein et al 1992). Services have in some cases developed a reputation as a pad provision service rather than a proactive treatment service. Modern continence services are actively raising their profile, aiming to be recognised for the development of nurse-led clinics

Box 11.2   An example of nurse-led clinics and joint clinics with other specialists involved in continence care

The integrated continence service model presented here is a successful model of a fully functioning integrated service with over 5 years' experience to share. The nurse-led and integrated clinics are an important part of the jigsaw which underpins the integrated service and a vital contribution to an integrated service but cannot be viewed in isolation. Developing the right level of nursing infrastructure is a priority but the service requires the support of local physiotherapists and other specialist nurses and consultants.

NURSE-LED TRIAGING CLINICS
The continence service has now become the first point of entry for people with bladder and bowel incontinence. We employ a service director and five continence advisers to cover five local authority boroughs (population size approximately 600 000; this equates to one nurse adviser per 100 000 population, a formula which has proved successful for the past 5 years). We also work closely with a urology and colorectal nurse specialist and two continence physiotherapists. The majority of our clinics, 16 in total, are nurse-led in order to triage patients in locally accessible clinics. These are geographically spaced around the county and held in community health clinics, acute and community hospitals and, in some cases, GP surgeries. The benefits of this triage/screening approach mean that the patient only needs to see a doctor in secondary care if they have failed to improve with conservative treatment.

NURSE-LED (NL) CLINICS
- Solely NL continence clinics in community and hospitals
- NL urodynamics clinics
- NL bowel clinics

- NL catheter clinics (urology)
- NL haematuria clinics (urology)
- NL enuresis clinics (school nurses)
The knowledge, skills and competencies required by nurses running these types of clinic are important prerequisites in the development of NL clinics.

INTEGRATED SPECIALIST CLINICS
- Joint continence clinics with a clinical nurse specialist (CNS) and urologist
- Joint continence clinics with multiple sclerosis (MS) nurse specialist and neurologist
- Joint continence clinics with geriatrician
- Pelvic floor clinics with consultant nurse, gynaecologist and physiotherapist
- Joint bowel clinics with a colorectal CNS and colorectal consultant surgeon
- 'One Stop' prostate assessment clinics with CNS and urologist
- Encopresis clinics with paediatrician, CNS and psychologist
- Joint urodynamics clinics with CNS, urologist and gynaecologist

RESOURCES
The clinics have access to and use the following equipment and aids to diagnosis:
- Bladder scanners
- Flow meters
- Urodynamics
- Bladder charts
- Urinalysis (testing sticks)
A number of the nurses have advanced certificates and skills to carry out nurse-led urodynamics. This is a valuable skill to support continence services.

and the implementation of preventative continence care based on early and effective conservative treatments or ongoing specialist referral where needed. Where pads are needed to contain urine leakage, patients must have a thorough assessment to ensure they receive the best product for their needs (see Ch. 10) and only when alternative approaches to care are inappropriate or unsuccessful.

The application of integrated care pathways (ICPs) for incontinence (Bayliss et al 2000a,b) offers a structured, consistent and readily auditable approach to assessment and treatment/care strategies. ICPs have been defined by Campbell et al (1998) as follows:

> Task oriented care plans which detail essential steps in the care of patients with a specific clinical problem and describes the patients' expected clinical course.

One of the main aims of introducing ICPs for continence is to enhance patients' access to nurse-led services, providing first level assessment and interventions which are managed predominantly by the patient and community nurse working in partnership and guided by the evidence-based pathway document (primary assessment) (see Ch. 2). If these interventions are inappropriate or fail to improve continence the patient should be referred for secondary assessment by the clinical nurse specialists.

Finally, if conservative treatments, with or without prescribed medications, fail to produce satisfactory symptom improvement, patients can be appropriately referred for specialist medical intervention in secondary care (tertiary assessment). Ultimately, this system has the potential to reduce the need for secondary care consultant referral as a first-line management, thus reducing the burden on secondary care waiting lists. Furthermore, it encourages continence promotion whilst discouraging excessive pad provision. In the words of Williams et al (2000):

> Most people with bladder or bowel problems are not sick; they do not need to go to hospital and there is evidence that 70–80% of patients can be successfully treated by nurses in accessible community clinics.

Clinical leadership

There can be no doubt that effective integration of continence services requires good leadership. Whatever their title (Director of Continence Services, Head of Continence Services, Clinical Lead), this individual must take the clinical leadership role, including budget management, in developing continence services across traditional boundaries where required, but with a major emphasis on community care. It is advisable that this service leader does not sit within a specialist directorate as continence is much broader than the medical specialties of urology, obstetrics and gynaecology, or geriatrics. However, they will need to develop robust relationships with the key medical consultants requiring their support and collaboration if integration, integrated clinics and multidisciplinary working are to be successful. It is vital that a flexible, open and collegiate approach is adopted, together with a change management strategy that fosters teamworking, new ways of working and innovative usage of scarce resources.

Investing time

The service leader will need to invest time in identifying and meeting with the key stakeholders, 'winning hearts and minds' to capture individuals' enthusiasm and support to work as part of the virtual team. In some cases this is not an easy task and is reliant on individual personality, confidence and drive, in conjunction with flexibility, knowledge, respect and credibility. However, without the collaboration of others in the multi-professional team, the integration is almost certainly doomed to failure. Certain professionals have a key integrative role in the network: the most obvious and often hardest to capture are the GPs, who hold continuing responsibility to integrate the overall treatment and care of the individual patients.

Planning and managing expectations

Integrated service development is a challenging initiative which demands a systematic, 'whole systems' approach. It takes time to achieve and calls for patience and unshakeable determination to overcome the setbacks that may occur. Development and implementation of plans and changes is best approached in manageable stages, acknowledging that this is a work in progress and is not a one-off 'job and finish' type project. It is important to agree realistic timeframes for evaluating and reporting progress so that expectations of all stakeholders are realistic and motivation remains high. However, there is a balance to be made between carefully planned, steady development and the need for a dynamic service which is able to respond to environmental changes and the service needs of the local population as required.

Ownership and motivation

The service leader will need to regularly host and chair an Integrated Continence Services Forum or similar group which draws together membership of key stakeholders from across the agencies and directorates to develop the joint working, audit strategies and service developments such as integrated clinics. Box 11.3 shows a series of steps and stages of development in the move towards integration of services.

The benefits of integrated working

Patients

Patients' views and outcomes are central to the organisation and delivery of integrated services and the overall benefit is that patients are seen by the 'right person at the right time, in the right place'. Generally, this is the continence adviser and/or physiotherapist, not necessarily the hospital consultant in the first instance. In other words, there is a planned 'streamlining of the patient's journey'. Development of local referral protocols, nurse-led clinics and joint working means that patients are seen promptly by the most appropriate clinician, removing artificial barriers between secondary and primary care and importantly between the nursing, physiotherapy and medical teams. Boxes 11.4 and 11.5 illustrate two case histories where patients have benefited from a joint working approach.

Box 11.5 Case study 2

Clarisse is a 49-year-old lady who was seen in the joint clinic that we run together with one of our consultant urologists. She was complaining of sudden onset of severe frequency, urgency (but no incontinence) and suprapubic discomfort. The frequency was so bad (half hourly) she felt she was living in the toilet and that it was ruling her life, to the point that she was off sick from work (6 months), feeling very depressed, and stating her life was a misery. On assessment by the nurse adviser, findings were normal, no blood or infection on urinalysis, no residual urine and a normal drinking pattern; her bladder chart confirmed half hourly voiding of very small quantities.

She was given the usual lifestyle healthy bladder advice with bladder training and we discussed her case with the urologist. It was decided not to investigate initially with urodynamics or flexible cystoscopy (if this had not been a joint clinic the patient would have been referred for a urology opinion and investigations) as the urologist felt a trial of amitriptyline was the best option in this case. We arranged close telephone contact but within 3 weeks Clarisse had telephoned us, saying her symptoms had miraculously resolved and she was feeling like a new woman again.

Services

Services that are heavily or solely reliant on medical consultants in secondary care as the first point of referral often suffer from 'log jams' or 'bottlenecks' created by long waiting lists for uro-dynamic investigations or for the initial consultation with a hospital urologist or gynaecologist. In many areas this is a real problem but it is one which can be relieved by taking the time to examine current services to identify what 'actually happens' rather than what people often 'think happens' and to identify inefficiencies, duplications and wasted time and money. There are many different ways to go about this but process mapping offers one powerful method which can help to unravel service complexities and facilitate stakeholders to work together to develop ways to solve problems (see 'Process mapping – what is it and what can it offer?' later in this chapter).

GOVERNMENT POLICY AND TARGETS RELATED TO CONTINENCE SERVICE DEVELOPMENT: HOW TO USE THEM

This section of the chapter provides reference to a number of useful and important government policies that relate to the development of integrated continence services and can provide clinicians with important information, guidance and resources to build a case for improving services for people with bladder and bowel conditions in community settings. Although incontinence does not have its own National Service Framework (NSF) or policy, there are milestones for integrated continence services mentioned in both the older persons' and children's NSFs (DH 2001a, 2004). *Good Practice in Continence Services* (DH 2000a) provides a strong underpinning framework for clinicians but is limited by a lack of authoritative status to direct service integration. The constant need to fight for higher priority recognition poses a real challenge to staff working in this area as continence services may not be seen as essential services by management. Consequently, clinical leaders and continence specialists need to work harder in finding the necessary 'hooks' on which to hang continence services – for example, the NSFs, NICE guidelines or policies relating to chronic conditions and policies calling for reduced referral and burden on secondary care (NICE 2004, 2006, WAG 2005, DH 2006).

Incontinence can and must be slotted into or 'hung' upon any of these policy hooks if health-care managers are to listen and invest in service redesign. It is up to continence specialists to make sure their voice is heard when competing for scarce health service resources on behalf of their patients.

The most recent government policy drivers calling for health service reform in England and Wales – *Our Health, Our Care, Our Say* (DH 2006) and *Designed for Life: Creating World Class Health and Social Care for Wales in the 21st Century* (WAG 2005) – have the potential to generate new opportunities for those providing local continence services, with added potential to align with the White Papers on long-term conditions (DH 2005), health promotion and improved quality of life. Implementation of these policies includes a shift in

Box 11.6   Sources of information to support developing services

- *Our Health, Our Care, Our Say* (DH 2006) (http://www.dh.gov.uk)
- *Designed for Life: Creating World Class Health and Social Care for Wales in the 21st Century* (WAG 2005) (http://www.wales.gov.uk)
- Scottish Intercollegiate Guidelines Network (SIGN 2004) (http:www.sign.ac.uk)
- *Good Practice in Continence Services* (DH 2000a) (http://www.dh.gov.uk)
- *Essence of Care: Patient Focused Benchmarking for Health Care Practitioners* (DH 2001b) (http://www.dh.gov.uk)
- *The National Service Framework for Older People* (DH 2001a) (http://www.dh.gov.uk)
- *The National Service Framework for Children, Young People and Maternity Services* (DH 2004) (http://www.dh.gov.uk)
- *The National Service Framework for Long-Term Conditions* (DH 2005) (http://www.dh.gov.uk)
- *Securing Good Health for the Whole Population* (HM Treasury 2004) (http://www.hm-treasury.gov.uk)
   - Local Wanless action plans have been produced by individual NHS Trusts and are available on most Trust websites
- *The NHS Plan: a Plan for Investment, a Plan for Reform* (DH 2000b) (http://www.dh.gov.uk)
- Is policy translated into action? (Thomas 2004) (http://www.rcn.org.uk)
- Action on urology/NHS Modernisation Agency (http://www.wise.nhs.uk)

funding from secondary care into primary care and this will promote opportunities for local service redesign. Some key policy documents are listed in Box 11.6 with brief summaries from selected papers in Box 11.7 to provide some indication of where continence service development can fit into both government and local health provision agendas.

UNDERSTANDING AND IMPROVING SERVICES

Although it may be relatively easy to recognise that a service could be improved, it is often much more difficult to determine exactly how, particularly when the patient's journey involves frequent and sometimes multiple involvement with a variety of different groups or individuals working within the healthcare service. Directives from those in senior positions may not work well on the ground and other staff directly involved in day-to-day delivery of the service may only see a part of the overall picture. One way to unravel these complexities is to use a process mapping model.

Process mapping – what is it and what can it offer?

Process mapping is an extremely effective way of capturing, recording and analysing complex activities in order to identify what works well and what doesn't and to produce a framework for moving forward. It provides a way of creating a visual 'map' of processes as they are now, which can then be used to help determine areas for improvement, in the context of better understanding of current bottlenecks and other barriers to efficiency and efficacy. When applied to service development in health care, process mapping offers a powerful way for multidisciplinary groups to understand the real problems which may be hindering improved service delivery, both from each other's perspective and importantly from the perspective of patients (Box 11.8). One of the main objectives of mapping is to get people talking to each other to share understanding of each other's roles and delivery capability. This interaction is most effective when people come together for a full day workshop (or two half-days as long as they are no more than 1 or 2 weeks apart). The end product of the session should be a highly visual, agreed and easy to understand process map.

The NHS Modernisation Agency provides a useful overview of process mapping and some guidance on its application to service development (www.modern.nhs.uk).

Using process mapping

If a process isn't documented it will be difficult, if not impossible, to improve. The term 'process' in this context refers to a series of connected steps to achieve a particular outcome. The process should have a name and be defined by a clear starting

Box 11.7 Summaries of selected government documents which offer some indication of where continence service development can fit into government and local healthcare agendas

GOOD PRACTICE IN CONTINENCE SERVICES (DH 2000)
This Guidance was produced by the Department of Health in 2000 in response to recognised inadequacies in incontinence care, and contains a number of recommendations for care which have been highlighted throughout this book. The Guidance can be downloaded from http://www.publications.doh.gov.uk/pdfs/continenceservices.pdf.

The Guidance provides an outline for integrated services that has been influential in changing the emphasis of continence care away from simply containment of incontinence towards management based on identification and treatment of the underlying causes. Continence specialists can use these recommendations to guide planning and management services which will ensure that every patient receives an appropriate continence assessment and optimal, tailored care based on evidence supporting best treatment and management choice.

OUR HEALTH, OUR CARE, OUR SAY: A NEW DIRECTION IN COMMUNITY SERVICES (DH 2006)
Health and social care working together in partnership
The model of the provision of care is changing with the publication of this governmental White Paper. It outlines how care will be moving into communities, with GPs empowered to commission services based on the needs of their local population and designing services around those needs which are safe, high quality and community based, ensuring easier access for patients. One way that this will be achieved is through the introduction of practice-based commissioning (PBC) which will give GPs more responsibility for local health budgets to deliver better health outcomes and well-being, with a focus on health promotion and disease prevention.

To support the development of targeted local services, the Department of Health is working with several of the Royal Colleges to define clinically safe pathways within primary care, one of which is in the area of urology. The model of care for urology outlines the potential to involve suitably trained non-specialists in the management and treatment of certain conditions. It also outlines that 'where appropriate, and with suitable diagnostic support, male and female bladder dysfunction can be locally managed in the community'.

Local health and social care commissioners have also been tasked with improving collaboration to create multidisciplinary networks in support of people with the most complex needs (development of personal health and social care plans and integrated social and health care records) to provide a more holistic approach to patient care. These activities aim to improve health promotion services, with prevention of the inappropriate use of specialist or acute health care and reducing unplanned admissions to hospital.

DESIGNED FOR LIFE: CREATING WORLD CLASS HEALTH AND SOCIAL CARE FOR WALES IN THE 21st CENTURY (WAG 2005)
The Welsh Assembly Government (WAG) has presented NHS organisations with the above White Paper, which sets out targets for healthcare redesign over the next 12 years. The document focuses on the need to provide local services in community settings, alleviating the burden on secondary care and focusing on quality measures which include patient experience, clinical outcomes, predicted and standardised data sets and the clinical governance process.

NATIONAL AUDIT OF CONTINENCE CARE FOR OLDER PEOPLE (ROYAL COLLEGE OF PHYSICIANS 2005)
The RCP audit carried out for the Healthcare Commission looked at the care of nearly 10 000 older people in England, Wales and Northern Ireland. It found that specialist NHS staff had good continence knowledge, but patients were often not examined thoroughly or given routine assessments. For most patients only the symptoms were managed, when in some cases there could be a cure. Only 59% of primary and 32% of secondary care sites had a written policy covering continence care for older people, despite the mandatory requirement in the *National Service Framework for Older People* (DH 2001a) to establish integrated continence services.

NATIONAL SERVICE FRAMEWORKS (NSFs)
The NSFs for both older people and for children (DH 2001a, 2004) recognise that continence services are a particularly important requirement for patients towards the extremes of the age spectrum (old and young). The Frameworks state that continence services should be readily available to all patients in need. They mandate the establishment of an integrated continence service and outline essential standards of care for this service, which include crossing interprofessional boundaries and encompassing both primary and secondary care. The NSF for long-term conditions (DH 2005) outlines 11 quality requirements, focusing on

Box 11.7   *Continued*

quality of life and rehabilitation issues relevant to continence (see Ch. 1).

CLINICAL GUIDELINE ON FALLS IN OLDER PEOPLE (NICE 2004)

Older people are recognised as a vulnerable group in the National Institute for Clinical Excellence (NICE) document and directive. Frequency, urgency and urge incontinence are identified as frequent and important contributory factors in falls among older people (Brown et al 2000).

URINARY INCONTINENCE: THE MANAGEMENT OF URINARY INCONTINENCE IN WOMEN (NICE 2006)

NICE and the National Collaborating Centre for Women's and Children's Health have published a clinical guideline which advises on the assessment, diagnosis and effective treatments for women with UI.

MANAGEMENT OF URINARY INCONTINENCE IN PRIMARY CARE (SIGN 2004)

This national guideline, from the Scottish Intercollegiate Guidelines Network, offers comprehensive guidance and treatment algorithms on the management of UI in the primary care setting. It aims to help identify opportunities and effective techniques within primary care for assessing and treating urinary incontinence in adults and to provide the primary care practitioner with an indication of factors which should lead to an onward referral (with acknowledgements to Pfizer Ltd, CARE programme).

Box 11.8   Benefits of process mapping

- Provides a way of capturing and documenting the way things are *actually* done during a process (e.g. patient's journey, ordering supplies, etc.) rather than what we may think is done
- Creates/facilitates a sense of ownership, responsibility and partnership by bringing together multidisciplinary teams/groups representing a wide range of roles/professions
- Produces an end product (process map) which is easy to understand and is highly visual
- Provides a clear base-line from which to measure and evaluate ongoing service improvement

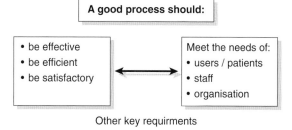

Figure 11.1   Characteristics of a good process.

point and an end point. It can be simple and short (e.g. from a patient's first contact with continence services to their initial assessment meeting) or long and complex (e.g. the whole patient journey from first contact to completion of treatment and discharge). Most processes are linked to others (e.g. processes for maintaining patient records or ordering supplies etc.). In the majority of cases there will be a number of different stakeholders who have some degree of involvement and a good process should aim to meet the needs of all stakeholders (Fig. 11.1). For this reason it is important to plan ahead carefully to ensure that there is representation from all key stakeholder groups at the process mapping meeting (Box 11.9).

Creating and documenting the 'map'

A good way of documenting the 'mapped process' is to use very large sheets of paper (brown paper or the reverse side of wallpaper works well) taped to the walls so that everyone in the group can see easily. The main steps in the process can be recorded in a series of blocks or boxes written directly on the paper. Issues and questions can be captured during the discussion by using post-it

Box 11.9   Using process mapping

1. Planning ahead – getting people involved
   - Preparation is very important. This includes getting the support of senior leaders in the organisation who may influence the implementation of changes resulting from the mapping process
   - Invite as wide a selection of people involved as possible (managers very often do not know the detail of what is actually done). Between 15 and 25 people is a good number; if there are more than this it can be difficult to manage and to ensure everyone feels engaged at all times. Outline the purpose and expectations of the event in advance
   - Define the objectives, scope and focus of the workshop. Don't try to do too much – it always takes longer than you think
2. Preparing for the workshop
   - One full day or two half days, preferably off-site
   - Plan to make it very visual
   - Use large rolls of brown paper or wallpaper which can be stuck onto walls, large coloured 'post-it' notes, flip-charts and marker pens
   - Independent facilitator
   - Someone to help record comments and ideas
3. On the day – getting started
   - Define the process – give it a name
   - Use flowcharting techniques and 'post-it' notes on large sheets of paper (see Fig. 11.2)
   - Initially every small step should be recorded:
     - if steps are variable use an '80% of the time' guide
     - don't try to solve problems until the process has been fully mapped and analysed
   - Use traffic light colours to identify the priorities on process steps and links (e.g. a red flag really needs fixing *now*)
   - 'Park' any issues where agreement can't be reached within 5 min and come back to them later (*don't forget!*)
4. Adding detail and digging down
   - Add communication medium – telephone, letter, e-mail
   - Add times taken to process steps – days, months, etc.
   - Use activity and role 'lane diagrams' to illustrate differing aspects – people, departments, organisations, etc. (see Figs 11.3 and 11.4)
   - Break down process steps into subprocesses for clarity and improvement work
   - Transfer to large sheets of paper and hang on wall for further comment and input
   - Get people to 'walk' the process steps to ensure all steps and data are captured
5. Analysing the process
   - Identify the number of steps in the process
   - Identify which ones:
     - don't add value
     - cause delays
   - Look for:
     - parallel processes
     - bottlenecks
     - clarity of 'ownership' and responsibility
     - what could be changed
   - Identify priorities for change and consider from perspectives of different stakeholders
6. Process improvement
   - Decide the basis for improvements: time, cost, efficient use of resources, etc.; this may be different for each step
   - Use the improvement cycle – Plan, Do, Study, Act (see Fig. 11.5)
   - 'Walk' through a process before implementing changes
   - Test changes on a small scale – get the people who actually do each step heavily involved
   - Agree review periods once the improvements are implemented (don't forget to switch off old process steps)
   - Try to have measures in place before process steps 'go live' (include automatic monitoring where possible)

notes stuck on to the main map (Fig. 11.2). Using a flowchart framework can be a useful way of recording processes which include alternative steps that depend on specific information and decision making. However, flowcharting is not essential and it is more important to employ a structure which 'works' for the group. A critical part of mapping is to identify who is currently responsible for each step. One way of recording this is to map activity/role lanes on to the process map (Fig. 11.3) and create an activity/role chart (Fig. 11.4).

Process name:

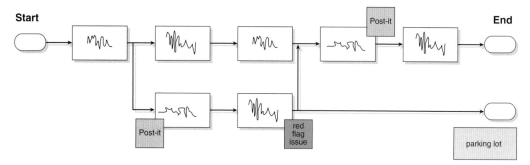

- identify tasks, one per 'Post-it' note (try different colours for different actions
- add arrows to show sequence
- 'Post-its' can be moved or added as the process is being defined
- use 'red flags' to identify issues which need urgent action
- use a 'parking lot' for issues to come back to later

Figure 11.2   Using stick-on 'post-its' to map processes.

Process name:

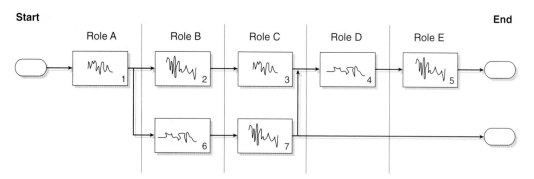

- understand who is responsible for each step / activity
- understand what inputs and outputs are appropriate for each step / activity

Figure 11.3   Using activity/role lanes.

These initial stages may take up the bulk of the process mapping meeting but there is no sense in trying to determine what to change and how until it is absolutely clear what the current process is. Once the map and current responsibilities have been agreed, the next step is to analyse where the present inefficiencies such as bottlenecks, duplications, other hold-ups or poor use of resources occur and to consider what can be done. It is always sensible to pilot major changes before embarking on them full scale and also to remember to 'turn off' old processes when they are no longer needed. Although it is not possible to provide detailed practical advice on using process

Box 11.10   Process mapping in action: developing integrated care pathways

Process mapping can be applied to the development and implementation of continence care pathways. As integrated care pathways (ICPs) are tools for improving care delivered to patients, it is clearly important that a firm understanding of what is actually happening currently is captured, understood and analysed by the whole clinical team, key stakeholders and patients from the outset. The process map will help to define:

- the sequence of steps and activities performed
- specific responsibilities for these steps and activities
- areas that lie outside the process but impact on it
- the relationships that exist between the different professionals in the process
- potential problem areas.

It is helpful for the ICP development team to set ground rules before the start of the exercise and emphasise that process mapping is about trying to really understand the patient's experience at various stages of their journey and not about blame for hold-ups or delays. Developing the map from the point of view of a clearly defined group of patients will keep the exercise focused and productive.

The process mapping session of the patient's journey should give the team:

- a key starting point from which to identify improvements
- the opportunity to bring together multidisciplinary teams from primary, secondary and tertiary settings, health and social care and, most importantly, patients and carers
- an overview of the whole process, often for the first time

- an insight into how many steps there are for the patient, how many times the patient is passed from one person to another (hand-off), the time taken for each step, steps which add no value to the patient, etc.
- an aid to effectively planning where to test improvement ideas and where they are likely to have the most impact
- brilliant ideas, from staff that really know the system and how it works
- an interactive event involving 'everyone'
- an end product – the map, which is clear and visible.

Once the current processes have been mapped and agreed by all stakeholders, the team can begin evaluating their practice against 'best' practice goals and start to ask themselves questions about the appropriateness of certain activities, tasks or investigations. This will facilitate the identification of opportunities for improvement and proposed changes in practice can be discussed and agreed. In this context ICPs can easily be viewed as a logical method of incorporating clinical effectiveness into practice and from this position the team can begin to determine how the process mapping information can be translated into the first draft of the ICP.

For example, a continence ICP could be developed in the following sections:

- Primary care: initial referral/assessment/management of incontinence
- A urinary incontinence pathway including treatment pathways for urge, stress and overflow incontinence
- A constipation and faecal incontinence pathway
- An assessment and management pathway for catheterised patients.

Activity/ responsibility	Role A e.g. continence advisor	Role B e.g. GP	Role C e.g. administrator	Role D e.g. urologist
1				
2				
3				
4				

Figure 11.4   An example of an activity/role lane diagram.

mapping within this book, some key pointers are offered in Box 11.9 with some further insights into process mapping in action in Box 11.10.

Continuous service improvement

Service development is an ongoing dynamic process and to ensure initial benefits are not only maintained but also improved upon, a continuous process improvement model such as the PDSA cycle can provide a tried and tested supporting framework (Fig. 11.5). There are four stages to a PDSA cycle:

Model for Continuous Improvement (PDSA)

What are we trying to accomplish?
How will we know a change is an improvement?
What changes can we make that result in improvements?

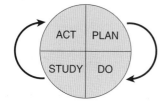

Figure 11.5 PDSA model for continuous improvement. Reproduced with permission from Langley et al (1996).

- *Plan*: Agree the next change to be tested or implemented and how to do it
- *Do*: Carry out the implementation and measure the impact
- *Study*: Study the data before and after the change and think about what was learnt
- *Act*: Determine the focus and components of the next change cycle

Evaluating services – audit and data collection

The base-line audit for an ICP is undertaken at the beginning of the project. The results will indicate not only where there are gaps in the service but also to what extent standards are currently being met. The audit will also form the basis of the evaluation of the ICP, as initial data can be compared with end of pilot data.

The steps involved in a base-line audit project are as follows:

1. *Form an audit team*: Which members of the ICP team are best placed to undertake this piece of work? A multidisciplinary team will be able to give a good perspective on what data are required and how to identify these within the notes. The team may decide that it would be appropriate to consult patients in planning the project; if so, you may need to obtain ethical approval. It is important that colleagues in positions of authority support the project and

have the commitment to see changes put into practice.

2. *Decide on the standards*: Your ICP will be based on national or local standards or consensus/custom-based best practice, or a combination of all three. It is crucial to measure key milestones or actions against appropriate standards so that the evaluation audit will be consistent. This is called variance analysis.

3. *Select an audit sample*: The team should agree whether to audit over a given period of time or choose a sample size from the patient population. There are ways of selecting samples of patients which you can be satisfied are representative of the larger group. Gathering data from an appropriate sample group is important as you must ensure that your data are sufficiently robust for your team to base decisions on. Your local audit facilitator can give you more advice about choosing your sample.

4. *Decide what data to collect*: Is your audit going to be retrospective or prospective? Are data going to be collected using an audit form or entered directly onto a computer? How will you track variances? A small pilot audit will ensure that your data collection tool works, especially if a team is collecting the data. The pilot may reveal that some of your questions are ambiguous, that the form is difficult to complete or that you are simply not getting the information you want. Ensure you allow sufficient time for data collection and modification of your initial data collection tool.

5. *Collect the data*: Only start collecting data when you have planned every detail of your audit, tested your methods and know how you are going to analyse the information collected. Make sure you are clear about exactly who is going to be responsible for doing what and when.

6. *Analyse the data*: Pull your data together in the most meaningful way and compare your results against your standards.

7. *Present your findings*: Present your findings to colleagues and agree an action plan of the way forward. The results will assist you in deciding any service redesign that is required at this stage of the ICP development.

8. *Evaluate your findings*: The baseline audit can clarify how to move forward but can also form

an indicator of the success of the ICP. Once the ICP is complete and implemented an infrastructure for continuous improvement should be put in place to consistently measure the performance of the ICP and the attainment of the standards.

CONCLUSIONS

The challenge to integrate and organise modern continence services is considerable but most services have enthusiastic and committed staff, who wish to do the best for their patients. This chapter has attempted to demonstrate that the achievement of a modern continence service is largely dependent upon organisational reform rather than large-scale financial investment. Whilst the majority of recommendations described here are reproducible elsewhere in similar types of organisation, their implementation requires recognition of the diversity that exists between healthcare organisations, local resources, geography, population and context for service delivery. This begins with understanding what happens in local services, understanding where the bottlenecks lie, and where and what the barriers may be. Process mapping has been described and recommended as a strategy to help to unravel service complexities and create ways to solve local organisational and service development problems.

The clinical and societal burden of incontinence places a mandate on continence specialists to promote optimal care and services to all patients with incontinence. Through the development of structured patient assessment plans and clinical management plans, by understanding the optimal use of available resources, through creation of care pathways and a sound knowledge of government policies, the continence specialist is well placed to orchestrate a strategy for the development of integrated services with the ultimate goal of improving continence management and overall service delivery.

KEY POINTS FOR PRACTICE

- Leadership is important to pull the disparate pieces of the jigsaw together: become a clinical champion, unleash your 'personal power'
- Always think big picture: develop a strategic plan for integration; map your service processes
- Acquire the necessary skills to develop both nurse-led triage and integrated continence clinics – they really do make a big difference to service provision
- Networking with stakeholders is vital: learn from others and understand their priorities; maintain teamwork and meet regularly
- Do not be 'territorial': share, enable, involve, motivate and empower others
- Become a political and strategic player: learn to speak the commissioner's language; be knowledgeable in government health policy
- Utilise audit and government documents when negotiating with service managers and commissioners
- Hone your influencing and negotiation skills
- Remember to keep the patient central to service development
- Do not give up: this agenda is not easy and it takes time to develop services in this way

References

Bayliss V, Cherry M, Locke R et al 2000a Pathways for continence care: background and audit. British Journal of Nursing 9(9):590–596

Bayliss V, Cherry M, Locke R et al 2000b Pathways for continence care: development of the pathway. British Journal of Nursing 9(17):1165–1172

Brown J, Vittinghoff E, Wyman J et al 2000 Urinary incontinence: does it increase risk for fall and fractures? Journal of the American Geriatrics Society. 48:721–725

Campbell H, Hotchkiss R, Bradshaw N et al 1998 Integrated care pathways. British Medical Journal 316:133–137

Department of Health 2000a Good practice in continence services. DH, London

Department of Health 2000b The NHS plan: a plan for investment, a plan for reform (Cm 4818-1). DH, London

Department of Health 2001a National Service Framework for older people. DH, London

Department of Health 2001b Essence of care: patient focused benchmarking for health care practitioners. DH, London

Department of Health 2004 National Service Framework for children, young people and maternity services. DH, London

Department of Health 2005 National Service Framework for long-term conditions. DH, London

Department of Health 2006 Our health, our care, our say. DH, London

Goldstein M, Hawthorn M E, Engburg S et al 1992 Urinary incontinence: why people do not seek help. Journal of Geriatric Nursing 18(4):15–20

Hands D 1999 Integrated care. In: Lugon M, Secker-Walker J (eds) Clinical governance: making it happen. Royal Society of Medicine Press, London

HM Treasury 2004 Securing good health for the whole population. HM Treasury, London. Online. Available: http://www.hm-treasury.gov.uk/consultations_and_legislation/wanless/consult_wanless04_final.cfm

Langley G, Nolan K, Nolan T et al 1996 The improvement guide; a practical approach to enhancing organisational performance. Jossey-Bass, San Francisco

Logan K, Proctor S 2003 Developing an interdisciplinary integrated continence service. Nursing Times 99(21):34–37

Milsom I, Abrams P, Cardozo L et al 2001 How widespread are symptoms of an overactive bladder and how are they managed? A population-based prevalence study. BJU International 87:760–766

National Institute for Clinical Excellence 2004 Clinical guideline for the assessment and prevention of falls in older people. Royal College of Nursing, London

National Institute for Health and Clinical Excellence 2006 Urinary incontinence: the management of urinary incontinence in women. Royal College of Obstetricians and Gynaecology Press, London

NHS Modernisation Agency The improvement leaders' guides. Online. Available: http://www.wise.nhs.uk/cmswise/default.htm

Pomfret I 2001 Reconfiguration of continence services. Journal of Community Nursing 15(7):28–32

Pritchard P, Hughes J 1995 Shared care: the future imperative? Nuffield Provincial Hospitals Trust. Royal Society of Medicine Press, London

Royal College of Physicians 2005 National audit of continence care for older people. RCP, London

Scottish Intercollegiate Guidelines Network 2004 Management of urinary incontinence in primary care. A national guideline. SIGN, Edinburgh

Speakman M J 1999 How to develop an integrated approach to continence care. In: Lucas M, Emery S, Beynon J (eds) Incontinence. Blackwell Science, Oxford

Thomas S 2004 Is policy translated into action? Royal College of Nursing/Continence Foundation, London. Online. Available: http://www.rcn.org.uk/members/downloads/policytranslatedaction.pdf

Thomas S, Billington A, Getliffe K A 2004 Improving continence services – a case study in policy influence. Journal of Nursing Management 12(4):252–257

Wanless D 2003 Securing good health for the whole population. DH, London

Welsh Assembly Government 2005 Designed for life: creating world class health and social care in the 21 century. WAG, Cardiff

Williams K, Assassa R P, Smith N K et al 2000 Development, implementation and evaluation of a new nurse-led continence service: a pilot study. Journal of Clinical Nursing 9:566–573

INDEX

C

Caecum 212
Caesarean section, elective 227
Caffeine 153
Calcium channel blockers *251*
Calcium ion channels 240, 242
Capsaicin 243–244
  intravesical 162
Carbachol 248
Carbalax suppositories 249
Care pathways
  evidence-based 42
  integrated 15–16
  see also integrated care pathways
Care plans for frail elderly people 139
Carers
  informal 11
  intermittent catheterisation 18
  perspectives 18
  residential care 11
Catheter(s) 260–286
  advice for patients 278
  antimicrobial surfaces 262, 271
  balloons 263, *264, 279*
  biofilms 270, *271*, 272
  changing 280
  coatings 262, 283
  complications *261*, 267–277
  dementia patients 150
  drainage equipment 263–265, 270, *273, 279*
  encrustation 267, 272–274, *275–276*, 276–277
  evaluation of care practice 286
  flushing 276
  indwelling 108
  inflammation 267–268
  information for patients 278
  maintenance solutions 274, 276, 277
  management 266–267
  materials 261–262, 271
  meatal cleansing 270
  patient support 277–278, *279*
  planned changes 274
  pressure necrosis 267–268
  recurrent blockage 272–274, *275–276, 276–277*
  risks *261*
  silver-alloy surface 262, 271, *273*
  sizes 262–263, 283–284
  tissue trauma 267–268
  troubleshooting 278, *279*
  types for intermittent self-catheterisation 283–284
  urinary bypassing *279*
  valves 266, 274
  see also indwelling catheters; intermittent catheterisation
Catheter-associated urinary tract infection (CAUTI) 262, 265, 267, 268–272
  antibiotics 271–272, *273*
  antiseptic therapies 271–272, *273*
  biofilms 270, *271*, 272
  fluid intake 272
  microorganisms 270, *271*
    access 269–270
Catheterisation 260–286
  complications 267–277
  documentation 286
  hygiene *273*
  long-term 164
  patient support 277–278, *279*
  proactive care 274
  quality of life 278
  sexual activity 278
  suprapubic 278, *279*–282
Cauda equina 223
Center for Applied Special Technology (CAST) 21
Chaining 187
Challenging behaviour 150, 180, 196–197
Chemotherapy
  cytotoxic drugs causing incontinence *251*
  prostate cancer 101
Child abuse 223
Childbirth 10
  faecal incontinence 5–6, 227, *229*
  incontinence 58
  trauma 5–6
  urine retention 36–37
  vaginal delivery 59, *60*
Children 113–133
  absorbent pad use 296
  biofeedback techniques 122
  bladder control 35, 114–117, 174
  bowel control 114–117, 174
  cognitive bladder training in the community 121–123
  constipation
    functional 127–132
    special needs children 117
  continence problem prevalence 177
  daytime wetting 117, 119–123
  detrusor instability 123
  diapers 296
  intermittent self-catheterisation 286
  nocturnal enuresis 5, *12*, 36, 123–127
  pelvic floor relaxation 123
  physical examination 120
  with special needs 116, 117

toilet training 114–117, 175–176
Chilli derivatives 243–244
Chlorhexidine 271, *273*
Cholinergic agonists 248
Clinical Guidelines on Falls in Older People (NICE, 2004) *318*
Clinics, joint *312*, 314, *315*
Clozapine 151
Cochrane Library 18
Codeine phosphate 249
Coeliac disease 209
Coffee, colonic activity stimulation 221
Cognitive bladder training in the community 121–123
Colon 211–212
  absorption 210, 212
  activity 209–210
  storage 210
  transit time studies 230
  vitamin synthesis 210
Colonoscopy 229–230
Colorectal cancer, early detection 231
Commercial companies 13
Commodes 289–291
Comorbid conditions
  elderly people 141
  older people 38
Complementary therapies 231–233
  homeopathic treatments causing incontinence *251*
Conduction aids 104, *105, 106*
Constipating agents 249
Constipation 203–206, 212
  assessment 130, 216, *217–218*
  causes 129, *205*
  children with special needs 117
  classification 204–205
  definition 204
  elderly people 204–205
    dietary factors 218, 220
  features 215–216
  fluid intake 220–221
  functional 127–132
  intellectual disability 193–196
  laxatives 221–223
  management 216, 218, 220–223
  medication 248–249
  multiple sclerosis 157
  neurological conditions of bowel 155
  prevalence 178
  slow transit 205–206
  stroke 157
  symptoms 215–216
  terminology 127–129
  treatment 130–132
  withholding 129